T0134511

# METHODS IN PHARMACOLOGY AND TOXICOLOGY

*Series Editor*
**James Y. Kang**
**Department of Medicine**
**University of Louisville School of Medicine**
**Prospect, Kentucky, USA**

For further volumes:
http://www.springer.com/series/7653

# Computer-Aided Drug Discovery

Edited by

## Wei Zhang

*Chemistry Department, Southern Research Institute,*
*Birmingham, AL, USA*

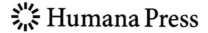 Humana Press

*Editor*
Wei Zhang
Chemistry Department
Southern Research Institute
Birmingham, AL, USA

ISSN 1557-2153          ISSN 1940-6053   (electronic)
Methods in Pharmacology and Toxicology
ISBN 978-1-4939-8065-9          ISBN 978-1-4939-3521-5   (eBook)
DOI 10.1007/978-1-4939-3521-5

Printed on acid-free paper

This Humana Press imprint is published by Springer Nature
The registered company is Springer Science+Business Media LLC New York

# Preface

Computational technologies have been applied in drug discovery for decades and are gaining increasingly in popularity, implementation, and appreciation due to the recent advances in computational methodologies and the fast growth of low-cost high performance computing techniques. Computer-aided drug discovery (CADD) has become a crucial component of modern drug discovery programs and is widely utilized to identity and optimize bioactive compounds for the development of new drugs. The intent of this book is to provide a practical guide for solving drug discovery-related problems using computational techniques.

CADD is a diverse discipline where various aspects of applied and basic research merge and stimulate each other. Computational strategies thus need to be frequently adjusted for different drug discovery purposes. A wide variety of computational approaches have been used in different stages of drug discovery and development, as well as in clinical studies. It is not possible to comprehensively cover such a broad field in one volume. Therefore, this book focuses on the methods that are commonly used in the early stage of drug discovery, including computer simulation, structure prediction, conformational sampling, binding site mapping, docking and scoring, in silico screening, and fragment-based drug design. In addition to the state-of-the-art theoretical concept, this book also includes step-by-step, readily reproducible computational protocols as well as examples of various CADD strategies. The limitations and potential pitfalls of different computational methods are discussed by experts, and tips and advice for their applications are suggested.

It has been a great privilege to work with the many experts in the CADD field. I very much appreciate the patience of the authors who carefully worked on their chapters and took into consideration my comments to make them a part of a coherent picture.

I would like to dedicate this book to my dearly beloved grandfather, whose wisdom, dedication, and passion for life has always been an inspiration for me.

*Birmingham, AL, USA*                                                                 *Wei Zhang*

# Contents

# Contributors

RAHUL BALASAHEB AHER • *Drug Theoretics and Cheminformatics Laboratory, Department of Pharmaceutical Technology, Jadavpur University, Kolkata, India*

MOSTAFA H. AHMED • *Department of Medicinal Chemistry, School of Pharmacy, Virginia Commonwealth University, Richmond, VA, USA; Institute for Structural Biology, Drug Discovery and Development, Virginia Commonwealth University, Richmond, VA, USA*

YURI ALEXEEV • *Leadership Computing Facility, Argonne National Laboratory, Argonne, IL, USA*

ALESSIO AMADASI • *Department of Food Science, University of Parma, Parma, Italy*

PRAVIN AMBURE • *Drug Theoretics and Cheminformatics Laboratory, Department of Pharmaceutical Technology, Jadavpur University, Kolkata, India*

ALEXANDER S. BAYDEN • *Department of Medicinal Chemistry, School of Pharmacy, Virginia Commonwealth University, Richmond, VA, USA; Institute for Structural Biology, Drug Discovery and Development, Virginia Commonwealth University, Richmond, VA, USA; CMD Bioscience, Inc., New Haven, CT, USA*

DEREK J. CASHMAN • *Department of Medicinal Chemistry, School of Pharmacy, Virginia Commonwealth University, Richmond, VA, USA; Institute for Structural Biology, Drug Discovery and Development, Virginia Commonwealth University, Richmond, VA, USA; Tennessee Technological University, Cookeville, TN, USA*

DELIANG L. CHEN • *Department of Medicinal Chemistry, School of Pharmacy, Virginia Commonwealth University, Richmond, VA, USA; Institute for Structural Biology, Drug Discovery and Development, Virginia Commonwealth University, Richmond, VA, USA; College of Chemistry and Chemical Engineering, Gannan Normal University, Ganzhou, Jiangxi, China*

EWA CHUDYK • *Evotec (UK) Ltd, Abingdon, Oxfordshire, UK*

PIETRO COZZINI • *Department of Food Science, University of Parma, Parma, Italy*

CHENXIAO DA • *Department of Medicinal Chemistry, School of Pharmacy, Virginia Commonwealth University, Richmond, VA, USA; Institute for Structural Biology, Drug Discovery and Development, Virginia Commonwealth University, Richmond, VA, USA*

GUOQIANG DONG • *Department of Medicinal Chemistry, School of Pharmacy, Second Military Medical University, Shanghai, People's Republic of China*

DMITRI G. FEDOROV • *Nanomaterials Research Institute, National Institute of Advanced Industrial Science and Technology (AIST), Tsukuba, Japan*

MICAELA FORNABAIO • *Department of Medicinal Chemistry, School of Pharmacy, Virginia Commonwealth University, Richmond, VA, USA; Institute for Structural Biology, Drug Discovery and Development, Virginia Commonwealth University, Richmond, VA, USA*

RYAN C. GODWIN • *Department of Physics, Wake Forest University, Winston-Salem, NC, USA*

NURIT HASPEL • *Department of Computer Science, University of Massachusetts Boston, Boston, MA, USA*

GLEN E. KELLOGG • *Department of Medicinal Chemistry, School of Pharmacy, Virginia Commonwealth University, Richmond, VA, USA; Institute for Structural Biology, Drug Discovery and Development, Virginia Commonwealth University, Richmond, VA, USA; Center for the Study of Biological Complexity, Virginia Commonwealth University, Richmond, VA, USA*

DAVID RYAN KOES • *Department of Computational & Systems Biology, School of Medicine, University of Pittsburgh, Pittsburgh, PA, USA*

LUHUA LAI • *College of Chemistry and Molecular Engineering, Peking University, Beijing, China*

MICHAEL P. MAZANETZ • *Evotec (UK) Ltd, Abingdon, Oxfordshire, UK*

RYAN MELVIN • *Department of Physics, Wake Forest University, Winston-Salem, NC, USA*

ANDREA MOZZARELLI • *Department of Medicinal Chemistry, School of Pharmacy, Virginia Commonwealth University, Richmond, VA, USA; Institute for Structural Biology, Drug Discovery and Development, Virginia Commonwealth University, Richmond, VA, USA; Department of Pharmacy, University of Parma, Parma, Italy*

VISHAL N.KOPARDE • *Department of Medicinal Chemistry, School of Pharmacy, Virginia Commonwealth University, Richmond, VA, USA; Institute for Structural Biology, Drug Discovery and Development, Virginia Commonwealth University, Richmond, VA, USA; Bioinformatics Computational Core Laboratories, Center for the Study of Biological Complexity, Virginia Commonwealth University, Richmond, VA, USA*

HARDIK I. PARIKH • *Department of Medicinal Chemistry, School of Pharmacy, Virginia Commonwealth University, Richmond, VA, USA; Institute for Structural Biology, Drug Discovery and Development, Virginia Commonwealth University, Richmond, VA, USA*

JIANFENG PEI • *Center for Quantitative Biology, Peking University, Beijing, China*

KUNAL ROY • *Drug Theoretics and Cheminformatics Laboratory, Department of Pharmaceutical Technology, Jadavpur University, Kolkata, India*

FREDDIE R. SALSBURYJR • *Department of Physics, Wake Forest University, Winston-Salem, NC, USA*

AURIJIT SARKAR • *Department of Medicinal Chemistry, School of Pharmacy, Virginia Commonwealth University, Richmond, VA, USA; Institute for Structural Biology, Drug Discovery and Development, Virginia Commonwealth University, Richmond, VA, USA*

J. NEEL SCARSDALE • *Institute for Structural Biology, Drug Discovery and Development, Virginia Commonwealth University, Richmond, VA, USA; Center for the Study of Biological Complexity, Virginia Commonwealth University, Richmond, VA, USA*

AMARDA SHEHU • *Department of Computer Science, George Mason University, Fairfax, VA, USA; Department of Bioengineering, George Mason University, Fairfax, VA, USA; School of Systems Biology, George Mason University, Manassas, VA, USA*

CHUNQUAN SHENG • *Department of Medicinal Chemistry, School of Pharmacy, Second Military Medical University, Shanghai, People's Republic of China*

FRANCESCA SPYRAKIS • *Department of Food Science, University of Parma, Parma, Italy; Department of Life Sciences, University of Modena and Reggio Emilia, Modena, Italy*

J. ANDREW SURFACE • *Department of Medicinal Chemistry, School of Pharmacy, Virginia Commonwealth University, Richmond, VA, USA; Institute for Structural Biology, Drug Discovery and Development, Virginia Commonwealth University, Richmond, VA, USA*

ASHUTOSH TRIPATHI • *Department of Medicinal Chemistry, School of Pharmacy, Virginia Commonwealth University, Richmond, VA, USA; Institute for Structural Biology, Drug Discovery and Development, Virginia Commonwealth University, Richmond, VA, USA*

CHEN WANG • *Changhai Hospital of Traditional Chinese Medicine, Second Military Medical University, Shanghai, People's Republic of China*

CHUNG F. WONG • *Department of Chemistry and Biochemistry and Center for Nanoscience, University of Missouri-Saint Louis, St. Louis, MO, USA*

CHENGFEI YAN • *Department of Physics and Astronomy, Dalton Cardiovascular Research Center, and Informatics Institute, University of Missouri, Columbia, MO, USA*

YAXIA YUAN • *College of Chemistry and Molecular Engineering, Peking University, Beijing, China; Center for Quantitative Biology, Peking University, Beijing, China*

SAHEEM A. ZAIDI • *Department of Medicinal Chemistry, School of Pharmacy, Virginia Commonwealth University, Richmond, VA, USA; Institute for Structural Biology, Drug Discovery and Development, Virginia Commonwealth University, Richmond, VA, USA*

WEILIN ZHANG • *Peking-Tsinghua Center for Life Sciences, AAIS, Peking University, Beijing, China*

XIAOQIN ZOU • *Department of Biochemistry, Dalton Cardiovascular Research Center, and Informatics Institute, University of Missouri, Columbia, MO, USA*

Methods in Pharmacology and Toxicology (2016): 1–30
DOI 10.1007/7653_2015_41
© Springer Science+Business Media New York 2015
Published online: 20 March 2015

# Molecular Dynamics Simulations and Computer-Aided Drug Discovery

## Ryan C. Godwin*, Ryan Melvin*, and Freddie R. Salsbury Jr.

## Abstract

Molecular dynamics simulations of biomolecules, proteins especially, have emerged as an important tool in the study of the conformational change, flexibility, and dynamics. These simulations, especially when combined with virtual screening, have been a tool in drug discovery. Herein, we cover the basics of molecular dynamics simulation, in the hopes that a reader would be able to intelligently conduct a simulation of their favorite protein(s), analyze the results in order to make hypotheses about the links between protein dynamics and conformation. We also discuss the integration between molecular dynamics and virtual screening, so that a reader could use the results of simulations to perform virtual screening for lead identification. Finally, we review several case studies to show what sort of information can be gained by simulation of biomedically interesting proteins, and how that may impact drug discovery, as well as a discussion of some areas in which simulation may prove more useful in the near future.

**Key words** Molecular dynamics, Simulations, Drug discovery, Markov analysis, Protein dynamics, Acmed

## 1  Introduction

Molecular dynamics simulations of biomolecules have been developed since the late 1970s and early 1980s (1) in order to harness the emerging power of computers to study the motions of proteins and other biopolymers, as well as to study the interactions of these biomolecules with small molecules, such as potential drugs. These computational techniques often complement experimental techniques such as Nuclear Magnetic Resonance (NMR) spectroscopy and X-ray crystallography. Observing dynamics or obtaining ensembles of conformations using these methods can be difficult. However, these experimental techniques often provide highly accurate structural information that computational methods can use as starting points to study biologically important molecules such as small molecule ligands, DNA, RNA and proteins. In particular, Molecular Dynamics (MD) simulations provide a

---

*Author contributed equally with all other contributors.

method to examine, in atomic detail if necessary, the kinetics and thermodynamics of important biomedical systems.

Since all-atom molecular dynamics simulations require the integration of Newton's equations of motion of each atom, usually including solvent and solvent ions, over short time-steps, typically on the femto-second timescale, these simulations can be rather computationally demanding. However, the growth of computer power especially in the late 1990s and early 2000s enabled these methods to be particularly predictive in studying protein dynamics, such as in investigating the impact of protein motions on catalysis and ligand binding (2–4). The latter studies have been especially influential as they have required considerable discussion of the interplay of conformational change, such as changes in active site geometries in DHFR (2) or metallo-beta-lactamases (3) and coupled protein fluctuations (4), which show that within a single protein conformation, long-range coupling networks exist and are sensitive to interactions with different ligands.

Even more recently, molecular dynamics simulations have proven useful in studying larger biological systems and in aiding in the drug discovery process by providing a predictive complement to experimental methods, contributing predictions for dynamics and structures not easily observed in vitro or in vivo. Such predictions are useful in pharmacology for understanding the interactions of drug candidates with biological systems on an atomic scale.

Molecular dynamics simulations also prove useful when considering proteins as ensembles of conformational states (5–10), as simulations explore ensembles and output large collections of structures, which sample the conformations that occur.

In part, the notion of generalized allostery comes out of the conceptualization of proteins as ensembles of states and the understanding of conformational changes occurring due to long-range coupling networks (9). If under certain conditions all proteins are indeed allosteric, it is possible to design drugs that will bind to allosteric sites. Such binding would force the protein into a certain conformation—or specific ensemble of conformations—thereby regulating the dynamics and interactions of the protein (9, 11). However, for any given protein, an appropriate ligand and corresponding binding site to induce the desired structural change must be found. This type of search is one for which molecular dynamics simulations are well suited. Much of the relevant scientific work in the 2000s was reviewed a few years ago (12). This chapter serves a few purposes. First, it expands upon and update that previous review, especially in light of the tremendous improvements in computational algorithms and hardware, such as GPU-enabled computing. Second, we describe the minimum theoretical and technical details necessary for setting up, executing, and analyzing MD simulations so that any who are interested in participating in computer-aided drug discovery may have the tools necessary for doing so.

## 2  Basics of Molecular Dynamics

### 2.1  Structures

The minimum structural information required to start a simulation is:

1. A list of all atoms involved in the simulation
2. Initial coordinates of these atoms

For a given system, with fixed protonation states, there is only one possible list of atoms; however, there are infinitely many possible initial coordinates. Of course, most of these combinations would have enormous energy and would be negligible members of the real, physical ensemble. To achieve realistic results, a physiological initial state needs to be considered. Folding a biopolymer from an unfolded state can rarely be achieved straightforwardly—the time scales are still too long—except for the smallest systems. Therefore, simulations usually start in a folded state; the set of coordinates that likely correspond to a minimum free energy state. Online databases–e.g., the protein databank (RCSB PDB—with 106,293 structures to date), which collect structures from X-ray crystallography and NMR spectroscopy (13)—are the normal sources for such initial structures. It is also possible sometimes to model the initial atomic coordinates based on the structure of other proteins with similar sequences via homology modeling (14). The extent to which this is accurate of course depends on how close the unknown protein is to the known proteins, which is generally not known. As such, simulations almost always start from structures obtained from the RCSB protein databank. A promising development that could have impact in the near future is the possibility of building up structures from a type of quantum mechanical method known as Density Functional Theory (DFT). Variants of this method have proven useful in materials science and computational chemistry (15).

### 2.2  Force Fields

Force fields are the potential energy functions used to calculate the accelerations of the atoms and subsequently update the coordinates and the velocities at each step of the simulation. This parameterization of the energy surface of a protein or other biopolymers is conceptually straightforward, but complicated in practice. In principle, the energy surface of even a small protein has 100,000s of dimensions even without solvent. However, since the aim is to simulate the dynamics of connected and folded proteins, this surface can be simplified using conventional terms from chemistry, such as bonds, angles, dihedrals, and other terms related to chemical connectivity, and long-range interactions as modeled by van der Waals interactions and electrostatics. Among the many force fields that exist, the most popular families of force fields include CHARMM (16), AMBER (17), and GROMOS (18). The energy equation from the CHARMM 27 force field is shown in Eq. (1), where $V$ is the total potential energy.

$$
\begin{aligned}
V &= \sum_{\text{bonds}} k_{\text{B}}(b - b_0)^2 + \sum_{\text{angles}} k_\theta(\theta - \theta_0)^2 + \sum_{\text{dihedrals}} k_\phi[1 - \cos(n\phi - \delta)] \\
&+ \sum_{\text{impropers}} k_\omega(\omega - \omega_0)^2 + \sum_{\text{UB}} k_{\text{u}}(u - u_0)^2 \\
&+ \sum_{i>j} \varepsilon_{ij}\left[\left(\frac{R_{\min_{ij}}}{r_{ij}}\right)^{12} - \left(\frac{R_{\min_{ij}}}{r_{ij}}\right)^6\right] + \sum_{i>j} \frac{q_i q_j}{4\pi\varepsilon_0 \varepsilon r_{ij}}
\end{aligned}
$$

(1)

Many of the bonded interactions are effectively modeled as simple harmonic oscillator potentials, including bonds, angles, the Urey-Bradley term, and impropers, i.e., the first, second, fourth, and fifth terms in Eq. (1). In each of these terms there are force constants that control the stiffness of the bonds, angles, impropers, and Urey-Bradley terms. In principle, every single such interaction can have its own minimum and force constant, but in practice there is a great of similarity. Bonds, the first terms, are 1–2 interactions that occur between all atoms that are directly connected via chemical bonds. Angles, the second term, are 1–3 interactions that occur between all atoms that share a common bonded atom. The impropers, the fourth term, are 1–4 interactions that occur between atoms that share common angles. They occur between some atoms, those in which dihedrals are insufficient to constrain the torsional angle. The Urey-Bradley term, the fifth term, is a 1–3 interaction energy, i.e., an interaction between atom pairs that share a common bonded angle, that some atom pairs have and is designed to control angle-bending for particularly stiff angles. Dihedrals, the third term, are 1–4 interactions between all atoms that share common angles and are modeled with a cosine approximation. The last two terms are the non-bonded interactions, and are modeled via the Lennard–Jones potential and the Coulomb potential, where every atom pair that does not occur in a bond, angle, or dihedral, possesses these long-range interactions. The nature of the $1/r$ Coulomb potential is a long-range interaction, and is computationally limiting, since it does not go rapidly to zero as the Lennard–Jones potential does over longer ranges. However, methods have been developed to approximate the Coulomb potential accurately over longer ranges, such as the particle mesh Ewald method (19).

Although force fields are complicated approximations, these models are constantly being vetted and compared to experiment to improve the force field parameterization for proteins, nucleic acids and lipids. The force fields have been refined over the years to correct issues where, for example, AMBER over-stabilized alpha-helices (20, 21) or CHARMM tended toward pi-helices (22). There is little consensus to suggest that one force field is better than the rest for protein simulations, and simulations performed on the same structure with different force fields generate consistent results, for example ref. (3) vs refs. (4) and (23). The success of these force fields has been recently highlighted when Martin Karplus, Michael Levitt, and Arieh Warshel won the 2013 Nobel Prize in Chemistry "*for the development of multiscale models for complex chemical systems*" (24).

**2.3 Simulation Programs**

Various simulation suites exist and the most popular include NAMD (25), CHARMM (26), AMBER (27), and GROMACS (28). These suites share common basic features but vary in their capacities and underlying philosophies.

The most user-friendly of these suites is NAMD, built upon C++ and TCL programming and scripting languages, but has the least functionality. However, it contains all the functionality needed for all-atom simulations. Conversely, the most versatile package is CHARMM, but it comes with a steep learning curve, and resembles a Fortran-based language. GROMACS is the only one of the four suites that is open source, and has been converted from its original FORTRAN implementation to C. Of these four packages, NAMD is the most capable of performing large, classical all-atom simulations on CPUs, and has been used to simulate particularly large proteins and protein complexes (for example (4, 29, 30)). GROMACS has the advantage of a large number of external tools for trajectory analysis; it is generally the second-fastest. CHARMM is the most flexible for analysis and for performing different simulations. For the simulations described in this chapter while running on CPUS, arguably the "best" combination would be to use NAMD to run simulations and CHARMM for analysis, while using GROMACS for both simulation and analysis would be a close second. However, over the last few years, GPU-enabled codes have emerged, especially ACEMD (31), which is similar to NAMD in its functionality. Until and unless other suites emerge that are as GPU-enabled, the ideal simulation technology at present is ACEMD on GPUs.

**2.4 Running a Simulation**

Given a particular biomolecular system of interest and a simulation package, the next step is to set up the simulation parameters. Many of these are default configuration parameters that should be understood.

First, a choice needs to be made as to which thermodynamic ensemble should be approximated. Since the isothermal–isobaric (NPT) ensemble has the Gibb's free energy as its thermodynamic potential, and usually corresponds to experimental conditions, this is currently the most common ensemble to simulate. Simulating the NPT ensemble requires using a thermostat and barostat to approximate constant temperature and constant pressure respectively.

Simulation packages typically offer the option to run other ensembles, minimally the canonical (NVT), and microcanonical (NVE) ensembles. Although it seems logical that one would simulate in the NPT ensemble for best agreement with experiments, it is not clear how different simulations are in these various ensembles.

To best represent physiological conditions, water molecules and ions that surround biomolecules in vivo are either explicitly or implicitly modeled in simulation; this is an important enough topic to warrant its only section below. In the most common case of explicit solvent and ions, periodic boundary conditions are implemented and then long-range electrostatic interactions are approximated using a particle mesh Ewald summation method with Fast Fourier transforms (32).

Embedded in each simulation code are numerical integration methods that are used to update the positions and velocities of each atom in the system from the accelerations determined by the force field for each simulated atom at each time-step. This time-step, or interval over which the forces are considered constant, and which determines how often configurations change, is an important consideration. If the time-steps are too small, computer time and disk space will be wasted. If the time-steps are too large, the simulation is no longer energy conserving and accuracy will suffer. However, simulation packages typically have good default choices of integrators, such as velocity Verlet (33) with time-steps of 1–2 fs.

After the simulation has been set up, usually a brief minimization is performed to remove any clashes between atoms. Post-minimization the system is simulated for a given number of time-steps—depending on the timescale necessary to address the biomedical problem as well as the computational power available. With current GPU-enabled codes, simulations on the 100s of nanosecond to microseconds are feasible depending on system size and patience of the user. Also, typically multiple simulations are performed where each atom starts with a different random velocity, taken from a Boltzmann distribution, to allow for better coverage of phase-space.

## 3    Solvation Techniques

In order to accurately simulate biomolecules, it is imperative to recreate the local environment as best as possible. As such, biomolecules are simulated in an aqueous environment to approximate physiological conditions. Modeling solvation is important, as it has been shown that solvent fluctuations can be directly related to protein motions (34, 35). Additionally, the layer of water surrounding the biopolymer, i.e., the water molecules closest to the sample, has properties different than that of the bulk solvent (36). It is clear that solvent interactions are critical to properly functioning biomolecules, and when simulating such systems, the choice of solvent approximation is an important issue. There are two main approaches to simulating solvents, with explicit or implicit solvent, and many models within each implementation. While none of these is perfect, some are advantageous particularly dependent on the simulation in question.

An explicit solvent is exactly that, including a box composed of an oxygen bound to two hydrogens, each with updated coordinates and velocities calculated at each time-step. These models are often characterized by the number of site interaction points considered and go from 2-site models up to 6-site models. TIP3P and TIP4P are common 3 and 4-site models, respectively (37, 38), that have been studied extensively (39, 40).

The simplest explicit water models assume rigid bonds and only calculate non-bonded interactions including van der Waals and electrostatic interactions. In many explicit models, water bonds are maintained via the SHAKE algorithm, in order to speed up calculations as these bonds are typically not interesting, yet are of high frequency (41).

Because explicit solvents can handle representative motions at a global and local scale, they are often preferred. Alternatives include implicit solvent approximations in which the electrostatic properties of the water are calculated approximately without including the explicit presence and motion of water molecules. This reduces the computational expense by removing explicit water atoms. Various implicit solvent models have been compared (42–44), and Generalized Born (GB) models (23) show the most promise of the implicit models (42, 43). The struggle is to reproduce the solvent behavior consistent with experiment, and while there has been some success (23, 45), comparison of the TIP3P water model to GB implicit models show an over-stabilization of secondary structure in implicit solvent models over explicit solvent models. Namely, it has been shown that alpha-helices are over stabilized in GB models over TIP3P (20), and ion pair interactions are sometimes over stabilized leading to the trapping of molecules in non-native states (39). Overall, implicit solvents reduce computational time, yet they pay a penalty in accuracy. However, explicit solvents, while generally more accurate, require additional computer resources. In the era of GPUs and parallelization of calculations, explicit models are preferable when possible, due to their accuracy.

Regardless of the solvation technique, in order to model in vivo or in vitro conditions, ions need to be added to the simulation. If the ions exist in the X-ray structure, then they can be added in explicit in the positions in the structure, as such ions are likely to be structurally important. Otherwise, there are automated processes for doing so in software packages such as VMD (46), which place sufficient ions randomly in the water box to match conditions desired; such as 0.15 M ionic strength with NaCl as is common to match experiment conditions, or just sufficient $Na^+$ or $Cl^-$ to neutralize the protein system.

## 4  Analysis Methods

Once simulations have been performed, they must be analyzed to check their validity and also to extract useful information. Since the results of a simulation are the coordinates of all the atoms in the system simulated over the timescale of the simulation, a wide variety of analysis methods can be applied to extract virtual any type of structural and provide the most dynamical information. Below, the most common–and typically the most useful—of these analysis methods are discussed.

*Simulation Check*: *Structural relaxation*
Given that simulations can run from hours to months depending on the system size and timescale desired, performing energy and structural checks shortly after starting a simulation minimizes time wasted on unstable or improperly setup simulations. If a simulation's log file has been configured to report energies, the user can read out the energies after a relatively small number of time-steps to see if the energies reported are reasonable. Similar checks can be performed on the pressure and temperature, which should be relatively constant for biological systems and fluctuate around the values set for the thermostat and barostat (usually 300 K and 1 atm, although 310 K can be used to better match physiological conditions). As an additional validity check, a user can calculate the Root Mean Square Deviation (RMSD) of a subset of the simulation's atoms. This measure quantifies how much the polymer of interest has changed from a reference structure over time. Such checks allow a user to judge the physical reasonableness—relative to the system and thermodynamic ensemble chosen—of a simulation (12). The reference structure is usually the initial structure that has been obtained from experimental work, in order to gauge the stability of the simulation and structure itself. Beyond understanding how realistic a simulation is, measures of energy, pressure, temperature and RMSD versus time are indicators of a successfully equilibrated system. An initial period of rapid change followed by relative stability with small fluctuations around a mean value indicates a successfully equilibrated system. For example, in Fig. 1, there is a rapid growth of RMSD in the first 100 ns. Afterward, the system reaches an equilibrated state with small fluctuations around a mean of about 5 Å.

This RMSD measures the average difference of all selected atoms from one frame to the next via

$$R_{\text{RMSD}} = \sqrt{\frac{1}{N}\sum_{i=1}^{N}\left(\vec{r}_i - \vec{r}_i'\right)^2}$$

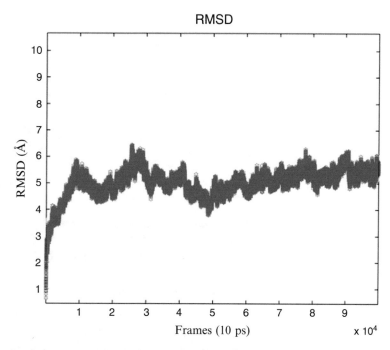

**Fig. 1** All-atom MD simulation of a Zinc-Finger structure has a 100 ns equilibration phase

where $N$ is the number of atoms in the selection, $r$ is the position vector $(x,y,z)$ of the atom at time $t$, and $r'$ is the position of the atom in the reference frame. Before a meaningful measure of RMSD (or any other quantity that depends on translational or rotational differences in position) can be made, the atoms of interest in the trajectory must first be aligned to some reference structure so as to remove the overall motion of the protein. Without this alignment, conformational changes will be conflated with rigid body motions of the protein that is the diffusion and overall rotation of the entire protein that occurs during the simulation. To align the atoms, analysis software, such as VMD or scripts in CHARMM or GROMACS, minimizes the RMSD of selected atoms between a reference structure and every frame in the trajectory using only rigid-body rotations and translations. This alignment focuses the analysis of protein conformations and dynamics.

*4.1   Clustering: Searching Conformation Space*

Given that simulations can run from hours to months depending on the system size and timescale desired, clustering analysis simplifies the comparison of structures output from an MD simulation by classifying thousands to ten thousands of frames into a smaller taxonomy with representative conformations. Figure 2 shows how finely these clusters can distinguish structures from simulations, while still reducing the complexity from, in the case, the structural information contained in a microsecond scale simulation to just 50 representative structures along with how often these structures are sampled. Two of which are depicted in Fig. 2 for illustrative purposes.

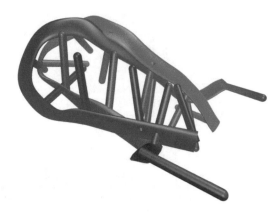

**Fig. 2** Two representative structures of a 10-residue FdUMP chain show small conformational differences between some clusters. From the *red* to the *blue* representative, F10's termini have spread apart

The clusters are defined by their size in a parameter space—typically pair-wise RMSDs between structures—so that clustering effectively partitions configuration space. Algorithms for deciding what conformations fall in a given cluster come in two categories, hierarchical clustering and nonhierarchical clustering. The method for determining the distance between clusters distinguishes algorithms within each category. Hierarchical clustering methods partition the conformation space into a tree by iteratively connecting neighboring elements in a dataset. Selecting a level at which to divide the tree forms clusters. Hierarchical clustering, Fig. 3, is simple and fast since once an element of the dataset has been placed in a cluster it is ignored for the remainder of the clustering process. Slower, nonhierarchical methods optimize each cluster based on some desired parameters set by the user. Nonhierarchical clustering, Fig. 4, allows for moving data among clusters as part of the optimization process, making them slower than their hierarchical counterparts (47, 48). Nonhierarchical, iterative methods are implemented in two popular analysis software packages, VMD (46) and CHARMM (49).

VMD uses a Quality Threshold (QT) clustering algorithm (47). The method begins by assembling a cluster based on every element in the dataset. For example, if an MD trajectory contains 10,000 frames, the first iteration of the QT algorithm will have 10,000 clusters. In this iteration the $N$th cluster begins with the $N$th frame and is compared with all other frames, regardless of whether those frames have already been placed in another cluster. The frame that causes the smallest increase in cluster diameter is accepted into the group. This process is repeated for the $N$th cluster until no frame can be added without taking the cluster diameter past the threshold specified by the user. At the end of this iteration,

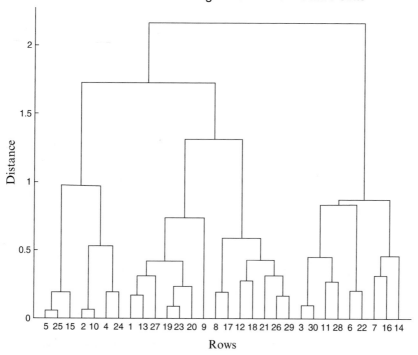

**Fig. 3** Once all data points are grouped in the clustering tree, a cutoff distance is chosen. Any lines that join at a distance equal to or greater than the cutoff distance are clustered; all other lines are unclustered. Row values are the representative cluster numbers

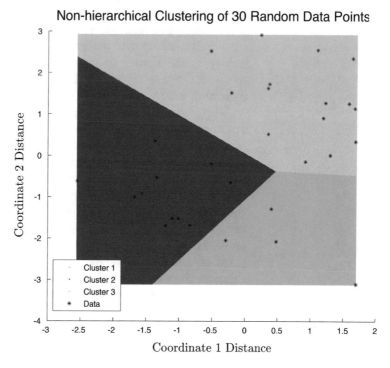

**Fig. 4** Non-hierarchical clustering interactively searches for partitions within conformation space that minimize the distance between clusters in each partition

all frames in the largest cluster are removed from consideration. This largest cluster is now fixed, and the process iterates until either no frames remain or the number of fixed clusters equals a target number of clusters set by the user. In the latter case the remaining frames are simply left unclustered. In VMD specifically, if $M$ is the target number of clusters, all unclustered frames are labeled as cluster $M + 1$. CHARMM uses the ART-2′ clustering Algorithm, which is based on a self-organizing neural network (50, 51). Similar to QT, this algorithm optimizes each cluster based on a constrained cluster radius. However, ART-2′ starts with one cluster rather than the largest possible number of clusters. The first of two phases in the clustering determines the number of clusters and their respective centers. To begin, ART-2′ selects the first frame of the trajectory as the center of a single cluster. Then, the Euclidean distance to each (in the space of the user-selected cluster parameter) frame is calculated. If the distance from the cluster center to a conformation is within the cutoff radius, that frame is added to the cluster and the cluster center is recalculated before comparison with the next frame. If the distance is outside the cutoff radius, the rejected frame is assigned as the center of a new cluster. The second phase of clustering is still done with Euclidean distance but is performed in multiple iterations; furthermore, at each iteration, the number of clusters and cluster centers are fixed. Once all frames are assigned to a cluster in a given iteration, the cluster centers are recalculated. Finally, the clustering assignment process is repeated. This cycle of the second phase continues until no changes occur between iterations. An obvious pitfall of this method is that the order of the frames influences the cluster assignment. Therefore, the user may wish to check the stability of the clusters by doing a second round of clustering with a randomized frame order (48).

Regardless of the clustering method used, the user must set input parameters based on some analysis criteria based on user preference. For example, when using VMD's RMSD clustering method, a cutoff distance and number of clusters must be set. These parameters should be chosen in such a way that balances the number of frames placed in clusters and the number of clusters themselves. Obviously, if the number of clusters is set to the number of frames, the user is guaranteed that all frames will be clustered. However, no information is gained in this example as the point of clustering is simplifying the analysis of the trajectory. To this end, the user may first decide a reasonable number of clusters, e.g., 50, to analyze and then adjust the cutoff parameter to minimize the number of unclustered frames. The strategy in that case is to begin with a low cutoff, e.g., 2 Å, and gradually increase it until the point when either VMD reports fewer clusters than the number desired or an increase results in no or a very small change in the number of unclustered frames. Such a procedure balances

approximations, but not requiring a large number of clusters to analyze while including as much of the simulation data available for in clusters for further analysis.

**4.2  Markov Analysis**    In addition to identifying representative structures of clusters, such as those in Fig. 2, plots of cluster vs frame, Fig. 5, can show the transitions among states. In this representation it is easy to identify long-lived states and to find the populations of different conformational states. However, it is also easy to miss short-lived stable states, and it is difficult to accurately see the transition states by eye. Accessing these transitions requires reconstructing the kinetics of the system, a task for which Markov State Models (MSMs) are well suited.

MSMs are network models that convey the rates of transition among states. These models typically assume the system is memoryless, though they can be generalized to systems with memory. For example, a memoryless process is a Markovian process of order 1. In this case, the state of a system at time-step $N$ depends only on the system's state at the previous time-step $N - 1$. To generalize to include memory, one uses a Markovian process of order $M$. In this case, the state of the system at time-step $N$ depends on the system's state at time-steps $N - M$, $N - (M - 1)$, ... and $N - 1$. Using

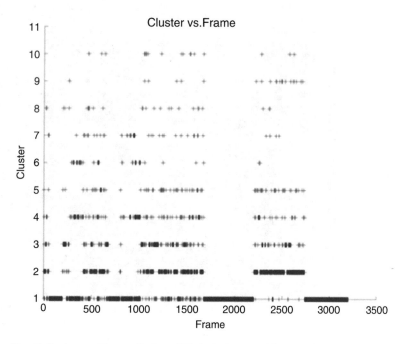

**Fig. 5** During a 16-μs all-atom MD trajectory, a 10-mer of FdUMP cluster analysis shows there is a preferred, low energy state with frequent transitions to higher energy states

these models requires defining states based on physical parameters, typically based on RMSD. For example, a state might consist of all structures within 2 Å of each other. In which case, these states are taken from clustering analysis. These Markov models also allow for further simplifications based on kinetic definitions of macrostates, which are combinations of microstates. A macrostate might be all microstates that transition among each other in less than 20 ps. Once these states are, it is possible to apply statistical mechanics to estimate various thermodynamics quantities, such as the free energy of a macrostate using kTlog($P$) where $P$ is the population of the states contained in a macrostate.

Recently, software packages for assisting in dynamics-based clustering and construction of MSM have been developed. Two such packages are EMMA (52) and MSMBuilder2 (53). The latter software package has a companion application, MSMExplorer, for visualizing MSMs (54).

A convenient way to convey the information in a MSM is with a rate matrix and heat map thereof, Fig. 6. There are three primary steps in the construction of such a matrix for an MD trajectory. First, order clusters by their corresponding frame number. This

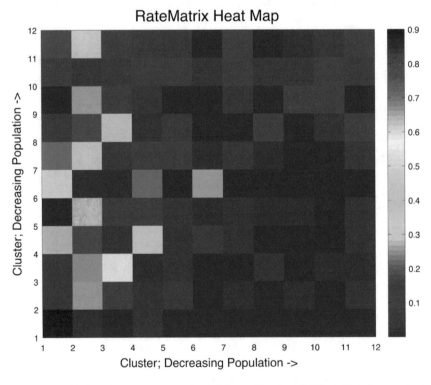

**Fig. 6** Whenever this FdUMP polymer enters cluster 1 (*blue* in Fig. 2), it is 90 % likely to remain there during the next time step (in this case 5 ns). This molecule frequently transitions from cluster 5 to cluster 2 and cluster 9 to cluster 2

sorted list is called a Markov chain. Next, count how often state $i$ is followed by state $j$ where both $i$ and $j$ run from 1 to the number of macrostates. Finally, place those counts in $A$, which is an $M \times M$ matrix, where $M$ is the number of states, and normalize each row so that it sums to unity. Now, the matrix is read "when the system is in state $i$, the probability it will transition to state $j$ in the next time-step is $Aij$." Using Markov State Models in this fashion quickly reduces the task of analyzing the kinetics of thousands to billions of conformations to reading an $M \times M$ matrix, where $M$ is much smaller than the number of frames in the trajectory. More details on such modeling are beyond the scope of this review, but a simple yet comprehensive review of them has been published (55).

**4.3 Analysis of Protein Motions and Dynamics**

Clustering combined with Markov analysis provide information about the configuration space accessed by a biopolymer during the timescale, typically nanosecond to microsecond, of the MD simulation. Markov analysis also provides information about kinetics via quantifying transitions between configurations. However, there is additional information contained in a simulation, including information about protein motions through analysis of dynamics via examination of fluctuations.

Dynamical studies of protein motions are important in understanding regulation and function of a cell. Naturally, cellular function is an extremely active process requiring a myriad of properly functional components. To use this information for predictive purposes, it behooves us to have some knowledge of the motions that dictate proper function and understand how physical laws drive motions. Simulations provide enough insight to hypothesize the important functional processes, as conformational changes have helped to identify drug targets, for example (...). Mechanisms such as protein–protein and protein–surface interactions have recently gained more traction in the drug targeting process (56).

Understanding how protein motions are affected by ligand binding and the impact that may have on proper function of a biomolecule suggest the importance of dynamics in the drug discovery process (57). However, there is a great deal of remaining investigation of the dynamics of protein, DNA, and RNA interactions, and dissecting these dynamics may yet inform the development of therapeutics.

Studies suggest that conformational changes at one site of a protein, for example, affect distant regions of a protein and its ability to bind properly, despite no noticeable changes in the binding region (58). This form of general or hidden allostery is a dynamical component often overlooked in the drug discovery process (9) and is proving useful in predicting functional molecular mechanisms (59).

**4.4 Root Mean Square Fluctuations**

Root mean square fluctuation (RMSF) is a useful analysis tool to examine the behavior of a protein with atomic precision across the whole trajectory by measuring the average mobility of each atom in the simulation. RMSFs are a measurement of time-averaged fluctuations from a reference frame, typically the first frame. The RMSF is a useful estimation of the rigidity of various parts of the biomolecule, with higher RMSF indicating a more flexible region. Values are typically on the order of a few to tens of Angstroms and are calculated using the following equation,

$$R_{\mathrm{RMSF}} = \sqrt{\frac{1}{T}\sum_{t_j=1}^{T}\left(\vec{r}_i(t_j) - \vec{r}_i'\right)^2}$$

Where $r$ is the $x$, $y$, $z$ coordinates of the atom, for example, and $r'$ is that of the reference structure. $T$ is the total number of frames, and $i$ represents the index over atoms and $j$ represents the index over time. Figure 7 provides an example of RMSFs for a small 28-residue zinc finger, NEMO (60). In this example, the flexibility of this protein is studied over different timescales, and surprisingly for such a small protein, the flexibility was radically increased on longer-time scales. The RMSFs plots also show changes in flexibility along the protein backbone, indicating regions of increased flexibility and regions of increased rigidity.

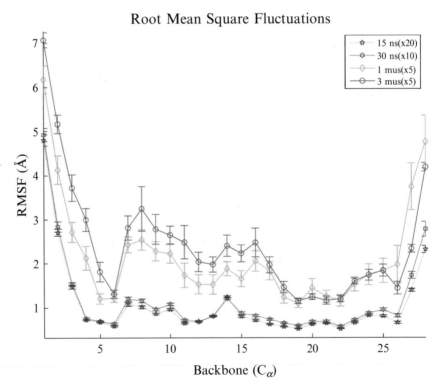

**Fig. 7** A plot of RMSF for each alpha carbon for four different timescales of simulations showing variation in flexibility on a residue basis

**4.5  Covariance and Correlation Analysis**

Whereas RMSFs provide information about flexibility at the atomic level, they provide no information about coupled motions. Covariances, or their normalized counterparts, correlations, however, provide an indication of coupled dynamics by indicating what parts of the system show correlated motions; these could be motions in the same direction, in the opposite directions, or most often, uncorrelated motions (61). Covariance analysis is a useful technique for detecting the motions of a protein that might, for example, be responsible for a particular interaction, or to elucidate long-range interactions within a sample that may be responsible for allosteric regulation or other functional behavior. If $r_i$ and $r_j$ are position vectors of two atoms in the sample, then the covariance is calculated using

$$\tilde{C}_{ij} = \sum_{\alpha=1}^{N} \frac{\left( \vec{r}_i^{\,\alpha} - \left\langle \vec{r}_i^{\,\alpha} \right\rangle \right) \cdot \left( \vec{r}_j^{\,\alpha} - \left\langle \vec{r}_j^{\,\alpha} \right\rangle \right)}{N}$$

Here $N$ indicates the total number of frames and alpha is the index over each frame of the trajectory. These covariances are then typically normalized into correlations by dividing by the square root of the product of $C_{ii}$ and $C_{jj}$, so that the diagonals are one; an atom always fluctuations with itself. In the molecular dynamics literature, correlation matrices, e.g., Fig. 8, are often referred to as covariance

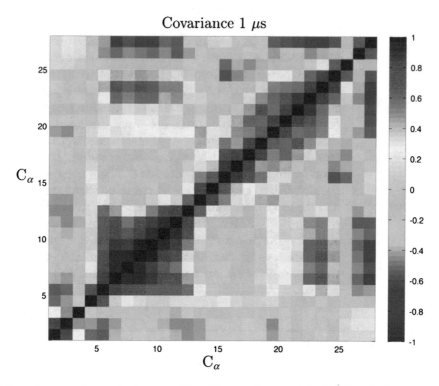

Covariance 1 $\mu$s

**Fig. 8** Alpha carbon covariances for the same 28-residue zinc finger protein, NEMO, as in Fig. 7, as simulated on the microsecond timescale

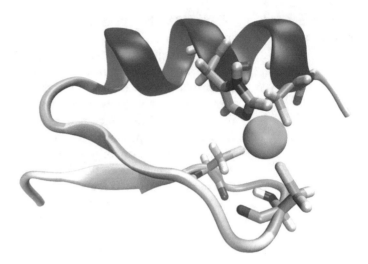

**Fig. 9** Cartoon drawing of NEMO. Based on the striker 2JVX from the RCSB. The alpha helix in *magenta*, the beta sheet in *yellow* with the zinc in vdW representation in *green*. The binding residues of the zinc are in a bonded representation

matrices, where they should properly be referred to as correlation matrices. The difference between the two is that a covariance matrix has not been normalized so that the diagonal elements are one, whereas a correlation matrix is a normalized version of the covariance matrix. Such correlation matrices aka normalized covariance matrices are useful in extracting the essential degrees of freedom often hypothesized responsible for the primary function of a system (62). Additionally, entropy estimates, and subsequently heat capacity, can be derived from the covariance matrix using harmonic approximations (63, 64). Figure 8 provides an example of correlations for the alpha carbons a small 28-residue zinc finger, NEMO (60). In this example, there are some unsurprising covariances, those within the secondary structural elements, the beta structure (residues 5–12), and the alpha helix (residues 16–24), but also shows correlated motions between the beta sheet and portions of the alpha helix, and anti-correlated motions between the beta-sheet and the loop connecting the helix and the sheet., c.f. Fig. 9 for the structure of NEMO. Whether these are due to zinc binding is a subject of further study, but this illustrates that non-trivial covariances can exist in even small proteins, and provides an example of the sort of information available from correlations plots, even by just visual inspection.

## 5    Small Molecule Docking

The analysis tools discussed so far provide information about the conformations, fluctuations and dynamics of a protein or other macromolecular system. Clustering and Markov analysis have particular uses also in syncing with small molecule docking for lead generations. Protein flexibility is a challenge for molecular docking. Rather than allow docking software to simulate small conformational changes, it is often more efficient to use MD software to assemble an ensemble of structures as initial structures for docking studies, since simulations of polymer flexing are squarely in the realm of MD. Once these conformations are selected from an MD trajectory, each one can be used as a starting structure for small molecule docking, for which there are multiple efficient software packages (65–72).

One such docking software, arguably the most efficient, that is popular in a wide variety of uses is AutoDock (73, 74). In 2004, an open source generation of the software was released—AutoDock Vina (75). Previous generation software focused on analytic approaches to docking. For example, AutoDock 4.2 calculated free energies of association for bound conformations using an empirical force field, Lamarckian Genetic Algorithm (76), and explicit modeling of side chains in receptors (77). While AutoDock Vina maintains some of these strategies, the energy function has been refined using machine learning and the PDBbind database (78, 79) of known binding affinities. The key advantage of Auto-Dock Vina is the calculation of both a scoring function and the gradient thereof. By calculating the gradient, the software knows which direction the next iteration of the search should move a given local set of atoms (75, 80–82). As a result, AutoDock Vina is far faster than previous software packages, while still retaining considerable precision.

In order to use docking software for identify potential lead candidates for drug discovery, ligand libraries must be used. While a small ligand library could be hand constructed using common molecular drawing and export software, a strategy to take advantage of the strength of molecular dynamics and of virtual screening would be to use a large general screening library of ligands. These can be obtained from various online chemical databases such as BindingDB (83), ChEMBL (84), DrugBank (85), PubChem (86), TCM Database@Taiwan (87), and ZINC (88, 89). This last database, ZINC, is arguably the best for general purpose docking and was originally developed with drug discovery in mind and has kept that focus while growing to sample 34,000,000 unique molecules from 134 commercial and 36 annotated catalogs. The attempt is to have a library of all commercially available compounds. This focus on drug discovery manifests itself in two ways. First, ZINC's structure files are generally selected for their biological relevance. Second, the subsets into which these structures are grouped have been curated with screening and discovery in mind so that datasets using standard definitions of "drug-like," "lead-like," and "fragment-like" are readily available for download. They also maintain subsets of these datasets containing "currently" available compounds;

usually updated every 6 months or so. Currently available means a delivery window of 0–10 weeks, with a target price of $100 or less per sample. Within each of the latter lead-like datasets, there are also different versions that have had different levels of similarity analysis performed on them. For example, one could download currently available lead-like molecules, from a set of 3,687,621 molecules at the time this was written. Or one could download a subset filtered at the 90 % similarity level—so that any two compounds that are more than 90 % similar are filtered out and only one selected—which is less than a tenth the size of the whole library; 322,638 molecules.

The ZINC database has other features that make it particularly useful for drug discovery using virtual screening. For example, to ensure the quality of structures and groupings, the creators of ZINC have what they term a "hit picking party" (89) from time to time, during which they run docking trials on structures in the ZINC database and compare the output structures to experimental data. Beyond providing structures for virtual screening, the physical compounds can be purchased through ZINC. For time-sensitive studies ZINC is able to sort purchasable compounds by estimated delivery time. While the physical compounds are sold commercially, searching for and downloading structure files are free services (89).

If it is not desirable to use a general library for virtual screening, for example, if there is a lead available and the goal is to refine or expand outward in the space of molecules, or if particular chemistries are desired, then libraries can be constructed combinatorially. That is particular core structures can be defined along with functional groups to modify those groups, and they can be combined computationally to generate a personalized library. There are commercial libraries that can be used for this purpose, but Simlib is a freely available code that can be used to easily generate libraries (90).

## 6  Timescale Considerations

It should not be surprising that longer timescale simulations require more computational resources, and choosing the appropriate timescale to simulate is an important consideration. The decision is motivated by the resources available and what is of biophysical interest. Nanosecond timescale simulations are valuable to elucidate low energy conformations and nearby fluctuations from that minimum. These simulations can be especially useful for identifying dynamical motion sufficient to hypothesize corresponding biological function (59, 91), and afford sufficient time to observe conformational changes such as motions of a lever arm, for example. These types of simulations may indeed be sufficient for lead identification (11, 92).

And yet, many important molecular processes occur at longer timescales, so if these are of primary interest, either for biological interest or to obtain rarer conformations for docking, then longer simulations are required. Larger conformational arrangements may require longer simulations as slower processes are responsible for some allosteric regulation or other conformational selection events (93). Even for small systems, such as a 28 residue zinc-finger motif, rare events, that are not available in shorter simulations, occur in the microsecond regime (60). These less-common events may well have significance for drug discovery, and the fact that they happen on the order of microseconds means they still happen 100s–1000s times per millisecond, and they may provide pockets for drug docking, as suggested by those who argue that allostery is an intrinsic property of all proteins (9).

# 7    Recent Applications of Molecular Dynamics and Docking

## 7.1    Molecular Dynamics and Docking: MSH2/6 and Rescinnamine

An example of pharmacological use of virtual screening via docking to clusters from MD simulations comes from a search for small molecules that would selectively bind to an apoptosis-inducing conformation of the MSH2/MSH6 proteins (92). These two proteins form a complex and recognize DNA defects resulting from improper replication. The proteins then enter either a repair conformation when the lesions are reparable or a death-signaling conformation when the lesions are irreparable (94–99). In both cases, this protein complex senses the defect or damage and recruits other proteins to either repair the defect or initiate cell death. It is also likely that there are multiple cell death pathways. The goal of this example study was to find cytotoxic agents that would bind to MSH2/MSH6 while the protein is in the death-signaling conformation, thereby triggering apoptosis (91, 99).

The researchers started with an X-ray structure of a complex of DNA and *Escherichia coli* MutS—a homolog of MSH—modified to include the cisplatin adduct cross linking DNA with hydrogens added via the CHARMM software package and solvated with TIP3P water using VMD's "Add Solvation Box" extension. They performed a 250 ps equilibration and subsequent 10 ns production run in NAMD with the CHARMM27 force field, having pressure set to 1.01325 bar and temperature to 300 K. Frames in the final trajectory were clustered using a 1 Å cutoff radius K-means clustering. They input the resulting ensemble of conformations into AutoDock 3 (see (76) for details of this version) for docking trials with a small library of commercially available compounds. They then tested the compounds with highest binding affinities for the E. coli MutS-DNA complex in vitro on MSH2/MSH6 and found that they could indeed use a selectively binding ligand to select out the death-signaling conformation of the proteins (92, 100).

Beyond their specific goal, this work demonstrated the predictive power of in silico molecular dynamics and virtual screening to select compounds for in vitro trials. Subsequent work building on this has focused on using nanoscale simulations to study further aspect of binding of damaged DNA to the human MSH2/6 (59, 101, 102).

### 7.2 Docking Without Molecular Dynamics

Docking trials on their own are powerful predictive tools for drug discovery. For example, they were used in the development of a novel phosphatidylinositol-3-kinase (PI3K) inhibitor that specifically targets prostate cancer (103). PI3K activity is currently understood to inhibit apoptosis of prostate cancer cells and allow them to continue multiplying even in local environments that would be unfavorable to healthy cells, specifically areas of low androgen concentration (104). In order to inhibit PI3K activity and allow induced apoptotic signaling, the researchers were searching for the most energetically favorable binding site on PI3K for a quercetin analog (LY294002). Using AutoDock 3 (76) with a pool of 30,000 initial dockings, the researchers found that the activated prodrug (L-O-CH2-LY294002) had a high affinity for PI3K's ATP binding site, leading them to conclude that the activated prodrug would indeed inhibit PI3K activity. They then confirmed experimentally that this compound was successful in inhibition and induced apoptosis in prostate cancer cells. Discovering this drug's affinity for PI3K's ATP binding site through 30,000 in vitro experiments would have been prohibitively expensive, in terms of both time and compound synthesis required, but was made tenable with the aid of in silico trials.

### 7.3 Sequence Similarity Motivates Drug Discovery with MD: Tamiflu and Relenza

A study of multiple drugs and their related proteins via MD simulation have proven useful in understanding how drug binding mechanisms work (29), and has implications for new drug discovery, as well as understanding mechanisms of drug resistance (105). In the Le study, the pathogenic avian H5N1 type-I neuraminidase, which is the target for drugs such as Tamiflu and Relenza, is compared to other sequence-similar proteins. These all-atom simulations investigated drug–protein interactions, including both conserved and unique interactions, with particular emphasis on hydrogen bonding and electrostatics. Their findings suggest how conserved networks of hydrogen bonds across the three structural variations elucidate a possible mechanism for how certain mutations might lead to drug resistance.

Such investigations on how mutations affect drug resistances or create genetic diseases are increasingly common, as conformational and dynamical changes comparing similar structures or systems highlight the specific mechanisms likely responsible for proper, or improper, function. This form of mechanism hypothesis is just one of the many ways MD simulations help to push the ability to generate effective drugs, namely, ones that are less susceptible to mutation based resistance.

## 8  Areas in Which Molecular Dynamics Shows Promise to Impact Drug Discovery

In addition to explicitly providing conformations, especially rarer conformations for ligand screening, there are multiple areas in which molecular dynamics appears poised to make an impact; these areas include protein–protein interfaces, an elusive, yet potentially profitable arenas for drug discovery, and in understanding more complex, longer-range allosteric interactions.

### 8.1  Protein–Protein Interfaces and Interactions via Molecular Dynamics: Peroxiredoxins

Another study involving molecular dynamics, enhanced by additional calculations, in this case electrostatic-based p$K$a calculations, have been ones on the peroxiredoxins (Prxs) shows how detailed p$K$a values, combined with MD simulation, can be combined to gain additional insight into the modeling chemical contributions to the oligomerization (106, 107). This family of proteins is responsible for catalyzing the reduction of hydrogen peroxide, alkyl hydroperoxides and peroxynitrite. They control levels of cytokine-induced peroxide and act as a regulator of signal transduction in mammals (108–110).

These interactions have proven elusive in the drug discovery process because of the complexity in finding information about specific sites for ligand binding (111), although progress is being made (56, 112). The transient nature of the PPI makes identification of regions for small molecule binding difficult to find, and understanding dynamics will be critical for effective predictions. Recent efforts combining NMR with MD have proven useful in this regard (112).

### 8.2  Molecular Dynamics and Long-Range Allostery: MetRS/tRNA Complexes

In a different research study, the authors used MD to probe action at a distance allostery involved in enzymatic reactions (113). They simulated E. coli methionyl-tRNA synthase (MetRS) with 9 ns long trajectories, using the CHARMM27 force field and a TIP3P explicit water model. Using RMSFs, they compared simulation results directly against experimental values from X-ray crystallography and compared global mobility for the different mutations. Additionally, covariance analysis helped reveal how certain amino acid substitutions alter the conformations and dynamics. Through this careful analysis of the results, the authors showed that substitution of a certain tryptophan residue (trp-461) results in specific changes in protein correlation and dynamics. Effects of this substitution to the local region are not surprising, but there is clear evidence that the mobility-correlated motions of a region 40–50 Å away are reduced in the absence of the conserving tryptophan. It appears that the conserved residue has function in addition to codon recognition that is mediating the conformational structures available to the protein. These simulations along with previous ones discussed (59, 91, 101, 102) show the utility of nanosecond scale simulations to study protein dynamics around the ground state of the folded structure.

Here we see another example of how MD is used to inform the drug discovery process. While this particular system might not have direct application for drug discovery, it is useful in showing how MD can help us realize the mechanism of action in these extremely complex, highly dimensional systems. It is difficult to conceive a better method of understanding elusive biomolecular processes, such as this type of hidden allostery, than MD simulations.

## 9  Further Reading

Although we have surveyed the basics of molecular dynamics as it pertains to drug discovery and discussed several illustrative studies, there are other articles which review different aspects of molecular dynamics simulations and their use in understanding drug–protein interactions, binding mechanisms, and protein–protein interactions. Additional case studies can be found in (12), and a discussion of homology modeling and a possible method for accelerating molecular dynamics can be found in (114).

The use of homology modeling in molecular simulation and drug discovery is somewhat controversial. However, homology has gained traction in recent years, as a means to alleviate the time consuming and expensive tasks of X-ray crystallography and NMR, especially in protein families for which there are many structures available (114). In addition becoming the basis for iterative processes for model refinement as more information becomes available, homology is commonly used for comparison of families of proteins for bioinformatics. As discussed in (114) homology has been used to help fill the gap between sequence and structure, for G-protein coupled receptors (GCPRs). They are among the most prominent targets for small molecule drugs, and, due to this abundance, they are a prime target for homology modeling as a means to structure based drug design. While there are roughly 100 GPCR structures in the PDB there are still many more in the family, and due to their popularity as a drug target for a variety of disease, this problem is particularly well suited to homology modeling, despite the difficulties (115, 116). There is even some evidence that homology modeling is more successful with GPCRs than de novo techniques (117). The success of homology modeling provides hope that computationally techniques will be able to draw upon the increasing number of experimental structures available to apply molecular dynamics and virtual screening techniques to the even larger protein universe, which is increasing even faster.

Additionally, Kalyaanamoorthy discusses implementations of enhanced sampling techniques to access longer timescales.

One such technique is promising, namely, that of random acceleration molecular dynamics (RAMD). Used for investigating ligand dissociation, RAMD applies a small, additional random force to the center of mass of the ligand allowing it to search the protein for potential egresses. This technique is appealing because it can provide ligand dissociation information on nanosecond timescales, it unbiasedly searches possible molecular channels, due to the stochastic nature of the extra force, and may be able to help identify key amino-acid residues in the ligand (un)binding process. Although a disadvantage of course is that this requires a structure with a ligand, but could be used, for example, to study conformational changes that occur due to ligand escape which could then be used to inform, or even to provide structures, for virtual screening. A complementary technique is steered MD (SMD) and it is analogous to an atomic force microscopy or optical tweezers, in silico. Much like RAMD, it could be used to look at small molecule dissociation. Both of these techniques show promise in further enabling drug discovery by using experimental structures with ligands, and providing information about the binding process.

One of the remaining challenges for the field is the perception of the scientific community. It seems that confidence in MD simulations has not gained the traction that it has in other scientific disciplines such as meteorology, fluid dynamics and astrophysics (118). Despite the success in other disciplines, MD simulations are often disregarded as insufficient, even though there is a wealth of data showing consistent results between simulation and experiment including many of the examples reviewed herein.

# References

1. Mccammon JA, Gelin BR, Karplus M (1977) Dynamics of folded proteins. Nature 267:585–590

2. Radkiewicz JL, Brooks CLI (2000) Protein dynamics in enzymatic catalysis: exploration of dihydrofolate reductase. J Am Chem Soc 122:225–231. doi:10.1021/ja9913838

3. Salsbury F (2001) Modeling of the metallo-$\beta$-lactamase from B. fragilis: structural and dynamic effects of inhibitor binding. Proteins 44:448–459

4. Salsbury FR, Crowder MW, Kingsmore SF, Huntley JJ (2009) Molecular dynamic simulations of the metallo-beta-lactamase from Bacteroides fragilis in the presence and absence of a tight-binding inhibitor. J Mol Model 15:133–145. doi:10.1007/s00894-008-0410-0

5. Kumar S, Ma B, Tsai C-J et al (2000) Folding and binding cascades: dynamic landscapes and population shifts. Protein Sci 9:10–19

6. Freire E (1999) The propagation of binding interactions to remote sites in proteins: analysis of the binding of the monoclonal antibody. Proc Natl Acad Sci 96:10118–10122

7. Kern D, Zuiderweg ER (2003) The role of dynamics in allosteric regulation. Curr Opin Struct Biol 13:748–757. doi:10.1016/j.sbi.2003.10.008

8. Pan H, Lee JC, Hilser VJ (2000) Binding sites in Escherichia coli dihydrofolate reductase communicate by modulating the conformational ensemble. Proc Natl Acad Sci U S A 97:12020–12025. doi:10.1073/pnas.220240297

9. Gunasekaran K, Ma B, Nussinov R (2004) Is allostery an intrinsic property of all dynamic proteins? Proteins 57:433–443. doi:10.1002/prot.20232

10. Tsai C, Ma B, Nussinov R (1999) Folding and binding cascades: shifts in energy landscapes. Proc Natl Acad Sci U S A 96:9970–9972

11. Vasilyeva A, Clodfelter JE, Rector B et al (2009) Small molecule induction of MSH2-dependent cell death suggests a vital role of mismatch repair proteins in cell death. DNA Repair (Amst) 8:103–113. doi:10.1016/j.dnarep.2008.09.008

12. Salsbury FR (2010) Molecular dynamics simulations of protein dynamics and their relevance to drug discovery. Curr Opin Pharmacol 10:738–744. doi:10.1016/j.coph.2010.09.016

13. Berman HM (2000) The protein data bank. Nucleic Acids Res 28:235–242. doi:10.1093/nar/28.1.235

14. Saxena A, Sangwan RS, Mishra S (2013) Fundamentals of homology modeling steps and comparison among important bioinformatics tools: an overview. Sci Int 1:237–252. doi:10.5567/sciintl.2013.237.252

15. Szalewicz K (2014) Determination of structure and properties of molecular crystals from first principles. Acc Chem Res 47:3266–3274. doi:10.1021/ar500275m

16. MacKerell A, Bashford D (1998) All-atom empirical potential for molecular modeling and dynamics studies of proteins. J Phys Chem 5647:3586–3616. doi:10.1021/jp973084f

17. Ponder JW, Case DA (2003) Force fields for protein simulations. Adv Protein Chem 66:27–85. doi:10.1016/S0065-3233(03)66002-X

18. Oostenbrink C, Villa A, Mark AE, Van Gunsteren WF (2004) A biomolecular force field based on the free enthalpy of hydration and solvation: the GROMOS force-field parameter sets 53A5 and 53A6. J Comput Chem 25:1656–1676. doi:10.1002/jcc.20090

19. Darden T, York D, Pedersen L (1993) Particle mesh Ewald: an N log(N) method for Ewald sums in large systems. J Chem Phys 12:10089–10092

20. Roe DR, Okur A, Wickstrom L et al (2007) Secondary structure bias in generalized Born solvent models: comparison of conformational ensembles and free energy of solvent polarization from explicit and implicit solvation. J Phys Chem B 111:1846–1857. doi:10.1021/jp066831u

21. García AE, Sanbonmatsu KY (2002) Alpha-helical stabilization by side chain shielding of backbone hydrogen bonds. Proc Natl Acad Sci U S A 99:2782–2787. doi:10.1073/pnas.042496899

22. Feig M, MacKerell AD, Brooks CL (2003) Force field influence on the observation of π-helical protein structures in molecular dynamics simulations. J Phys Chem B 107:2831–2836. doi:10.1021/jp027293y

23. Lee MS, Salsbury FR, Brooks CL (2002) Novel generalized born methods. J Chem Phys 116:10606. doi:10.1063/1.1480013

24. The 2013 Nobel Prize in Chemistry

25. Phillips JC, Braun R, Wang W et al (2005) Scalable molecular dynamics with NAMD. J Comput Chem 26:1781–1802. doi:10.1002/jcc.20289

26. Brooks B, Brooks C (2009) CHARMM: the biomolecular simulation program. J Comput Chem 30:1545–1614. doi:10.1002/jcc.21287.CHARMM

27. Case DA, Cheatham TE, Darden T et al (2005) The Amber biomolecular simulation programs. J Comput Chem 26:1668–1688. doi:10.1002/jcc.20290

28. Hess B, Kutzner C, van der Spoel D, Lindahl E (2008) GROMACS 4: algorithms for highly efficient, load-balanced, and scalable molecular simulation. J Chem Theory Comput 4:435–447. doi:10.1021/ct700301q

29. Le L, Lee E, Schulten K, Truong TN (2009) Molecular modeling of swine influenza A/H1N1, Spanish H1N1, and avian H5N1 flu N1 neuraminidases bound to Tamiflu and Relenza. PLoS Curr 1:RRN1015. doi:10.1371/currents.RRN1015

30. De Meyer FJ-M, Venturoli M, Smit B (2008) Molecular simulations of lipid-mediated protein-protein interactions. Biophys J 95:1851–1865. doi:10.1529/biophysj.107.124164

31. Harvey M, Giupponi G, Fabritiis G (2009) ACEMD: accelerating biomolecular dynamics in the microsecond time scale. J Chem Theory Comput 5:1632

32. Schlick T (2010) Molecular modeling and simulation: an interdisciplinary guide: an interdisciplinary guide. Springer Science & Business Media, New York, NY

33. Frenkel D, Smit B (2001) Understanding molecular simulation: from algorithms to applications. Academic, San Diego, CA

34. Fenimore PW, Frauenfelder H, Mcmahon BH, Parak FG (2002) Slaving: solvent fluctuations dominate protein dynamics and functions. Proc Natl Acad Sci U S A 99:16047–16051

35. Frauenfelder H, Fenimore PW, Young RD (2007) Protein dynamics and function: insights from the energy landscape and solvent slaving. IUBMB Life 59:506–512. doi:10.1080/15216540701194113

36. Tarek M, Tobias DJ (2000) The dynamics of protein hydration water: a quantitative comparison of molecular dynamics simulations and neutron-scattering experiments. Biophys J 79:3244–3257. doi:10.1016/S0006-3495 (00)76557-X

37. Berendsen HJC, Postma JPM, van Gunsteren WF, Hermans J (1981) Interaction models for water in relation to protein hydration. In: Pullman B (ed) Intermolecular forces. Springer, Berlin, pp 331–342

38. Jorgensen WL, Chandrasekhar J, Madura JD et al (1983) Comparison of simple potential functions for simulating liquid water. J Chem Phys 79:926. doi:10.1063/1.445869

39. Zhou R (2003) Free energy landscape of protein folding in water: explicit vs. implicit solvent. Proteins 161:148–161

40. Mark P, Nilsson L (2001) Structure and dynamics of the TIP3P, SPC, and SPC/E water models at 298 K. J Phys Chem A 105:9954–9960. doi:10.1021/jp003020w

41. Ryckaert J, Ciccotti G, Berendsen H (1977) Numerical integration of the cartesian equations of motion of a system with constraints: molecular dynamics of n-alkanes. J Comput Phys 341:327–341

42. Knight JL, Brooks CL (2011) Surveying implicit solvent models for estimating small molecule absolute hydration free energies. J Comput Chem 32:2909–2923. doi:10.1002/jcc.21876

43. Pu M, Garrahan JP, Hirst JD (2011) Comparison of implicit solvent models and force fields in molecular dynamics simulations of the PB1 domain. Chem Phys Lett 515:283–289. doi:10.1016/j.cplett.2011.09.026

44. Zhou R, Berne B (2002) Can a continuum solvent model reproduce the free energy landscape of a β-hairpin folding in water? Proc Natl Acad Sci U S A 99:12777

45. Lee MS, Feig M, Salsbury FR, Brooks CL III (2003) New analytic approximation to the standard molecular volume definition and its application to generalized born calculations. J Comput Chem 24:1348

46. Humphrey W, Dalke A, Schulten K (1996) VMD: visual molecular dynamics. J Mol Graph 14:33

47. Heyer L, Kruglyak S, Yooseph S (1999) Exploring expression data: identification and analysis of coexpressed genes. Genome Res 9:1106–1115

48. Karpen M, Tobias D, Brooks C III (1993) Statistical clustering techniques for the analysis of long molecular dynamics trajectories: analysis of 2.2-ns trajectories of YPGDV. Biochemistry 32:412–420

49. Brooks BR, Bruccoleri RE, Olafson BD et al (1983) CHARMM: a program for macromolecular energy, minimization, and dynamics calculations. J Comput Chem 4:187–217. doi:10.1002/jcc.540040211

50. Carpenter GA, Grossberg S (1987) A massively parallel architecture for a self-organizing neural pattern recognition machine. Comput Vis Graph Image Process 37:54–115. doi:10.1016/S0734-189X(87)80014-2

51. Pao Y-H (1989) Adaptive pattern recognition and neural networks. Addison-Wesley Longman Publishing Co., Inc., Boston, MA

52. Senne M, Schütte C, Noé F (2012) EMMA: a software package for Markov model building and analysis. J Chem Theory Comput 8:2223–2228

53. Beauchamp K, Bowman G (2011) MSMBuilder2: modeling conformational dynamics on the picosecond to millisecond scale. J Chem Theory Comput 7:3412–3419. doi:10.1021/ct200463m.MSM Builder2

54. Cronkite-Ratcliff B, Pande V (2013) MSMExplorer: visualizing Markov state models for biomolecule folding simulations. Bioinformatics 29:950–952. doi:10.1093/bioinformatics/btt051

55. Pande V, Beauchamp K, Bowman G (2010) Everything you wanted to know about Markov State Models but were afraid to ask. Methods 52:99–105. doi:10.1016/j.ymeth.2010.06.002.Everything

56. Kozakov D, Hall DR, Chuang G-Y et al (2011) Structural conservation of druggable hot spots in protein-protein interfaces. Proc Natl Acad Sci U S A 108:13528–13533. doi:10.1073/pnas.1101835108

57. Peng JW (2009) Communication breakdown: protein dynamics and drug design. Structure 17:319–320. doi:10.1016/j.str.2009.02.004

58. Mauldin RV, Carroll MJ, Lee AL (2009) Dynamic dysfunction in dihydrofolate reductase results from antifolate drug binding: modulation of dynamics within a structural state. Structure 17:386–394. doi:10.1016/j.str.2009.01.005

59. Negureanu L, Salsbury FR (2012) Insights into protein - DNA interactions, stability and allosteric communications: a computational study of mutSα-DNA recognition complexes. J Biomol Struct Dyn 29:757–776. doi:10.1080/07391102.2012.10507412

60. Godwin RC, Gmeiner WH, Salsbury FR (2015) Importance of long-time simulations

for rare event sampling in zinc finger proteins. J Biomol Struct Dyn (In press). doi:10.1080/07391102.2015.1015168

61. Ichiye T, Karplus M (1991) Collective motions in proteins: a covariance analysis of atomic fluctuations in molecular dynamics and normal mode simulations. Proteins 11:205–217

62. Amadei A, Linssen A, Berendsen HJC (1993) Essential dynamics of proteins. Proteins 17:412–425

63. Schäfer H, Mark AE, Van Gunsteren WF (2000) Absolute entropies from molecular dynamics simulation trajectories. J Chem Phys 113:7809–7817. doi:10.1063/1.1309534

64. Andricioaei I, Karplus M (2001) On the calculation of entropy from covariance matrices of the atomic fluctuations. J Chem Phys 115:6289–6292. doi:10.1063/1.1401821

65. Huang Z, Wong C (2009) Docking flexible peptide to flexible protein by molecular dynamics using two implicit-solvent models: an evaluation in protein kinase and phosphatase systems. J Phys Chem B 113:14343–14354. doi:10.1021/jp907375b.Docking

66. Knegtel RM, Kuntz ID, Oshiro CM (1997) Molecular docking to ensembles of protein structures. J Mol Biol 266:424–440. doi:10.1006/jmbi.1996.0776

67. Claussen H, Buning C, Rarey M, Lengauer T (2001) FlexE: efficient molecular docking considering protein structure variations. J Mol Biol 308:377–395. doi:10.1006/jmbi.2001.4551

68. Lin J-H, Perryman AL, Schames JR, McCammon JA (2002) Computational drug design accommodating receptor flexibility: the relaxed complex scheme. J Am Chem Soc 124:5632–5633. doi:10.1021/ja0260162

69. Frembgen-Kesner T, Elcock AH (2006) Computational sampling of a cryptic drug binding site in a protein receptor: explicit solvent molecular dynamics and inhibitor docking to p38 MAP kinase. J Mol Biol 359:202–214. doi:10.1016/j.jmb.2006.03.021

70. Tatsumi R, Fukunishi Y, Nakamura H (2004) A hybrid method of molecular dynamics and harmonic dynamics for docking of flexible ligand to flexible receptor. J Comput Chem 25:1995–2005. doi:10.1002/jcc.20133

71. Lin J, Perryman A (2003) The relaxed complex method: accommodating receptor flexibility for drug design with an improved scoring scheme. Biopolymers 68:47–62

72. Totrov M, Abagyan R (1997) Flexible protein-ligand docking by global energy optimization in internal coordinates. Proteins 220:215–220

73. Goodsell DS, Olson AJ (1990) Automated docking of substrates to proteins by simulated annealing. Proteins 8:195–202. doi:10.1002/prot.340080302

74. Goodsell D (1996) Automated docking of flexible ligands: applications of AutoDock. J Mol Recognit 9:1–5

75. Trott O, Olson AJ (2010) Software news and update AutoDock Vina: improving the speed and accuracy of docking with a new scoring function, efficient optimization, and multithreading. J Comput Chem 31:455–461. doi:10.1002/jcc

76. Morris G, Goodsell D (1998) Automated docking using a Lamarckian genetic algorithm and an empirical binding free energy function. J Comput Chem 19:1639–1662

77. Morris G, Huey R (2009) AutoDock4 and AutoDockTools4: automated docking with selective receptor flexibility. J Comput Chem 30:2785–2791. doi:10.1002/jcc

78. Wang R, Fang X, Lu Y, Wang S (2004) The PDBbind database: collection of binding affinities for protein-ligand complexes with known three-dimensional structures. J Med Chem 47:2977–2980. doi:10.1021/jm030580l

79. Wang R, Fang X, Lu Y et al (2005) The PDBbind database: methodologies and updates. J Med Chem 48:4111–4119. doi:10.1021/jm048957q

80. Abagyan R, Totrov M, Kuznetsov D (1994) ICM—a new method for protein modeling and design: applications to docking and structure prediction from the distorted native conformation. J Comput Chem 15:488–506

81. Blum C, Roli A, Sampels M (2008) Hybrid metaheuristics: an emerging approach to optimization. Springer, New York, NY

82. Nocedal J, Wright SJ (1999) Numerical optimization. Springer, New York, NY

83. Liu T, Lin Y, Wen X et al (2007) BindingDB: a web-accessible database of experimentally determined protein-ligand binding affinities. Nucleic Acids Res 35:D198–D201. doi:10.1093/nar/gkl999

84. Gaulton A, Bellis LJ, Bento AP et al (2012) ChEMBL: a large-scale bioactivity database for drug discovery. Nucleic Acids Res 40:D1100–D1107. doi:10.1093/nar/gkr777

85. Knox C, Law V, Jewison T et al (2011) DrugBank 3.0: a comprehensive resource for "omics" research on drugs. Nucleic Acids Res 39:D1035–D1041. doi:10.1093/nar/gkq1126

86. Li Q, Cheng T, Wang Y, Bryant S (2010) PubChem as a public resource for drug discovery. Drug Discov Today 15:1052–1057. doi:10.1016/j.drudis.2010.10.003. PubChem

87. Chen C (2011) TCM Database@ Taiwan: the world's largest traditional Chinese medicine database for drug screening in silico. PLoS One 6:e15939. doi:10.1371/journal.pone.0015939

88. Irwin JJ, Shoichet BK (2005) ZINC - a free database of commercially available compounds for virtual screening. J Chem Inf Model 36:177–182. doi:10.1002/chin.200516215

89. Irwin JJ, Sterling T, Mysinger MM et al (2012) ZINC: a free tool to discover chemistry for biology. J Chem Inf Model 52:1757–1768. doi:10.1021/ci3001277

90. Schüller A, Hähnke V, Schneider G (2007) SmiLib v2.0: a Java-based tool for rapid combinatorial library enumeration. QSAR Comb Sci 26:407–410. doi:10.1002/qsar.200630101

91. Salsbury FR, Clodfelter JE, Gentry MB et al (2006) The molecular mechanism of DNA damage recognition by MutS homologs and its consequences for cell death response. Nucleic Acids Res 34:2173–2185. doi:10.1093/nar/gkl238

92. Vasilyeva A, Clodfelter JE, Gorczynski MJ, et al. (2010) Parameters of reserpine analogs that induce MSH2/MSH6-dependent cytotoxic response. J Nucleic Acids, Article ID 162018, doi: 10.4061/2010/162018

93. Lange O, Lakomek N, Farès C (2008) Recognition dynamics up to microseconds revealed from an RDC-derived ubiquitin ensemble in solution. Science 320:1471–1475

94. Stojic L, Brun R, Jiricny J (2004) Mismatch repair and DNA damage signalling. DNA Repair (Amst) 3:1091–1101. doi:10.1016/j.dnarep.2004.06.006

95. Fishel R, Wilson T (1997) MutS homologs in mammalian cells. Curr Opin Genet Dev 7:105–113

96. Kolodner RD, Marsischky GT (1999) Eukaryotic DNA mismatch repair. Curr Opin Genet Dev 9:89–96. doi:10.1016/S0959-437X(99)80013-6

97. Bellacosa A (2001) Functional interactions and signaling properties of mammalian DNA mismatch repair proteins. Cell Death Differ 8:1076–1092. doi:10.1038/sj.cdd.4400948

98. Kunkel TA, Erie DA (2005) DNA mismatch repair. Annu Rev Biochem 74:681–710. doi:10.1146/annurev.biochem.74.082803.133243

99. Drotschmann K, Topping RP, Clodfelter JE, Salsbury FR (2004) Mutations in the nucleotide-binding domain of MutS homologs uncouple cell death from cell survival. DNA Repair (Amst) 3:729–742. doi:10.1016/j.dnarep.2004.02.011

100. Abdelhafez OM, Amin KM, Ali HI, Abdalla M, Ahmed EY (2014) RSC Adv 4:11569–11579. doi:10.1039/c4ra00943f

101. Negureanu L, Salsbury FR (2012) The molecular origin of the MMR-dependent apoptosis pathway from dynamics analysis of MutSα-DNA complexes. J Biomol Struct Dyn 30:1–15. doi:10.1080/07391102.2012.680034

102. Negureanu L, Salsbury FR (2014) Nonspecificity and synergy at the binding site of the carboplatin-induced DNA adduct via molecular dynamics simulations of the MutSα-DNA recognition complex. J Biomol Struct Dyn 32:969–992. doi:10.1080/07391102.2013.799437

103. Baiz D, Pinder T, Hassan S (2012) Synthesis and characterization of a novel prostate cancer-targeted phosphatidylinositol-3-kinase inhibitor prodrug. J Med Chem 55:8038–8046. doi:10.1021/jm300881a

104. Cohen MB, Rokhlin OW (2009) Mechanisms of prostate cancer cell survival after inhibition of AR expression. J Cell Biochem 106:363–371. doi:10.1002/jcb.22022

105. Woods CJ, Malaisree M, Pattarapongdilok N et al (2012) Long time scale GPU dynamics reveal the mechanism of drug resistance of the dual mutant I223R/H275Y neuraminidase from H1N1-2009 influenza virus. Biochemistry 51:4364

106. Yuan Y, Knaggs MH, Poole LB et al (2010) Conformational and oligomeric effects on the cysteine pK(a) of tryparedoxin peroxidase. J Biomol Struct Dyn 28:51–70. doi:10.1080/07391102.2010.10507343

107. Salsbury FR, Yuan Y, Knaggs MH et al (2012) Structural and electrostatic asymmetry at the active site in typical and atypical peroxiredoxin dimers. J Phys Chem B 116:6832–6843. doi:10.1021/jp212606k

108. Rhee SG, Kang SW, Jeong W et al (2005) Intracellular messenger function of hydrogen peroxide and its regulation by peroxiredoxins. Curr Opin Cell Biol 17:183–189. doi:10.1016/j.ceb.2005.02.004

109. Sue GR, Ho ZC, Kim K (2005) Peroxiredoxins: a historical overview and speculative preview of novel mechanisms and emerging

concepts in cell signaling. Free Radic Biol Med 38:1543–1552. doi:10.1016/j.fre eradbiomed.2005.02.026

110. Wood ZA, Schroder E, Robin Harris J, Poole LB (2003) Structure, mechanism and regulation of peroxiredoxins. Trends Biochem Sci 28:32–40. doi:10.1016/S0968-0004(02) 00003-8

111. Kube S, Weber M (2007) A coarse graining method for the identification of transition rates between molecular conformations. J Chem Phys 126:024103. doi:10.1063/1. 2404953

112. Bernini A, Henrici De Angelis L, Morandi E et al (2014) Searching for protein binding sites from Molecular Dynamics simulations and paramagnetic fragment-based NMR studies. Biochim Biophys Acta 1844:561–566. doi:10.1016/j.bbapap.2013.12.012

113. Budiman ME, Knaggs MH, Fetrow JS, Alexander RW (2007) Using molecular dynamics to map interaction networks in an aminoacyl-tRNA synthetase. Proteins 68:670–689. doi:10.1002/prot.21426

114. Kalyaanamoorthy S, Chen Y-PP (2014) Modelling and enhanced molecular dynamics to steer structure-based drug discovery. Prog Biophys Mol Biol 114:123–136. doi:10. 1016/j.pbiomolbio.2013.06.004

115. Kobilka BK (2007) G protein coupled receptor structure and activation. Biochim Biophys Acta 1768:794–807. doi:10.1016/j. bbamem.2006.10.021

116. Patny A, Desai PV, Avery MA (2006) Homology modeling of G-protein-coupled receptors and implications in drug design. Curr Med Chem 13:1667–1691. doi:10.2174/ 092986706777442002

117. Bhattacharya S, Lam AR, Li H et al (2013) Critical analysis of the successes and failures of homology models of G protein-coupled receptors. Proteins 81:729–739. doi:10. 1002/prot.24195

118. Borhani DW, Shaw DE (2012) The future of molecular dynamics simulations in drug discovery. J Comput Aided Mol Des 26:15–26. doi:10.1007/s10822-011-9517-y

Methods in Pharmacology and Toxicology (2016): 31–64
DOI 10.1007/7653_2015_47
© Springer Science+Business Media New York 2015
Published online: 13 August 2015

# A Review of Evolutionary Algorithms for Computing Functional Conformations of Protein Molecules

## Amarda Shehu

## Abstract

The ubiquitous presence of proteins in chemical pathways in the cell and their key role in many human disorders motivates a growing body of protein modeling studies to unravel the relationship between protein structure and function. The foundation of such studies is the realization that knowledge of the structures a protein accesses under physiological conditions is key to a detailed understanding of its biological function and the design of therapeutic compounds for the purpose of altering misfunction in aberrant variants of a protein.

Dry laboratory investigations promise a holistic treatment of the relationship between protein sequence, structure, and function. Significant efforts are made in the dry laboratory to map protein conformation spaces and underlying energy landscapes of proteins. The majority of such efforts employ well-studied computational templates, such as Molecular Dynamics and Monte Carlo. The focus of this review is on a third emerging template, stochastic optimization under the umbrella of evolutionary computation. Algorithms based on such a template, also known as evolutionary algorithms, are showing promise in addressing fundamental computational challenges in protein structure modeling and are opening up new avenues in protein modeling research. This review summarizes evolutionary algorithms for novice readers, while highlighting recent developments that showcase current, state-of-the-art capabilities for experts.

**Keywords:** Protein structure modeling, Conformation space, Energy landscape, Conformational search, Stochastic optimization, Evolutionary computation, Evolutionary algorithms

## 1  Introduction

Proteins are ubiquitous macromolecules in the cell as central components of cellular organization and function. Many diseases are due to misbehaving proteins, including critical human diseases, such as cancer, amyotrophic lateral sclerosis, Alzheimer's, and other neurodegenerative disorders. The list of known gene mutations resulting in aberrant proteins misfunctioning in the cell is now growing [1, 2]. An important class of human diseases is due to proteins failing to adopt their native, biologically active, three-dimensional (3D) structures with which they bind to small molecules or dock other macromolecules, giving rise to molecular interactions that make up all chemical reactions in the cell. While many such failures are deleterious, others lead to protein misfunction [3–9]. Elucidating the long-lived structure or set of structures that an aberrant protein assumes and employs to interact with other molecules in the cell is key not only to a detailed understanding of how mutations impact function but also to pharmaceutical efforts to design effective compounds for blocking interactions of aberrant structures.

Investigations in the wet laboratory have elucidated by now over a hundred thousand active or functional structures of diverse proteins. As of May 2015, there are 108,957 protein structures in the Protein Data Bank (PDB) [10]. Increasingly, the focus is on rapidly resolving functional structures of possible protein constructs of decoded genomes and structures of misbehaving proteins due to sequence mutations. Investigations in the dry laboratory are demonstrating their capability to complement wet-laboratory research and greatly enhance our understanding of the relationship between protein sequence, structure, and function. The role of dry-laboratory investigations is also expected to increase with the recently discontinued Protein Structure Initiative [11].

The foundation of dry-laboratory investigations is on the early experiments by Anfinsen, who demonstrated that a denatured protein spontaneously self-assembles into its native structure [12]. The mechanistic treatment, which advocates that the native 3D structure of a protein determines its function, and that in turn the amino-acid sequence determines to a great extent the native 3D structure, is by now the basis of a growing body of protein research aiming to model structures and structural deformations relevant for biological function [13–15].

The most publicized work in protein modeling research is that on the protein structure prediction (PSP) problem, where the goal is to predict a structural representative of the active, functional state of a protein. The more challenging version of this problem, is known as de novo PSP (also referred to as ab initio PSP or *template-free* modeling, where de novo or *free* indicates the absence of a known structural template after which to model the unknown structure of the target protein sequence). While early investigations in silico pursued protein structure modeling with classic templates, such as Molecular Dynamics (MD), by now the most successful methods for de novo PSP build on the Metropolis Monte Carlo (MC) template [16]. These methods aim to reveal the breadth of long-lived (and possibly functional) structures of a given protein sequence, as doing so constitutes a holistic treatment of the relationship between protein sequence, structure, and function. The holistic treatment also promises a detailed and comprehensive view of all possible long-lived structures a mutated protein sequence may assume to misbehave in the cell. However, at present, the computational demands of a holistic treatment are impractical for most existing methods due to the high-dimensionality of the protein conformation space [17].

The focus of this review is on an emerging group of methods known as evolutionary algorithms (EAs). EAs approach the problem of protein structure modeling under the umbrella of stochastic optimization and employ techniques from Evolutionary Computation (EC) to effectively find solutions of variable spaces with numerous and possibly interdependent variables. Though adaptations of EAs for the de novo PSP problem have been regularly pursued for decades, recent developments in computational structural biology regarding protein geometry and energetics have led to novel EAs with increased performance not only in terms of computational time but also in prediction quality. EAs are also gaining ground as effective tools to circumvent outstanding challenges in protein structure modeling and advance our ability to reveal detailed structure spaces of the healthy versions, wild-type sequences of a protein, and the unhealthy, aberrant variants.

This review appeals to both experts and novices. A short prime is provided first on protein geometry and energetics. Connections are then made between protein structure modeling and stochastic optimization. A summary of EAs for de novo PSP is provided next, highlighting recent developments for experts. A growing group of EAs is also presented to showcase their ability to map structure spaces of the healthy and aberrant versions of a protein. The review concludes with a summary of outstanding challenges and opportunities for the EC community in protein structure modeling.

## 2   Protein Geometry and Energetics

### 2.1   Protein Geometry

A protein molecule consists of one or more polypeptide chains. A polypeptide chain is comprised of many peptides, or reduced amino acids, bound in a serial fashion through covalent bonds. Many polypeptide chains can be held together through non-covalent interactions in quaternary structures of protein assemblies or complexes. In this review, we focus on protein molecules comprised of only one chain. Single-chain proteins are predominantly the subject of PSP and structure modeling in general (structure modeling of protein complexes is known as protein–protein docking and is beyond the subject of this review).

Amino acids are the fundamental building blocks of proteins and come in 20 different naturally occurring types. They are assigned 20 different names, which have abbreviated three-letter and one-letter codes. An amino acid consists of a central group of heavy atoms that is shared among all amino acids, a sidechain group of atoms that gives an amino acid its unique chemical properties (and its type), and hydrogens. The commonly shared group of atoms consists of N, CA, C, and O. These are known as the backbone atoms. If one follows the thread of these atoms through the peptide bonds that links the terminal backbone C of one amino acid to the terminal backbone N atom of another, a skeleton or backbone can be traced that gives a protein chain its connectivity. The side chains dangle off the backbone and both guide and constrain its motions. Figure 1a draws the native structure of a protein in 3D, highlighting the backbone. A short fragment of a few amino acids is drawn in greater detail in Fig. 1b.

*2.1.1 Representation of a Protein Chain: Conformation Space*

While the covalent bonds provide local rigidity, the protein chain (both backbone and side chains) is highly flexible. This intrinsic flexibility necessitates introducing the concept of a conformation, which refers to the spatial arrangement of the atoms in a protein chain. An all-atom conformation refers to the fact that detailed information is available at all times regarding all atoms. Not all atoms need to be explicitly modeled. Many algorithms for PSP primarily model the backbone, and once a set of (functional) conformations likely to comprise the native state of a protein are available, sidechain atoms are packed in optimal configurations with sidechain packing techniques. When not all the atoms of an amino acid are modeled explicitly by neglecting some atoms or grouping atoms together in pseudo-atoms, the conformation is said to employ a reduced, or coarse-grained representation of a protein chain. Research into effective reduced representations for protein conformations is active [18].

A conformation does not need to be represented internally in a computer code as a list of atomic coordinates. Generally, a conformation is a list of instantiated variables or parameters. These variables can be discrete, such as positions on a lattice or bits encoding positions or angles, or continuous, such as Cartesian coordinates or angles. The former are known as discrete representations, and the latter as continuous representations. There are advantages and disadvantages with either, as summarized briefly below.

*Discrete Representations: Atoms on a Lattice*

The earliest representations of protein chains were on a 2D or 3D lattice. Typically, only the CA atom of each amino acid is explicitly modeled and restricted to lie on the lattice [19]. The lattice restricts bonded atoms to neighboring cells and allows both fast integer-math evaluations of conformational energies, as well as enumeration of all self-avoiding walks on the lattice [20–22]. On-lattice deterministic search algorithms were useful to elucidate various organizing principles of amino acids during folding; the number of amino acid types was often restricted to 2, hydrophobic (H) vs. hydrophilic/polar (P), resulting in the popular HP model, to allow calculations on chains of more than a dozen amino acids. On-lattice representations allowed also obtaining a theoretical understanding of the PSP problem and facilitated various complexity results [23–25]. While the majority of conformation sampling algorithms nowadays has moved away from on-lattice models, significant research on EAs for PSP still employs them.

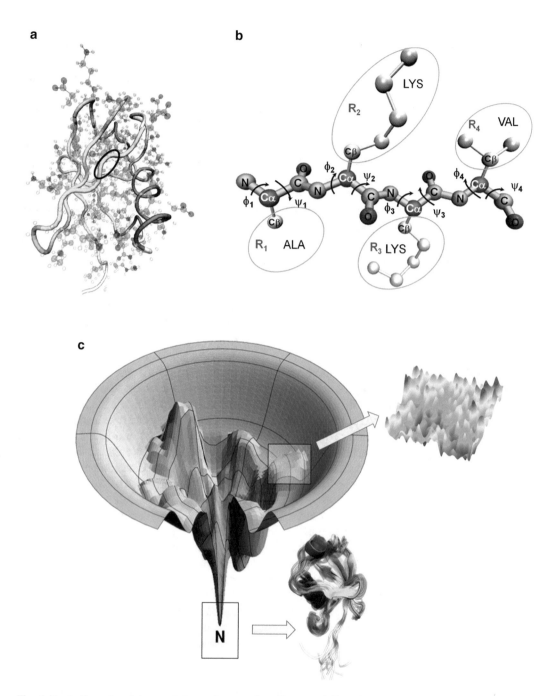

**Fig. 1** Illustration of protein geometry and energetics. *Top panel*: The 3D structure shown on the *left* (**a**) is a wet-laboratory snapshot of the biologically active state of the ubiquitin protein. The Visual Molecular Dynamics (VMD) [136] is used for rendering. The backbone is drawn in *opaque*, with the local secondary structures drawn in different colors and side chains in transparent to easily visualize the backbone. A small fragment from amino acid at position 47 to position 52 in the 76aa chain of ubiquitin is *highlighted* in greater detail on the *right* (**b**). The chain is drawn in the *ball-stick* representation with VMD. Backbone atoms in each amino acid are annotated. The side chain atoms are drawn in *silver*. The $\varphi$, $\psi$ dihedral angles are shown, as well. *Bottom panel* (**c**): A model energy surface with a single deepest basin is illustrated here, adapted from ref.[34]. The surface is nonlinear and multimodal. The deepest basin is populated by conformations of the biologically active state, illustrated here by superimposing over one another conformations of the ubiquitin NMR ensemble deposited in the PDB under ID 1d3z

Several types of lattice models are pushed forward in the EC community, such as triangular, cubic, and face-centered-cubic. In general, the top-performing algorithms for PSP employ off-lattice representations. The reason is that on-lattice representations sacrifice a lot of structural detail and have been shown to reproduce the backbone of a known native structure with accuracy no greater than half the lattice spacing [26]; some lattice representations have also been shown to bias towards specific secondary structures [27]. It is worth noting that on-lattice representations are nowadays the only computationally reasonable representations for very large proteins of hundreds of amino acids [28].

**Continuous, Off-Lattice Representations**

The majority of MC-based conformation sampling algorithms for PSP employ continuous representations, where atoms are not forced to occupy a limited number of positions on a 2D or 3D lattice. Two popular representations are the Cartesian-based and the angular-based ones. There are advantages and disadvantages with either.

**Cartesian-Based Representations**

Cartesian-based representations are straightforward for conducting energetic calculations, as summarized below, because most protein energy functions contain terms that are distance-based. Cartesian-based representations are also typically computationally demanding. In naive cartesian-based representations, the number of variables (Cartesian coordinates) for a protein chain of $N$ atoms is $3N$. A small protein chain contains hundreds of atoms. Cartesian-based representations do not allow trivial satisfying explicit constraints on locations of atoms, such as those imposed by covalent bonds. While covalently bound atoms do oscillate, large oscillations carry heavy energetic penalties. So, it is often computationally desirable to preserve the lengths of covalent bonds in computed conformations. However, a computer algorithm that modifies cartesian-based variables to compute new conformations will move atoms independently of one another and break bonds. Less naive cartesian-based representations that preserve local constraints exist, and they often build on statistical analysis techniques to define variables that encode collective motions of atoms.

**Angular-Based Representations**

In addition to covalent bonds, there are other local constraints in native protein structures whose violation results in high energetic penalties. Optimal valence angles (between two consecutive covalent bonds) observed to remain constant and depend only on the types of atoms involved in protein functional conformations would also be changed if one were to employ Cartesian-based representations. Instead, angular-based representations that model only dihedral angles (*see* Fig. 1b for an illustration of such angles) save on both the number of variables (on average, there are $3N/7$ dihedral angles in a protein chain of $N$ atoms [29]) and the number of constraints that are violated. The only constraints that angular-based representations cannot readily satisfy are long-range ones resulting from energetically constrained motions of non-bonded atoms. Typically, the violation of such constraints is evaluated through energy functions. Increasingly, while Cartesian-based representations are employed by MD-based methods for simulating the dynamics of a protein molecule, angular-based representations are the preferred ones in MC-based methods and those particularly designed for de novo PSP. Angular-based representations necessitate that a transformation occur from angles to cartesian coordinates [30] in order to evaluate a computed conformation with specified energy function.

**Distance Functions for Conformations**

Measuring the distance between two conformations is key to the ability to report the performance of a PSP algorithm to reproduce a known native structure. Depending on the representation employed, several distance functions can be useful. For instance, Hamming and Manhattan distance can be useful for discrete representations, such as on-lattice ones. Continuous representations allow the employment of Euclidean-based distance functions. The majority of PSP algorithms that employ off-lattice representations make use of the popular RMSD function to measure the distance between two conformations.

**Root-Mean-Squared-Deviation (RMSD)**

RMSD is a Euclidean-based dissimilarity metric to measure the distance between two conformations. Given two conformations $C$ and $C^*$ of $N$ atoms, where $p_i(C)$ indicates the position of atom $i$ in conformation $C$, $\mathrm{RMSD}(C, C^*) = 1/N \sum_{i=1}^{N} |p_i(C) - p_i(C^*)|^2$. Prior to measuring the RMSD between a computed conformation and the native structure, an algebraic procedure is carried out that determines the optimal superimposition removing differences due to rigid-body motions in 3D (translations and rotations of the whole conformation) [31]. The term "least" is sometimes explicitly added, as in least RMSD (lRMSD), to indicate that the conformations have undergone rigid-body motions so as to report their lowest RMSD from the known native structure. It is generally understood that even when RMSD is reported, it is lRMSD. It is also worth noting that even conformation sampling algorithms that use continuous, angular-based representations make use of RMSD to report results. The homogeneous transformations encoded by the angles in a conformation represented as a list of angles can be accumulated to obtain the Cartesian coordinates of the atoms over which angles are defined. While angular-based distance functions are available, they are not widely adopted in structure modeling literature.

## 2.2 Protein Energetics

Current protein energy functions are based on molecular mechanics, summing over favorable and unfavorable atomic interactions (and possibly with surrounding solvent) to associate a potential energy value with a conformation. Interactions between atoms are classified as bound (local, due to covalent bonds) or non-bound (nonlocal due to non-covalent interactions). Local interactions concern bonds, bond angles, and the periodicity of dihedral angles. Nonlocal interactions are divided based on their physical nature, electrostatic (measured through the Coulomb) or van der Waals (measured through the Lennard–Jones—LJ function). The latter interactions are estimated via distance-based power terms responsible for the computational cost and nonlinearity of protein energy functions. Equation 1 shows the functional form of the CHARMM potential energy function [32].

$$
\begin{aligned}
E_{\text{CHARMM}} = {} & \sum_{\text{bonds}} k_b (b - b_0)^2 + \sum_{\text{UB}} k_{\text{UB}} (S - S_0)^2 + \sum_{\text{angles}} k_\theta (\theta - \theta_0)^2 \\
& + \sum_{\text{dihedrals}} k_\chi \left(1 + \cos\left(n\chi - \delta\right)\right) + \sum_{\text{impropers}} k_{\text{imp}} (\varphi - \varphi_0)^2 \\
& + \sum_{\text{impropers}} k_{\text{imp}} (\varphi - \varphi_0)^2 + \sum_{\text{non-bond}} \varepsilon_{ij} \left[ \left(\tfrac{R_{\min}}{r}\right)^{12} - \left(\tfrac{R_{\min}}{r}\right)^{6} \right] \\
& + \sum_{\text{non-bond}} \frac{q_i q_j}{\varepsilon r}
\end{aligned}
$$

$$(1)$$

In Eq. 1, the $k_*$ terms are constants, and the $*_0$ terms are ideal values of variables. The Urey Bradley (UB) term is calculated over pairs of atoms separated by two covalent bonds (known as the 1,3 interaction), and $S$ is the distance between the atoms. The $n$ and $\delta$ variables in the fourth term are the multiplicity and the phase angle, respectively. In CHARMM, improper dihedral angles are penalized according to the formula shown in the fifth term. The sixth term measures the LJ interactions: $r_{ij}$ measures the Euclidean distance between two non-bonded atoms (that are not covered by the UB term), $\varepsilon_{ij}$ is the LJ well depth, and $R_{\min ij} = (R_{\min i} + R_{\min j})/2$ is the minimum interaction radius between the atoms, measured as half the sum of the known van der Waals radii. The LJ term in CHARMM has a 12–6 functional form, whereas other physics-based functions may have a 12–10 functional form. The final term measures electrostatic interactions via the Coulomb functional form: $q_i$ measures the known partial charge of atom $i$, and $\varepsilon$ is the dielectric constant encoding the type of environment (vacuum, solvent).

Different energy functions may have different functional forms and even employ a different list of terms; for instance, some treat hydrogen interactions differently. This is particularly the case for knowledge-based functions, which may also contain additional terms based on statistically observed interactions calculated over databases of protein structures. Whether physics-based, knowledge-based, or hybrid functions that combine both physics-based and knowledge-based terms, current protein energy functions are semiempirical. In addition to decisions on how many terms and what the terms should capture, important decisions are made to weight the contribution of each term so as to reproduce experimental measurements on specific subsets of protein structures. Moreover, most energy functions limit interactions to pairwise ones. Energy functions that calculate multibody interactions often outperform pairwise-based functions in reproducing experimental kinetic data, but their computational cost remains high to be practical for most protein structure modeling algorithms [18].

*2.2.1  Protein Energy Surfaces*

If one were to organize all conformations of a protein chain on horizontal axes and the potential energy corresponding to each conformation in a vertical axis, the view that would emerge would be a funnel-like (multidimensional) energy surface [33, 34]. If one were to find few collective (also referred to as reaction) coordinates that discriminate among the important structural states, projecting the surface onto these coordinates would give rise to the energy landscape, where thermodynamically available states would be easily discerned as basins [35]. A classic landscape is shown in Fig. 1c.

Horizontal cuts would reveal energetic states (and thus conformations of comparable potential energies). The width of these cuts goes down as energy decreases in a true protein energy surface. This width is captured in the concept of entropy, which measures the degree to which a protein chain can assume different conformations while maintaining the same potential energy (within a $dE$). An entropy value can be associated with each energetic state; thermodynamically stable states are those with low free energy $F$, measured as $F = <E> - TS$, where $<E>$ is the average potential energy over the conformational ensemble corresponding to the state, $T$ is temperature, and $S$ is entropy. Evolutionary bias has been found to be the reason for why the native state in naturally occurring proteins has lowest free energy [12].

Long-lived states in proteins correspond to deep and wide basins. The exact details of the contribution of potential energy versus entropy are what determine whether a basin corresponds to the most thermodynamically stable (longest-lived) and thus the native state of a protein or a semi-stable state. In many proteins, complex energy surfaces are emerging, where more than one structural state is employed in conformational switch mechanisms that modulate function and gives rise to rich functionality. In many aberrant versions of a protein, energy barriers between stable and semi-stable states drastically change and modify the underlying detailed structural mechanism regulating function, resulting in misfunction.

In view of complex protein energy surfaces, conformational search algorithms need to elucidate not just one putative global minimum but map the breadth of low-energy conformations corresponding to local minima in the underlying energy surface. Visualization of this surface via a low-dimensional energy landscape may reveal a multitude of basins that are worth considering, whether the goal is to select from them the one corresponding to the predicted native state or understand the mechanisms through which a protein and its aberrant versions may make use of more than one basin for function modulation and misfunction.

## 3    PSP as an Optimization Problem

Whether cartesian-based or angular-based representations are employed, it is generally expected that the representation of a protein chain of hundreds of amino acids will result in hundreds of variables. Thus, the conformation space is expected to be high-dimensional. The space can be discretized, but the number of variables makes enumeration impractical as a way of computing conformations of a protein chain. It is worth noting that in the early days, when short polypeptide chains were being investigated to extract physical principles of protein folding, bonded atoms were forced to occupy neighboring cells in a 2D or 3D lattice [19]. Combinatorial techniques could be employed to enumerate conformations of short protein chains [20–22], but finding the lowest-energy conformation on a lattice has been proved to be NP-hard [23–25]. While lattice representations allow tackling very large proteins of several hundred amino acids, PSP methods designed for small-to-medium size proteins not exceeding 200 amino acids can afford to produce higher-quality conformations with more accurate backbones by employing off-lattice representations.

When off-lattice representations are considered, the conformation space is expected to be vast, high-dimensional, and continuous. As described later, discretization can still be employed (as in the popular molecular fragment replacement technique), but the exponential explosion in the number of resulting conformations makes enumeration impractical. As a result, only stochastic or probabilistic algorithms can be employed to essentially sample the conformation space one conformation at a time. Such algorithms essentially build sample-based representations of conformation spaces. Since the goal is to map low-energy regions of the underlying energy surface where deep and wide basins may be found that correspond to the native, longest-lived structural state, such algorithms implement stochastic optimization of complex, nonlinear, and multimodal energy functions.

Stochastic optimization algorithms forsake completeness, as no guarantees can be made even on their ability to find, for instance, the global minimum energy conformation or GMEC (a term coined by Scheraga and colleagues [36]). It is worth noting that the GMEC may not correspond to the native structure, after all. One reason is due to inaccuracies in energy functions. The global minimum of even state-of-the-art all-atom energy functions can be more than 4 Å off the true native structure [37]. Another reason is due to the thermodynamic argument that the native state is not necessarily the one with the lowest energy but the one that compromises between potential energy and entropy. A deep but narrow basin may not only be an artifact in an energy function but also possibly a kinetic trap. The native basin may be deep enough and wide enough to prevent fast escapes and allow structural flexibility at equilibrium.

There are currently three groups of stochastic optimization methods. The first group builds on the MD template and essentially follows the negative gradient of a given energy function to find local minima. The second group builds on the MC template and makes use of repeated moves or perturbations to hop between conformations while generally lowering potential energy. The third group of methods and the subject of this review, EAs, builds on the EC template and shares many characteristics in its core functional units with MC-based methods. Indeed, MC-based methods can be classified as special EAs. We summarize the popular MD and MC templates before proceeding with EAs in the next section in order to better appreciate the algorithmic differences among these three groups of methods.

MD-based methods simulate the dynamics of a physics-based system. An MD trajectory is initiated from a protein conformation and systematically searches the conformation space one conformation at a time by numerically solving Newton's equations of motion. These are integrated to obtain a conformation $C_{t+\delta t}$ at time $t + \delta t$ from a current conformation $C_t$ at time $t$ in the trajectory. All atoms in $C_t$ are modified in the direction of the calculated forces, allowing the MD trajectory to essentially follow the slope of the potential energy function. Newton's equations of motions are used to update the position and velocity of each atom in time. While velocity is initialized at some random value, accelerations are computed from the (negative) gradient of the potential energy function. Repeated application of the equations of motions dictates that a small timestep $\delta t$ in the order of 12 fs be used so that the calculated gradient at each conformation in the trajectory closely follow the curvature of the potential energy function. The small timestep limits the breadth of conformation space that an MD trajectory can explore. Significant advances in dedicated, specialized hardware for MD simulations, parallelizations, and other enhanced sampling techniques have pushed the capability of MDs and their ability to capture molecular processes in the order of micro-to-milliseconds [38–40].

It remains hard for MD trajectories to reach the length and time scales needed to follow transitions between unfolded and folded states, or vice versa, or between other stable states. Moreover, gradient calculations are more easily conducted in cartesian space, which results in a vast search space. Modifications to conduct MD search over the space of dihedral angles have been proposed [41–43]. In essence, an MD trajectory realizes local search, and it is bound to converge to a local minimum in the energy surface. For these reasons, most methods with high sampling capability employ a thermodynamic rather than a kinetic treatment in the interest of computational efficiency. MC-based methods fall in this category.

In contrast to MD, conformations in an MC trajectory are not obtained by following the slope of the energy function but are the direct result of designed moves. The moves change values of the underlying variables and do not have to be physically realistic as long as they are coupled with the Metropolis criterion $e^{-dE/T}$; $dE$ is difference in energy between the conformation resulting from the move, and $T$ (effective temperature) is a scaling parameter that determines whether an energetic increase can be accepted or not. The result is a series of conformations that still converges to a local minimum but has the ability to cross over energetic barriers by controlling $T$. The MC template has higher sampling capability than the MD one, as moves can be designed to allow larger jumps in conformation space. However, because designed moves do not have to encode realistic (physics-based) motions, any information on whether and when the protein chain can diffuse from a computed conformation to another (thus, actual timescale information) is lost.

## 4  EAs for PSP and Mapping Energy Landscapes

We first summarize the unifying template of EAs and show how MC can be regarded as a specialized EA. We then provide a summary of EAs for PSP, organizing it around principal algorithmic components. Recent EAs with high performance on PSP are highlighted in greater detail. The section concludes with an exposition of a recent group of EAs that go beyond the narrow focus of single-structure prediction in PSP and instead mapping the breadth of functionally relevant structures and corresponding basins in the energy landscape.

## 4.1 Unifying Template of EAs for PSP

The realization that protein energy functions are nonlinear and multimodal, and that PSP can be cast as a global optimization problem has motivated many researchers in the EC community to approach PSP with specialized EAs. One of the first works demonstrating the promise of EAs for PSP proposes a genetic algorithm (GA) [44]. Several lattice-based and off-lattice EAs have been proposed since then. Before summarizing the developments in a little over a decade, the unifying template that EAs follow is summarized first.

The basic EA template mimics the process of evolution and natural selection to find local minima of a complex objective/fitness function. The template evolves a population of conformations (generally referred to as individuals) over a number of generations. A mechanism needs to be specified to generate the initial population, which can consist of conformations sampled at random over the employed variables (especially in the context of PSP, where only the amino-acid sequence is provided) or conformations provided by domain experts, such as wet-laboratory investigators, corresponding to known structures (in other applications that go beyond PSP and aim to map energy landscapes).

The population is allowed to evolve over generations such that individual (conformations in EAs for protein structure modeling) with low potential energy values (high fitness) are repeatedly selected and improved upon. In each generation, a selection mechanism is specified to select parent conformations for producing new conformations (offspring). The mechanism can be based on energies or other measures, incorporating various heuristics on what is more likely to lead to low-energy (high fitness) and possibly (structurally) diverse offspring. Popular selection mechanisms are truncation-based, fitness-proportional, tournament-based, and others [45]. The injection of structural diversity in the selection mechanism is particularly important to diversify a population and often credited with avoiding premature convergence to select local minima.

Once parents are selected, asexual perturbation or reproductive operators that modify/mutate one parent at a time or sexual operators that combine parents through crossover are invoked to compute new individuals, offspring. A survival mechanism determines which individuals survive to the next generation. In nonoverlapping or generational survival mechanisms, the offspring replace the parents. In overlapping ones, a subset of individuals from the combined parent and offspring pool are selected. Survival mechanisms may be based on fitness or consider other criteria (such as structural similarity of conformations) in order to steer the algorithm over the generations to optima of the fitness landscape.

EAs that employ crossover in addition to the mutation operator are often referred to as genetic algorithms, or GAs. EAs that additionally incorporate a meme, which is a local search/improvement operator to optimize a child and effectively map it to a nearby local minimum, are referred to as hybrid or memetic EAs (MAs). The employment of multiple objective functions as opposed to a single fitness function results in multi-objective EAs (MOMAs). Specific variants that build over GA are respectively referred to as MGAs and MOGAs.

Customized EAs for PSP contain many other evolutionary strategies and metaheuristics, such as the employment of a hall of fame to preserve "good" solutions, tabu search to improve the performance of a meme, coevolving memes, niching, crowding, twin removal for population diversification, structuring of the solution space to facilitate distributed implementations capable of exploiting parallel computing architectures, and more. The combination of all these strategies and more (Ref. [45] provides a comprehensive review on EAs for stochastic optimization) give rise to different, powerful EAs.

EAs have been demonstrated effective for sampling low-energy protein conformations. Though MC-based methods for PSP are generally more accepted and popular in computational structural biology, EAs have less of a chance of getting stuck at local minima compared to MC search [44]. Recent adaptations of EAs that employ state-of-the-art domain-specific knowledge on proteins, such as off-lattice, coarse-grained, angular representations of protein chains, state-of-the-art protein energy functions, and the popular molecular fragment replacement technique in perturbation and improvement operators, have been demonstrated to be competitive with state-of-the-art MC-based methods [37, 46–49].

## 4.2 Performance Measurements of EAs for PSP

There are typically two measurements used to assess the performance of an EA. When the goal is to compare the addition of novel algorithmic components and heuristics in a customized EA for PSP against a baseline EA, performance is assessed based on the lowest energy reached by each algorithm over the course of the execution. The termination criterion is set in terms of number of generations or total energy evaluations allowed. The latter allows for fair comparison of EAs with MAs. The second performance metric assesses the ability of the algorithm to compute the known global optimum, that is, the known native structure of a protein. The metric of choice is the least RMSD metric summarized in Section 2. The lowest RMSD from the native structure over conformations obtained by a conformation sampling algorithm is recorded and reported as the closest that the algorithm comes to the known native structure. In EAs, this calculation is often carried out over all conformations ever computed (over all generations) as opposed to only those in the final population or those in the hall of fame (if a hall of fame is employed). The reason for doing so is that it is not uncommon for a good solution to be lost in later generations.

### 4.3 MC as 1 + 1 EA: Basin Hopping as a Specialized MA

We now provide further understanding on why EAs are promising avenues to approach PSP by first demonstrating that they encapsulate MC-based methods.

MC can be cast as a 1 + 1 EA. Since an MC trajectory is a series of conformations, where $C_{i+1}$ is the result of applying a move on $C_i$ in the trajectory, an MC trajectory of $n$ conformations can be viewed as an EA of $n$ generations. In each generation $i$, the only individuals $C_i$ is subjected to a perturbation operator that employs a designed move, and the result of that operator is conformation $C_i + 1$. A nonoverlapping, generational model replaces $C_i$ with $C_{i+1}$; that is, $C_{i+1}$ is the only conformation retained in the population of the next generation. This is a standard MC algorithm. In a specialized version, known as the Metropolis MC, a probabilistic criterion is employed to determine whether $C_{i+1}$ is retained in the trajectory or another attempt/move needs to be made on $C_i$. Even Metropolis MC can be viewed as a 1 + 1 EA. Instead of the generational model, the parent and offspring are combined, and a probabilistic criterion is employed to determine which one survives in the next generation.

An interesting adaptation of Metropolis MC has been proposed to address PSP in the computational structural biology community. The adaptation concerns additionally subjecting each generated conformation $C_{i+1}$ to an energetic minimization technique that maps $C_{i+1}$ to a local minimum in the energy surface. The conformation representing the local minimum, $C_{i+1*}$ is the one considered for addition into the trajectory through the Metropolis criterion. Essentially, the MC trajectory is a series of local minima, or basins, and the algorithm has also been referred to as basin hopping (BH). BH is a specialized EA. The energetic minimization can be considered a local improvement iterator, thus making BH a 1 + 1 MA.

The history of BH in computational structural biology is rich and can be traced to work by Wales and Doye on obtaining the LJ minima of small atomic clusters [50]. When considering that BH is an MC with minimization, its roots go even deeper to the "MC with minimization" methods proposed by Scheraga and colleagues [36, 51]. Simultaneous work on BH for addressing challenging real-life problems has appeared in the AI community. In particular, in the EC community, BH is also known as Iterated Local Search and is popular for solving discrete optimization problems [52].

Recently, BH algorithms has seen a comeback in computational structural biology. BH algorithms essentially differ in how they implement the perturbation and improvement operators. For instance, the perturbation predominantly modifies atomic coordinates, and minimization is either a gradient descent or a Metropolis MC at low temperature [37, 53–55]. Application for PSP in ref. [49] shows that Cartesian-based representations are the culprit of decreased efficiency and efficacy on capturing the native structure on protein sequences longer than 75 amino acids. Adaptations of BH algorithms to employ angular-based representations and the fragment replacement technique in the perturbation operator have resulted in competitive performance with top MC-based conformational sampling algorithms in PSP. We highlight one such algorithm below. The reader is referred to ref. [56] for a review on BH algorithms for protein structure modeling.

*4.3.1 Highlight: Basin Hopping for PSP*

Work in ref. [46] extends the applicability of BH for PSP in proteins more than 120 amino acids long. This is mainly a result of employing the molecular fragment replacement technique in the perturbation operator. The technique is popular with the top conformational sampling algorithms for PSP and other structure-related problems and central to their performance [46, 47, 57–66]. Its popularity is due to the fact that it allows rapidly computing conformations with credible secondary structures. Below we briefly summarize it.

Molecular Fragment Replacement

The basic idea is to bundle together consecutive dihedral angles of $k$ amino acids ($k$ is typically 3 and 9). The segment $[i, i + k - 1]$ in the protein chain is referred to as a fragment, and the dihedral angles corresponding to the fragment are referred to as the fragment configuration. A move consists of replacing values of all these angles simultaneously with values obtained from a precompiled library (often referred to as a library of fragment configurations). The library is precompiled from known, nonredundant protein structures. The chain of each structure is excised in overlapping fragments, and configurations are stored organized by their amino-acid sequence. Making a move on a conformation $C$ to generate a new conformation consists of the following three steps: a position $i$ in the protein chain/sequence is sampled at random. A fragment $[i, i + k - 1]$ is then defined. The library is queried with the amino-acid sequence of the fragment. Configurations of fragments with the identical (or similar) sequence are then collected, and one is selected at random to replace that of the fragment in conformation $C$. Details on constructing fragment configuration libraries are presented in ref. [67]. A representative PSP package that employs MC-based conformational sampling algorithms with the molecular fragment replacement technique is the Rosetta package [68].

PSPBH with Molecular Fragment Replacement

The BH-based algorithm in ref. [46] samples local minima within 5–6 Å at most of the native structure on diverse proteins and is thus competitive with MC-based state-of-the-art sampling algorithms for PSP. Work in ref. [46] shows a strong correlation between RMSD to the native structure and RMSDs between consecutive local minima. Based on this finding, later work in ref. [47] introduces techniques to control the distance between consecutive local minima and thus further improve proximity to the native structure. Work in ref. [47] also shows that simple greedy search in the local improvement operator is just as effective but more efficient that MC-based improvement.

**4.4 Population-Based Off-Lattice and On-Lattice EAs for PSP**

We now summarize state-of-the-art population-based EAs and algorithmic components responsible for recent advances.

The popularity of lattice-based representations in the early 1980s in protein structure modeling motivated development and adaptations of EAs for a simplified instantiation of the PSP problem. Significant work in the EC community on PSP still employs a lattice-based HP model of a protein chain, where an amino acid is modeled as a bead in 2D or 3D, two types of beads are considered (hydrophobic/H versus hydrophilic/P), and amino acid beads are positioned on a 2D or 3D lattice. In essence, the PSP problem is simplified, and the objective becomes finding an on-lattice self-avoiding walk that minimizes the interaction energy among amino-acid beads. Lattice-based representations facilitate the design of simple perturbation operators and are amenable to simplistic energy functions for summing up interactions and scoring conformations. The employment of lattice-based representations reduces the typical computational demands of PSP and allows focusing on algorithmic design and analysis, particularly regarding an optimal the interplay of exploration versus exploitation. A comprehensive review of on-lattice EAs can be found in ref. [69]. In the following, we review salient search strategies demonstrated effective on on-lattice and off-lattice EAs and then highlight recent developments that position EAs as competitors with top MC-based PSP conformation sampling algorithms.

*4.4.1 Hybridization to Balance Global and Local Search*

In the EC community it is well understood that, for complex optimization problems, simple EAs are not sufficient for achieving the necessary balance between exploration and exploitation. As a consequence, there continues to be an interest in developing more complex EAs capable of achieving this balance on complex fitness landscapes rich in local minima. One direction concerns the design and implementation of hybrid EAs that combine population-based global search techniques with domain-specific local search methods.

There are a variety of ways in which local search methods have been embedded in EAs. MA is the most well-known hybridization approach, based on the idea that a top level EA manages a population of local searches (memes) with the goal of maintaining a diverse set of memes (exploration) while exploiting efficient local search methods with memes. Other less well-known approaches include Baldwinian EAs, Lamarkian EAs, cultural algorithms, and genetic local search [70–73]. MAs have been first adapted for conformation sampling in PSP for toy or short peptides, employing the lattice-based HP model [74–79].

Work on on-lattice EAs has demonstrated that the addition of local searches or memes is particularly effective when crossover is employed to combine features from multiple previously sampled conformations [80]. In a rugged landscape, offspring obtained through crossover are highly likely to have low fitness. This is particularly the case for protein conformations, where variable coupling makes it difficult to obtain offspring that readily satisfy implicit energetic constraints imposed by long-range interactions. Studies show that the use of short memes improves the ability of an MA to sample low-energy conformations [81]. This in turn allows reaching significantly lower-energy conformations in a shorter amount of time and has been demonstrated both in on-lattice and off-lattice MAs [74–79, 82, 83].

In ref. [80], where the meme is a hill-climbing local search, the MA is shown both more efficient and more effective at finding near-native conformations over a standard EA. A recent study in ref. [84], which extends the EA-based Harmony algorithm to use a hybrid local search shows similar improvements over the original algorithm. However, improvements are often reported in terms of energetic values reached, with lower values taken as indication of higher exploration capability [85, 86]. While such a metric is important for comparing novel algorithmic ingredients to baseline EAs, in itself it is not indicative of the utility of sampled conformations for PSP. In the computational structural biology community, the focus is often on the ability of a conformation sampling algorithm to reach the known native structure; that is, the metric underpinning performance is RMSD or other distance-based metrics between sampled conformations and the known native structure. When judged by this metric, many on-lattice EAs fall short when compared to the state-of-the-art MC-based conformation sampling algorithms that have moved beyond lattice models. In addition, due to the popularity of a legacy benchmark dataset, the majority of on-lattice MAs are tested on proteins no longer than 61 amino acids. On longer chains, prediction quality suffers; for instance work in ref. [84] reports the inability to find conformations below 6 Å RMSD to known native structures on chains longer than 60 amino acids [84].

**Highlight: Population-Based, Off-Lattice MAs for PSP**

MAs capable of reaching similar or better prediction quality than state-of-the-art MC-based conformation sampling algorithms incorporate key domain-specific insight on proteins. These include off-lattice, backbone-based angular representations, state-of-the-art energy functions, such as the suite of Rosetta energy functions, and the popular molecular fragment replacement technique in perturbation operators and memes [46, 48, 87, 88]. Work in ref. [82] introduces a fixed-size MA that makes use of such domain-specific insights. The greedy local search that constitutes the meme makes use of the fragment replacement technique; conformations are evaluated with the Rosetta score3 function, and elitism is employed to pitch the

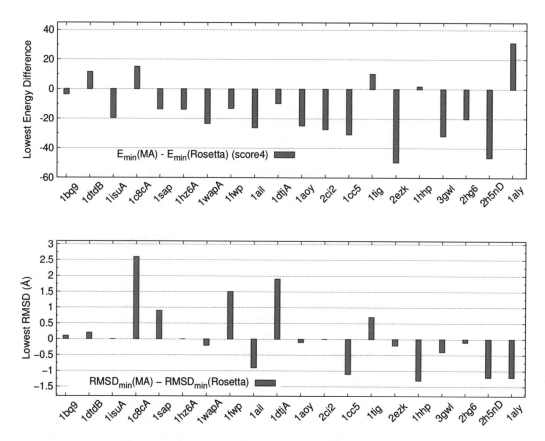

**Fig. 2** Illustration of performance of state-of-the-art MAs for PSP. *Top panel*: Given the same computational budget, the lowest energy value (measured with the score4 energy function in Rosetta) reached by the on-lattice MA in ref. [128] and the multi-start MC-based conformation sampling algorithm in Rosetta are measured. The *y* axis shows the difference. Bars below the 0 line indicate where MA reaches lower energy regions in the variable space. MA does so for 75 % of the 20 different protein sequences used for the comparison. The PDB IDs of the native structures of these sequences are shown on the *x* axis. Results combine many independent runs of each algorithm under comparison. *Bottom panel*: The *y* axis shows the difference in the lowest RMSD reached by many runs of each algorithm to the known native structure. The difference shows that MA is competitive with the conformation sampling algorithm in Rosetta even on the unforgiving RMSD metric

top offspring against the top parents. The survival mechanism is truncation-based. A representative result of the performance of this MA is provided in Fig. 2, which shows that this MA beats the (multi-start) MC-based conformation sampling algorithm employed in the popular Rosetta structure prediction protocol in terms of exploration capability while achieving similar or lower RMSDs to the known native structure. Work in ref. [82] additionally considers injecting crossover into this MA and studies the interplay between various crossover operators and the local search. A novel crossover operator is proposed that preserves local structural features and results in offspring with fewer constraint violations.

With the realization that the local search/improvement operator is key to obtaining optimal conformations, significant efforts are spent in designing customized operators for both on-lattice and off-lattice EAs for PSP. Due to the demonstrated superiority of the molecular fragment replacement technique in MC-based conformation sampling algorithms, related efforts in off-lattice EAs have pursued memes that are hill climbers, MC local search, Metropolis MC local search over fragment replacement moves [46–48, 82, 87–89].

Work in on-lattice EAs has also revealed a variety of effective memes for EAs on 2D square and triangular, and 3D cubic, triangular, and FCC lattices. The majority of memes for lattices employ the concept of move sets, such as diagonal moves and tilt moves [90], moves that preserve local, secondary structures [91], pull moves [92, 93], end moves, corner moves, three-bead and end flip for single-point moves and crankshaft for double point moves [94], rotation moves [23]. In particular, recent work in ref. [95] investigates in detail the geometric properties of the 3D FCC lattice and proposes several local search operators that build on lattice rotation and generalized move sets to achieve optimal conformations much faster than baseline EAs.

Another interesting direction in MAs is the coevolving of memes. Early work in MAs for PSP pursued dynamically modifying memes. The idea is that a single static local search may not be effective for all protein sizes and topologies or stages of an EA. Work in ref. [96] proposes an on-lattice GA with a Metropolis MC-based local search (an HP lattice model is employed). Temperature in the Metropolis criterion is varied in a reactive scheme so that the method balances between exploration and exploitation. When the population of conformations is deemed diverse, the temperature is lowered to focus on exploitation of local minima. As the population converges, the temperature is increased to shift the focus on exploration. The method is reported to find high-fitness conformations faster than a baseline EA. Extensions in ref. [97] coevolve memes alongside conformations (variables such as length of the local search and type of mutation are added to the variables employed to represent a conformation) [97]. Coevolving memes is shown to improve both time performance and fitness of computed conformations over baseline EAs [97–99].

### 4.4.2 Evolutionary Strategies to Avoid Premature Convergence

The issue of premature convergence or stalling due to loss of population diversity, long known in the EC community to accompany GAs, has also been observed in adaptations for PSP. The GA crossover and mutation operators can become ineffective over time, leading to growing similarity among individuals in a population [100, 101]. Stalling is an expected phenomenon, as earlier generations are expected to cover a broader search space while later generations are expected to converge to specific regions in the fitness landscape. With growing similarity in a population, the crossover operator becomes implicitly controlled and fails to produce offspring that are significantly different from their parents. In effect, the crossover operator produces more twins.

Stalling is responsible for GAs getting frequently trapped in local minima [102]. This is exacerbated for longer protein sequences and is credited as one of the major reasons why GAs, though effective, are not competitive with state-of-the-art MC-based conformation sampling algorithms for PSP [103].

Some of the earliest work addresses this phenomenon by using genotypic diversity for selection and replacement of individuals in a population [104]. The original on-lattice GA proposed in ref. [96] is extended in ref. [104] so that parents selected for crossover have maximal genotypic difference, measured via the Manhattan distance metric. Experiments show that significantly lower energy values are obtained over the original GA [104].

In other studies, a twin removal approach is employed instead. Twins are energetically and structurally similar conformations and they are determined based on phenotypic distance measured via Hamming distance or distance over contact maps [105]. There are several twin removal strategies. One strategy is to periodically remove and replace twins with new conformations sampled at random [77, 105, 106]. Other strategies relax the definition of twins to include not only identical but also highly correlated individuals [107]. Work in ref. [107] shows that such an approach significantly improves performance of a number of on-lattice, GA-based methods. Crowding, a strategy originally introduced in ref. [108], can also be seen as a specific implementation of twin removal, though restricted to an offspring replacing an individual most similar to itself [109]. Another strategy known as niched-penalty [110] does not explicitly remove similar individuals but imposes a penalty to discourage their participation as parents for producing offspring for the next generation. Though promising, the strategy has yet to be evaluated in EAs for PSP.

Another popular approach for increasing diversity in EAs for PSP is to avoid redundant conformations all together. This approach, known as tabu search, keeps track of conformations recently visited by the local search to avoid their revisitation by other local searches [28]. Work in ref. [111] employs a subset of already-sampled conformations to avoid revisitation at the global level in an MA. Comparison of these two distinct employments of tabu search to avoid revisitation shows that tabu search at the global level is more effective than at the local level on HP-lattice models [111]. Customizations of tabu search for on-lattice EAs are regularly pursued [112, 113]. Integrations of tabu search in off-lattice MAs are also beginning to be pursued, though currently limited to HP toy models [114, 115].

### 4.4.3 Multi-objective Optimization in EAs for PSP

Casting PSP as a multi-objective rather than a single-objective PSP problem is proving powerful and effective at avoiding premature convergence and overall improving the performance of EAs regarding their ability to reproduce known native structures.

Multi-objective optimization (MOO) lies in the ability to decouple and group terms in an energy function in a few categories considered as separate objectives. MOO originates from the Pareto analysis in economic theory on simultaneous optimization of conflicting objectives. Casting PSP as an MOO problem is particularly suitable, because terms in protein energy functions compete with one another. For instance, slight fluctuations in the backbone of a protein conformation may simultaneously lower the value of the energy terms measuring local interactions but increase the value of the terms measuring nonlocal interactions.

A simple way to cast PSP as an MOO is to do so in the survival mechanism through the concept of dominance. Suppose that the terms in a protein energy function are grouped into two categories, NB (non-bonded) and B (bonded). A conformation $C_i$ is said to dominate $C$ when the value of every category in $C_i$ is strictly less than the value of the corresponding category in $C$. This is known as strong dominance (weak dominance allows equivalent values). If strong dominance is employed, the number of conformations that dominate a conformation $C_i$ is known as the Pareto count of $C_i$. Non-dominated conformations (those with Pareto count 0) constitute the Pareto front of a set of conformations. A Pareto rank can also be associated with a conformation $C_i$ by counting the number of conformations that $C_i$ dominates (conformations in the Pareto front have Pareto rank 0 by definition).

Before highlighting several EAs that treat PSP as an MOO problem, it is worth noting that the concept of Pareto dominance has been shown useful also for *decoy selection* techniques that select a subset of computed conformations for further refinement and then decide among those which ones represent the unknown native state in true blind prediction setting. The majority of current decoy selection techniques in PSP make use of RMSD-based clustering of conformations; typically, the cluster with the largest number of members is predicted as the native state.

MOO analysis provides an alternative route. Recent work has shown that the Pareto front or various thresholds of Pareto counts are effective at reducing the ensemble of sampled conformations while retaining near-native ones [47]. The selection of the Pareto knees is also shown effective [116, 117]. In ref. [117], a knee-based selection technique retains conformations within 0.3 Å of the actual best conformation in the ensemble (best in terms of RMSD to the native structure). Work in ref. [118] provides contradictory results and shows that including knees makes little difference. Testing is conducted on short peptides up to 20 amino acids long, which probably do not benefit from MOO analysis.

Decoupling energy terms into separate objectives and employing MOO reduces the complexity of the energy landscape in short polypeptides by reducing the number of local minima [119]. MOO has already been integrated in on-lattice EAs for conformation sampling [120, 121]. MOO in off-lattice EAs decomposes terms of all-atom energy functions, such as CHARMM and AMBER [122, 123]. Typically, terms of the energy function are grouped in two categories, with one category consisting of the LJ term that measures non-bonded interactions, and the other category summing up all other terms. Doing so in the fast messy Genetic Algorithm (fmGA), which represents dihedral angles as 10bit strings, is shown to result in lower-energy conformations over the baseline fmGA for short protein chains of 514 amino acids [122, 123]. Other studies employ three rather than two categories and show that doing so results in more conformations closer to the native structure. Testing is limited, however, to a short peptide and a medium-length protein [124–126].

**Highlight: State-of-the-Art 1 + 1 MOMA for PSP**

Work in ref. [127] integrates MOO in a 1 + 1 EA, using the same CHARMM bonded vs. non-bonded categories as work in refs. [122, 123]. Conformations in the Pareto front are recorded in an archive or hall of fame, and secondary structure prediction from a given amino-acid sequence and sidechain rotamer libraries are used to bias sampling toward physically relevant conformations. At each generation, the offspring and parent compete for survival. If neither dominates the other, the one which dominates more of the archive survives. Later work extends the IPAES and shows it effective on several longer protein chains up to 70 amino acids [117]. Conformations below 5 Å lRMSD to the known native structure are found for sequences up to 70 amino acids in length, and results are shown to outperform several other MOO EAs and standard EAs on shorter chains, as well. Some representative results are shown in Fig. 3.

**Highlight: State-of-the-Art Population-Based MOMAs and MOMGAs for PSP**

Work in ref. [128] integrates MOO in the population-based MAs and MGAs proposed and shown competitive in ref. [82] to the Rosetta MC-based conformation sampling algorithm. Three categories are defined that group together terms of the Rosetta score4 function; the first category measures short range hydrogen bonding, the second measures long-range hydrogen bonding; and the third term summing the rest of the terms. It is worth noting that the employment of backbone dihedral angles as variables preserves bond lengths and valence angles; thus, energetic differences between conformations are due to non-bonded interactions. A novel truncation selection mechanism is employed, which sorts

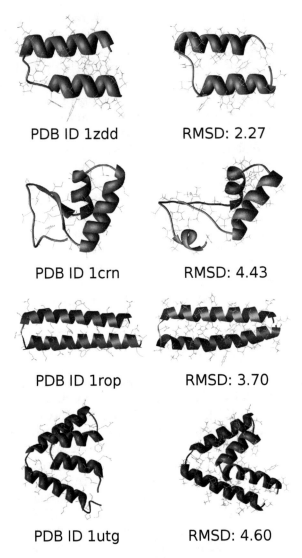

PDB ID 1zdd          RMSD: 2.27

PDB ID 1crn          RMSD: 4.43

PDB ID 1rop          RMSD: 3.70

PDB ID 1utg          RMSD: 4.60

**Fig. 3** Illustration of best models obtained by a state-of-the-art MOMA. Four proteins of varying sizes from 34 to 70 amino acids are chosen to illustrate the high quality of the lowest-RMSD conformations obtained by the MOGA algorithm presented in ref. [117]. The *left panel* shows the native structure and its PDB ID, whereas the *right panel* shows the computed lowest-RMSD conformation for each protein and its CA RMSD (calculated over CA atoms) from the native structure. Rendering is done with Pymol, showing secondary structures of the backbone and drawing side chains with *thin lines*. Figures are kindly provided by Giuseppe Nicosia and Giuseppe Narzisi

parent and offspring at the end of each generation first by their Pareto rank and then by total energy (for conformations with the same Pareto rank). The injection of this MOO technique is compared against the baseline MA and MGA algorithms originally introduced in ref. [82], resulting in the MOMA and MOMGA algorithms presented in ref. [128]. The addition of Pareto count

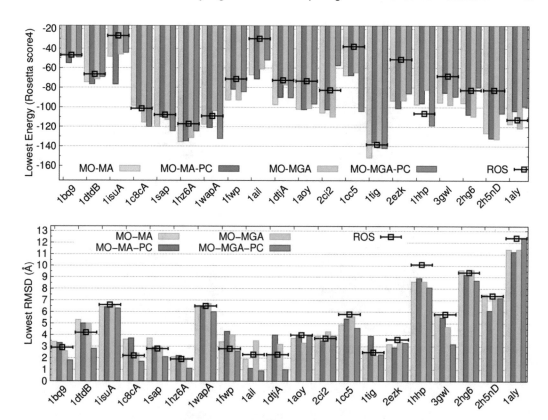

**Fig. 4** Illustration of performance of state-of-the-art MOM(G)As for PSP. The performance of MOMA and MOMGA presented in ref. [128] and MOMAPC and MOMGAPC presented in ref. [129] is shown here, compared to the MC-based conformation sampling in Rosetta, on 20 proteins. The PDB IDs of the native structures of these sequences are shown on the x axis. The *top panel* shows the lowest energy reached by each algorithm. The *bottom panel* shows the lowest RMSD to the native structure reached by each algorithm. Results combine many independent runs of each algorithm under comparison

in the truncation-based mechanism is also tested (conformations are first sorted by Pareto rank, then Pareto count, then total energy). The resulting extensions are referred to as MOMAPC and MOMGAPC [129]. Figure 4 shows that these four algorithms outperform the multi-start MC-based conformation sampling algorithm in Rosetta and represent the state of the art in off-lattice EAs for PSP. Figure 5 showcases the capability of these algorithms by rendering the lowest-RMSD (best) conformations obtained by these algorithms on a variety of proteins and comparing these to the best conformations found by multi-start MC-based conformation sampling algorithm in Rosetta.

**4.5 EAs for Mapping Protein Energy Landscapes**

EAs obtain a discrete representation of the potential energy surface of a protein chain. It is thus easy to see the promise of EAs for more than PSP. A central challenge in molecular biology is to understand functional changes upon single-point mutations in proteins.

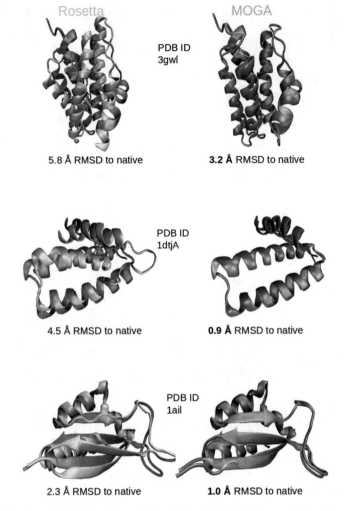

**Fig. 5** Illustration of best models obtained by a state-of-the-art MOGA. Three proteins of varying sizes from 70 to 106 amino acids are chosen to illustrate the high quality of the lowest-RMSD conformations obtained by the MOGA algorithm presented in ref. [128]. The *left panel* superimposes the best conformation produced by the MC-based conformation sampling algorithm in Rosetta (drawn in *lemon green*) over the known native structure (drawn in *gray*). The *right panel* superimposes the best conformation produced by MOGA (drawn in *orange*) over the native structure. The PDB IDs of each native structure are shown. The RMSD of each lowest-RMSD conformation to the known native structure is shown for each algorithm on each of the three selected proteins. The reported RMSD is computed over backbone atoms. Rendering is performed with VMD [136], using the NewCartoon graphical representation that shows the local secondary structures

EAs hold significant promise for providing a detailed characterization of structure spaces and underlying energy landscapes, which currently challenge methods based on MC and those based on MD. However, a truly de novo setting currently proves too challenging, given that the objective is to retain diversity and map multiple basins of a protein's energy landscape. In recent work, EA-based methods are proposed to map multi-basin energy landscapes of complex proteins over 100 amino acids long. These methods make use of known, experimentally available long-lived structures of healthy (wild type) and aberrant versions of a protein. These structures are leveraged to transform a discrete problem into a continuous one, subjecting them to Principal Component Analysis to reveal a few collective variables constituting the search space for the EA. In refs. [109, 130], mutation operators are defined over the variables and a family based crowding mechanism is used to retain diverse conformations longer. The evaluation operator lifts individuals from the reduced representation to an all-atom representation prior to subjecting them to a meme for improvement; the latter uses a simulated annealing MC local search currently implemented as the *relax* protocol in Rosetta.

An implementation of the above method is available in http://www.cs.gmu.edu/~ashehu/?q=OurTools. Applications on several proteins up to 165 amino acids long show that this MA is able to reveal multiple basins of proteins known switch between different structural states for function. In particular, work in ref. [131] builds on this MA and introduces a method that is capable of mapping energy landscapes of wild-type and oncogenic sequences of the H-Ras catalytic domain and explaining via comparison of the landscapes the reasons for functional changes. While these methods explicitly seed the initial population with experimentally available structures, an adaptation of the popular CMAES technique is introduced in ref. [132] employs these structures only to extract the reduced search space via PCA and initialize the multivariable distribution.

## 5   Future Prospects

As stochastic optimization now represents the only computationally feasible approach to PSP, work on improving the capability of EAs for PSP is expected to continue. Work on on-lattice EAs is expected to advance PSP for very large protein chains of several hundred amino acids. On protein chains of up to 200 amino acids, the goal is to increase prediction accuracy, and in this domain, more returns are expected from off-lattice EAs that make use of state-of-the-art protein energy functions.

While this review highlighted several evolutionary techniques adapted from the EC community to address the exploration vs. exploitation issue in the multimodal protein energy landscapes, there are other opportunities to design more complex EAs. As the review has highlighted, there are several known mechanisms for population diversification that have yet to be adapted and tested for PSP. There are opportunities to further investigate dynamic, coevolving memes, particularly for more complex local searches. There is a growing interest in the EC community to dynamically make decisions on allocation of computational resources to computation-heavy memes [133].

Other evolutionary strategies for structurization of EAs also present interesting new avenues to enhance exploration capability. Interestingly, structured EAs have been debuted in macromolecular modeling but have been limited to sequence-function prediction problems [134]. Further investigation of multi-objective optimization and Pareto-based measures is expected to improve accuracy, particularly in the context of inherently approximate protein energy functions. Finally, given the importance of injecting domain-specific insight in EAs for PSP, efforts on designing novel, representation-specific perturbation operators are expected to improve performance.

As this review has highlighted, the potential of EAs beyond PSP for the more general and challenging problem of mapping protein energy landscapes is only beginning to be realized [109, 130–132, 135]. Evolutionary strategies that hold off premature convergence are key to the ability of EAs to reproduce a multitude of possible basins in a complex landscape.

EC researchers tempted by the richness and complexity of scientific questions posed by protein structure modeling now have strong foundations to venture into this domain. Work in protein structure modeling is challenging, as it often requires researchers to attain working knowledge in a new discipline. For those willing to do so, however, the payoff is significant. It is worth considering that, while at the moment EAs are not the top methods for PSP and modeling of single protein chains, there is one domain where they have dominated and replaced MC-based algorithms. In protein–ligand binding and protein–protein docking, the top algorithms are complex EAs. The hope is that in a few years, one will be able to say the same for PSP and protein structure modeling in general.

## Acknowledgement

Funding for this work is provided in part by the National Science Foundation (Grant No. 1421001 and CAREER Award No. 1144106) and the Thomas F. and Kate Miller Jeffress Memorial Trust Award.

## References

1. Hamosh A, Scott AF, Amberger JS, Bocchini CA, McKusick VA (2005) Online Mendelian Inheritance in Man (OMIM), a knowledge-base of human genes and genetic disorders. Nucleic Acids Res 1(33):D514–D517

2. Stenson PD, Mort M, Ball EV, Shaw K, Phillips A, Copper DN (2014) The Human Gene Mutation Database: building a comprehensive mutation repository for clinical and molecular genetics, diagnostic testing and personalized genomic medicine. Hum Genet 133(1):1–9

3. Ratovitski T, Corson LB, Strain J, Wong P, Cleveland DW, Culotta VC et al (1999) Variation in the biochemical/biophysical properties of mutant superoxide dismutase

1 enzymes and the rate of disease progression in familial amyotrophic lateral sclerosis kindreds. Hum Mol Genet 8(8):1451–1460

4. DiDonato M, Craig L, Huff ME, Thayer MM, Cardoso RM, Kassmann CJ et al (2003) ALS mutants of human superoxide dismutase form fibrous aggregates via framework destabilization. J Mol Biol 332 (1):601–615

5. Soto C (2003) Unfolding the role of protein misfolding in neurodegenerative diseases. Nat Rev Neurosci 4(1):49–60

6. Soto C (2008) Protein misfolding and neurodegeneration. JAMA Neurol 65(2):184–189

7. Uversky VN (2009) Intrinsic disorder in proteins associated with neurodegenerative diseases. Front Biosci 14:5188–5238

8. Neudecker P, Robustelli P, Cavalli A, Walsh P, Lundstrm P, ZarrineAfsar A et al (2012) Structure of an intermediate state in protein folding and aggregation. Science 336 (6079):362–366

9. Fetics SK, Guterres H, Kearney BM, Buhrman G, Ma B, Nussinov R et al (2015) Allosteric effects of the oncogenic RasQ61L mutant on RafRBD. Structure 23 (3):505–516

10. Berman HM, Henrick K, Nakamura H (2003) Announcing the worldwide Protein Data Bank. Nat Struct Biol 10(12):980

11. Reardon S (2013) Large NIH, projects cut. Nature 503(7475):173–174

12. Anfinsen CB (1973) Principles that govern the folding of protein chains. Science 181 (4096):223–230

13. Boehr DD, Wright PE (2008) How do proteins interact? Science 320(5882):1429–1430

14. Dill KA, Ozkan B, Shell MS, Weikl TR (2008) The protein folding problem. Annu Rev Biophys 37:289–316

15. Boehr DD, Nussinov R, Wright PE (2009) The role of dynamic conformational ensembles in biomolecular recognition. Nat Chem Biol 5(11):789–796

16. Zhang Y (2014) Interplay of ITASSER and QUARK for template-based and ab initio protein structure prediction in CASP10. Proteins 82(Suppl 2):175–187

17. Amaro RE, Bansai M (2014) Editorial overview: theory and simulation: tools for solving the insolvable. Curr Opin Struct Biol 25:4–5

18. Clementi C (2008) Coarse-grained models of protein folding: toy models or predictive tools? Curr Opin Struct Biol 18:10–15

19. Taketomi H, Ueda Y, Go N (1975) Studies on protein folding, unfolding and fluctuations by computer simulation: the effect of specific amino acid sequence represented by specific inter-unit interactions. Int J Pept Prot Res 7 (6):445–459

20. Hinds DA, Levitt M (1994) Exploring conformational space with a simple lattice model for protein structure. J Mol Biol 243 (4):668–682

21. Kolinski A, Skolnick J (1994) Monte Carlo simulations of protein folding. I. Lattice model and interaction scheme. Prot Struct Funct Genet 18(4):338–352

22. Ishikawa K, Yue K, Dill KA (1999) Predicting the structures of 18 peptides using Geocore. Protein Sci 8(4):716–721

23. Unger R, Moult J (1993) Finding lowest free energy conformation of a protein is an NP-hard problem: proof and implications. Bull Math Biol 55(6):1183–1198

24. Hart WE, Istrail S (1997) Robust proofs of NP-hardness for protein folding: general lattices and energy potentials. J Comp Biol 4 (1):1–22

25. Crescenzi P, Goldman D, Papadimitriou C, Piccolboni A, Yannakakis M (1998) On the complexity of protein folding. J Comput Biol 5(3):423–465

26. Reva BA, Finkelstein AV, Sanner MF, Olson AJ (1996) Adjusting potential energy functions for lattice models of chain molecules. Prot Struct Funct Genet 25(3):379–388

27. Park BH, Levitt M (1995) The complexity and accuracy of discrete state models of protein structure. J Mol Biol 249(2):493–507

28. Dotu I, Cebrian M, Van Hentenryck P, Clote P (2011) On lattice protein structure prediction revisited. IEEE Trans Comp Biol Bioinform 8(6):1620–1632

29. Abayagan R, Totrov M, Kuznetsov D (1994) ICM a new method for protein modeling and design: applications to docking and structure prediction from the distorted native conformation. J Comput Chem 15(5):488–506

30. Zhang M, Kavraki LE (2002) A new method for fast and accurate derivation of molecular conformations. Chem Inf Comp Sci 42 (1):64–70

31. McLachlan AD (1972) A mathematical procedure for superimposing atomic coordinates of proteins. Acta Crystallogr A 26 (6):656–657

32. Brooks BR, Bruccoleri RE, Olafson BD, States DJ, Swaminathan S, Karplus M (1983) CHARMM: a program for macromolecular energy, minimization, and dynamics calculations. J Comput Chem 4(2):187–217

33. Onuchic JN, LutheySchulten Z, Wolynes PG (1997) Theory of protein folding: the energy landscape perspective. Annu Rev Phys Chem 48:545–600

34. Dill KA, Chan HS (1997) From Levinthal to pathways to funnels. Nat Struct Biol 4(1):10–19

35. Onuchic JN, Wolynes PG (1997) Theory of protein folding. Curr Opin Struct Biol 14:70–75

36. Li Z, Scheraga HA (1987) Monte Carlo minimization approach to the multiple minima problem in protein folding. Proc Natl Acad Sci U S A 84(19):6611–6615

37. Verma A, Schug A, Lee KH, Wenzel W (2006) Basin hopping simulations for all-atom protein folding. J Chem Phys 124(4):044515

38. LindorffLarsen K, Piana S, Dror RO, Shaw DE (2011) How fast-folding proteins fold. Science 334(6055):517–520

39. Vendruscolo M, Dobson CM (2011) Protein dynamics: Moore's law in molecular biology. Curr Biol 21(2):R68–R70

40. Piana S, LindorffLarsen K, Shaw DE (2013) Atomic-level description of ubiquitin folding. Proc Natl Acad Sci U S A 110(15):5915–5920

41. Stein EG, Rice LM, Bruenger AT (1997) Torsion-angle molecular dynamics as a new efficient tool for NMR structure calculation. J Magn Reson 124(1):154–164

42. Rice LM (2004) Bruenger AT.277290. Prot Struct Funct Bioinf 19(4):277–290

43. Chen J, Im W, Brooks C (2005) Application of torsion angle molecular dynamics for efficient sampling of protein conformations. J Comput Chem 26(15):1565–1578

44. Unger R (2004) The genetic algorithm approach to protein structure prediction. Struct Bond 110:153–175

45. De Jong KA (2006) Evolutionary computation: a unified approach. MIT Press, Boston, MA

46. Olson B, Shehu A (2012) Evolutionary-inspired probabilistic search for enhancing sampling of local minima in the protein energy surface. Proteome Sci 10(10):S5

47. Olson B, Shehu A (2013) Rapid sampling of local minima in protein energy surface and effective reduction through a multi-objective filter. Proteome Sci 11(Suppl1):S12

48. Saleh S, Olson B, Shehu A (2013) A population-based evolutionary search approach to the multiple minima problem in de novo protein structure prediction. BMC Struct Biol 13(Suppl1):S4

49. Prentiss MC, Wales DJ, Wolynes PG (2008) Protein structure prediction using basin hopping. J Chem Phys 128(22):225106

50. Wales DJ, Doye JPK (1997) Global optimization by Basin-Hopping and the lowest energy structures of Lennard-Jones clusters containing up to 110 atoms. J Phys Chem A 101(28):5111–5116

51. Nayeem A, Vila J, Scheraga HA (1991) A comparative study of the simulated-annealing and Monte Carlo with minimization approaches to the minimum energy structures of polypeptides: [Met]enkephalin. J Comput Chem 12(5):594–605

52. Lourenco HR, Martin OC, Stutzle T, Glover F, Kochenberger G (eds) (2002) Iterated local search. Kluwer Academic Publishers, Norwell, MA

53. Abagyan R, Totrov M (1994) Biased probability Monte Carlo conformational searches and electrostatic calculations for peptides and proteins. J Mol Biol 235(3):983–1002

54. Mortenson PN, Evans DA, Wales DJ (2002) Energy landscapes of model polyalanines. J Chem Phys 117(3):1363–1376

55. Iwamatsu M, Okabe Y (2004) Basin hopping with occasional jumping. Chem Phys Lett 399:396–400

56. Olson B, Hashmi I, Molloy K, Shehu A (2012) Basin hopping as a general and versatile optimization framework for the characterization of biological macromolecules. Adv AI J 2012:674832

57. Bradley P, Misura KMS, Baker D (2005) Toward high-resolution de novo structure prediction for small proteins. Science 309(5742):1868–1871

58. Rohl CA, Strauss CE, Misura KM, Baker D (2004) Protein structure prediction using Rosetta. Methods Enzymol 383:66–93

59. Brunette TJ, Brock O (2009) Guiding conformation space search with an all-atom energy potential. Prot Struct Funct Bioinf 73(4):958–972

60. DeBartolo J, Colubri A, Jha AK, Fitzgerald JE, Freed KF, Sosnick TR (2009) Mimicking the folding pathway to improve homology-free protein structure prediction. Proc Natl Acad Sci U S A 106(10):3734–3739

61. Shehu A, Olson B (2010) Guiding the search for native-like protein conformations with an ab-initio tree-based exploration. Int J Robot Res 29(8):1106–1127

62. Simoncini D, Berenger F, Shrestha R, Zhang KYJ (2012) A probabilistic fragment-based protein structure prediction algorithm. PLoS One 7(7):e38799

63. Handl J, Knowles J, Vernon R, Baker D, Lovell SC (2011) The dual role of fragments in fragment-assembly methods for de novo protein structure prediction. Prot Struct Funct Bioinf 80(2):490–504

64. Shmygelska A, Levitt M (2009) Generalized ensemble methods for de novo structure prediction. Proc Natl Acad Sci U S A 106 (5):94305–95126

65. Shehu A, Kavraki LE, Clementi C (2009) Multiscale characterization of protein conformational ensembles. Prot Struct Funct Bioinf 76(4):837–851

66. Molloy K, Shehu A (2013) Elucidating the ensemble of functionally-relevant transitions in protein systems with a robotics-inspired method. BMC Struct Biol 13(Suppl 1):S8

67. Han KF, Baker D (1996) Global properties of the mapping between local amino acid sequence and local structure in proteins. Proc Natl Acad Sci U S A 93(12):5814–5818

68. LeaverFay A, Tyka M, Lewis SM, Lange OF, Thompson J, Jacak R et al (2011) ROSETTA3: an object-oriented software suite for the simulation and design of macromolecules. Methods Enzymol 487:545–574

69. Hoque M, Chetty M, Sattar A (2009) Genetic algorithm in ab initio protein structure prediction using low resolution model: a review. In: Biomedical data and applications, vol 224. Springer, Berlin, pp 317–342

70. Hart WE, Krasnogor N, Smith JE (eds) (2004) Recent advances in memetic algorithms. Vol 166 of Studies in fuzziness and soft computing. Springer, Heidelberg

71. Ong YS, Keane AJ (2004) Meta-Lamarckian learning in memetic algorithms. IEEE Trans Evol Comp 8(2):99–110

72. Ong YS, Krasnogor N, Ishibuchi H (2004) Special issue on memetic algorithms. IEEE Trans Syst Man Cybernet B 37(1):2–5

73. Ong Y, Lim M, Neri F, Ishibuchi H (2004) Special issue on emerging trends in a soft computing: memetic algorithms. Soft Comp 13:739–740

74. Lopes HS, Scapin MP (2005) An enhanced genetic algorithm for protein structure prediction using the 2D hydrophobic-polar model. In: Intl Conf on artificial evolution. Springer, Berlin, pp 238–246

75. Berenboym I, Avigal M (2008) Genetic algorithms with local search optimization for protein structure prediction problem. In: International conference on genetic evolutionary computation (GECCO). ACM, New York, NY, pp 1097–1098

76. Islam M (2009) Novel memetic algorithm for protein structure prediction. In: AI 2009: Advances in Artificial Intelligence. Springer, Berlin

77. Chira C, Horvath D, Dumitrescu D (2010) An evolutionary model based on hill-climbing search operators for protein structure prediction. In: Evolutionary computation, machine learning and data mining in bioinformatics. Springer, Berlin, pp 38–49

78. Tsay J, Su S (2011) Ab initio protein structure prediction based on memetic algorithm and 3D FCC lattice model. In: International conference on bioinformatics and biomedicine (BIBM). IEEE, Washington, DC, pp 315–318

79. Su S, Lin C, Ting C (2011) An effective hybrid of hill climbing and genetic algorithm for 2D triangular protein structure prediction. Proteome Sci 9(Suppl 1):S19

80. Cooper L, Corne D, Crabbe M (2003) Use of a novel Hill-climbing genetic algorithm in protein folding simulations. Comput Biol Chem 27(6):575–580

81. Cotta C (2003) Protein structure prediction using evolutionary algorithms hybridized with backtracking. In: Artificial neural nets problem solving methods. Springer, Berlin, p 1044

82. Olson B, Jong KAD, Shehu A (2013) Off-lattice protein structure prediction with homologous crossover. In: Intl Conf Genet Evol Comput (GECCO). ACM, New York, NY, pp 287–294

83. Olson B (2013) Evolving local minima in the protein energy surface. PhD thesis, George Mason University, Fairfax, VA

84. AbualRub MS, AlBetar MA, Abdullah R, Khader AT (2012) A hybrid harmony search algorithm for ab initio protein tertiary structure prediction. In: Network modeling and analysis in health informatics and bioinformatics. Springer, Berlin, pp 1–17

85. Tantar AA, Melab N, Talbi E (2008) A grid-based genetic algorithm combined with an adaptive simulated annealing for protein structure prediction. Soft Comp 12 (12):1185–1198

86. Goldstein M, Fredj E, Gerber R, Benny RB (2011) A new hybrid algorithm for finding the lowest minima of potential surfaces: approach and application to peptides. J Comput Chem 32(9):1785–1800

87. Olson B, Shehu A. Populating local minima in the protein conformational space. In: IEEE Intl Conf on Bioinf and Biomed, Atlanta, GA, 2011, pp 114–117

88. Saleh S, Olson B, Shehu A. A population-based evolutionary algorithm for sampling minima in the protein energy surface. In: IEEE Intl Conf on Bioinf and Biomed Workshops (BIBMW), Philadelphia, PA, 2012, pp 64–71

89. Olson B, Shehu A. Efficient basin hopping in the protein energy surface. In: IEEE Intl Conf on Bioinf and Biomed, Philadelphia, PA, 2012, pp 119–124

90. Hoque T, Chetty M, Dooley LS (2006) A guided genetic algorithm for protein folding prediction using 3D hydrophobic-hydrophilic model. In: 2006 I.E. congress on evolutionary computation, CEC 2006. IEEE, Washington, DC, pp 2339–2346

91. Huang C, Yang X, He Z (2010) Protein folding simulations of 2D HP model by the genetic algorithm based on optimal secondary structures. Comput Biol Chem 34 (3):137–142

92. Bockenhauer HJ, Dayem UA, Kapsokalivas L, Steinhofel K (2008) A local move set for protein folding in triangular lattice models. In: LNCS: algorithms in bioinformatics, vol 11. Springer, Berlin, pp 369–381

93. Lesh N, Mitzenmacher M, Whitesides S (2003) A complete and effective move set for simplified protein folding. In: Seventh annual Intl Conf on Res in Comp Mol Biol (RECOMB). ACM, New York, NY, pp 188–195

94. Dill KA, Bromberg S, Yue K, Fiebig KM, Yee DP, Thomas PD et al (1995) Principles of protein folding – a perspective from simple exact models. Protein Sci 4(4):561–602

95. Tsay J, Su S (2013) An effective evolutionary algorithm for protein folding on 3D FCC HP model by lattice rotation and generalized move sets. Proteome Sci 11(Suppl 1):S19

96. Krasnogor N, Smith J (2000) A memetic algorithm with self-adaptive local search: TSP as a case study. In: Intl Conf Genet Evol Comput (GECCO). ACM, New York, NY, pp 987–994

97. Krasnogor N, Blackburne B, Burke E, Hirst J (2002) Multi-meme algorithms for protein structure prediction. In: Parallel problem solving from nature (PPSN) VII, Lecture notes in computer science. Springer, Berlin, pp 769–778

98. Smith JE (2003) Protein structure prediction with coevolving memetic algorithms. In: Congress on evolutionary computation (CEC), vol 4. IEEE, Washington, DC, pp 2346–2353

99. Smith JE (2005) The coevolution of memetic algorithms for protein structure prediction. In: Recent advances in memetic algorithms. Springer, Berlin, pp 105–128

100. Fogel DB (2005) Evolutionary computation: toward a new philosophy of machine intelligence, 3rd edn. Wiley IEEE Press, New York, NY

101. Deb K, Goldberg DE (1989) An investigation of niche and species formation in genetic function optimization. In: Intl Conf Genet algorithms. ACM, New York, NY, pp 42–50

102. Deb K, Goldberg DE (1994) Simple subpopulation schemes. In: Evol Prog Conf. ACM, New York, NY, pp 296–397

103. Corne DW, Fogel GB (2004) An introduction to bioinformatics for computer scientists. In: Fogel GB, Corne DW (eds) Evolutionary computation in bioinformatics. Elsevier, India, pp 3–18

104. Bazzoli A, Tettamanzi A (2004) A memetic algorithm for protein structure prediction in a 3D lattice HP model. In: Applications of evolutionary computing, vol 3005. Springer, Berlin, pp 1–10

105. Chira C (2011) A hybrid evolutionary approach to protein structure prediction with lattice models. In: IEEE congress on evolutionary computation. IEEE, Washington, DC, pp 2300–2306

106. Chira C, Horvath D, Dumitrescu D (2011) Hill-Climbing search and diversification within an evolutionary approach to protein structure prediction. BioData Min 4(1):23

107. Hoque MT, Chetty M, Lewis A, Sattar A (2011) Twin removal in genetic algorithms for protein structure prediction using low-resolution model. IEEE Trans Comp Biol Bioinf 8(1):234–245

108. De Jong KA (1975) An analysis of the behavior of a class of genetic adaptive systems. University of Michigan, Ann Arbor, MI

109. Clausen R, Shehu A. A multiscale hybrid evolutionary algorithm to obtain sample-based representations of multi-basin protein energy landscapes. In: ACM Conf Bioinf and Comp Biol (BCB), Newport Beach, CA, 2014, pp 269–278

110. Deb K, Agrawal S (1999) Niched-penalty approach for constraint handling in genetic algorithms. In: Artificial neural nets and genetic algorithms. Springer, Berlin, pp 235–243

111. Swakkhar S, Hakim Newton MA, Pham DN, Sattar A (2012) Memory-based local search for simplified protein structure prediction. In: ACM conference on bioinformatics, computational biology and biomedicine (ACMBCB). ACM, New York, NY, pp 1–8

112. Liu J, Sun Y, Li G, Song B, Huang W (2013) Heuristic-based tabu search algorithm for folding two-dimensional AB off-lattice model proteins. Comput Biol Chem 47:142–148

113. Zhou C, Hou C, Zhang Q, Wei X (2013) Enhanced hybrid search algorithm for protein structure prediction using the 3DHP lattice model. J Mol Model 19(9):3883–3891

114. Zhang X, Wang T, Luo H, Yang JY, Deng Y, Tang J et al (2010) 3D Protein structure prediction with genetic tabu search algorithm. BMC Syst Biol 4(Suppl 1):S6

115. Zhou C, Hou C, Wei X, Zhang Q (2014) Improved hybrid optimization algorithm for 3D protein structure prediction. J Mol Model 20(7):2289–2300

116. Becerra D, Sandoval A, Restrepo-Montoya D, Nino LF (2010) A parallel multi-objective ab initio approach for protein structure prediction. In: Intl Conf on bioinformatics and biomedicine (BIBM). IEEE, Washington, DC, pp 137–141

117. Cutello V, Narzisi G, Nicosia G (2006) A multi-objective evolutionary approach to the protein structure prediction problem. J R Soc Interface 3(6):139–151

118. Narzisi G, Nicosia G, Stracquadanio G (2010) Robust bioactive peptide prediction using multi-objective optimization. In: 2010 International conference on biosciences. IEEE, Washington, DC, pp 44–50

119. Handl J, Lovell S, Knowles J (2008) Investigations into the effect of multiobjectivization in protein structure prediction. In: Parallel problem solving from nature – PPSN X. Springer, Berlin, pp 702–711

120. Garza-Fabre M, Rodriguez-Tello E, Toscano-Pulido G (2012) Multi-objectivizing the HP model for protein structure prediction. In: Evolutionary computation in combinatorial optimization. Springer, Berlin, pp 182–193

121. Garza-Fabre M, Toscano-Pulido G, Rodriguez-Tello E (2012) Locality-based multi-objectivization for the HP model of protein structure prediction. In: International conference on genetic evolutionary computation (GECCO). ACM, New York, NY, pp 473–480

122. Day RO, Zydallis JB, Lamont GB, Pachter R (2002) Solving the protein structure prediction problem through a multi-objective genetic algorithm. Nanotechnology 2:32–35

123. Day RO (2002) A multiobjective approach applied to the protein structure prediction problem. MS thesis, Air Force Institute of Technology, March 2002. Sponsor: AFRL/Material Directorate

124. Calvo JC, Ortega J (2009) Parallel protein structure prediction by multi-objective optimization. In: Euromicro Intl Conf on parallel, distributed and network-based processing. IEEE, Washington, DC, pp 268–275

125. Calvo JC, Ortega J, Anguita M (2011) PITAGORASPSP: including domain knowledge in a multi-objective approach for protein structure prediction. Neurocomputing 74 (16):2675–2682

126. Calvo JC, Ortega J, Anguita M (2011) Comparison of parallel multi-objective approaches to protein structure prediction. In: Supercomputing. Springer, Berlin, pp 253–260

127. Cutello V, Narzisi G, Nicosia G (2005) A class of pareto archived evolution strategy algorithms using immune inspired operators for ab initio protein structure prediction. In: Applications of evolutionary computing. Springer, New York, NY, pp 54–63

128. Olson B, Shehu A. Multi-objective stochastic search for sampling local minima in the protein energy surface. In: ACM Conf on Bioinf and Comp Biol (BCB), Washington, DC, 2013, pp 430–439

129. Olson B, Shehu A. Multi-objective optimization techniques for conformational sampling in template-free protein structure prediction. In: Intl Conf on Bioinf and Comp Biol (BICoB), Las Vegas, NV, 2014

130. Clausen R, Shehu A (in press) A data-driven evolutionary algorithm for mapping multibasin protein energy landscapes. J Comput Biol

131. Clausen R, Ma B, Nussinov R, Shehu A (in press) Mapping the conformation space of wildtype and mutant H-Ras with a memetic, cellular, and multiscale evolutionary algorithm. PLoS Comput Biol

132. Clausen R, Sapin E, De Jong KA, Shehu A (2015) Evolution strategies for exploring

protein energy landscapes. In: International conference on genetic evolutionary computation (GECCO). ACM, New York, NY

133. Ong YS, Lim M, Wong K (2006) Classification of adaptive memetic algorithms: a comparative study. IEEE Trans Syst Man Cybernet B 36(1):2–5

134. Kamath U, Kaers J, Shehu A, De Jong KA (2012) A spatial EA framework for parallelizing machine learning methods. In: Coello C, Cutello V, Deb K, Forrest S, Nicosia G, Pavone M (eds) Parallel problem solving from nature PPSN XII, vol 7491, Lecture notes in computer science. Springer, Berlin, pp 206–215

135. Sapin E, Clausen R, De Jong KA, Shehu A (2015) Mapping multiple minima in protein energy landscapes with evolutionary algorithms. In: International conference on genetic evolutionary computation (GECCO). ACM, New York, NY

136. Humphrey W, Dalke A, Schulten K (1996) VMD Visual molecular dynamics. J Mol Graph Model 14(1):33–38, http://www.ks.uiuc.edu/Research/vmd/

Methods in Pharmacology and Toxicology (2016): 65–84
DOI 10.1007/7653_2015_56
© Springer Science+Business Media New York 2015
Published online: 18 November 2015

# Incorporating Receptor Flexibility into Structure-Based Drug Discovery

## Chung F. Wong

## Abstract

Biological receptors are not completely rigid molecules. They can adopt many different structures at physiologically relevant temperatures. Different drugs can bind to different ensembles of conformations of these receptors. Reliably predicting to which conformations of a receptor a compound might bind well calls for the proper account of receptor flexibility. Researchers have developed various computational methods to deal with this aspect of drug discovery. Some of these methods are still too expensive to be used extensively in practice. Ensemble docking has emerged as one of the most popular practical approaches. This chapter summarizes basic principles and common techniques underlying ensemble docking, illustrates its use with several examples, and concludes with suggestions for future improvements.

Keywords: Computer-aided drug design, Ensemble docking, Molecular dynamics, Normal mode, Conformational transition paths, Homology modeling, Virtual screening, Enrichment factor, Boltzmann-enhanced discrimination of receiver operating characteristics (BEDROC)

## 1 Introduction

As biological molecules can adopt a wide range of conformations at physiologically relevant temperatures, reliable computational models need to take such flexibility into account to predict to which conformations drug candidates might bind well. Different methods have been developed to incorporate receptor flexibility into computational models to address this aspect of drug discovery. Many of these methods are still computationally too expensive to be applied to evaluate a large number of compounds. Therefore, this chapter focuses on ensemble docking as a special class of flexible-receptor docking that has become popular and practical in virtual screening.

Before ensemble docking was introduced, molecular docking was largely done by docking rigid or flexible compounds to rigid receptors [1–3]. This can produce many false negatives as some compounds might bind to the conformations of the receptors that are thermally accessible but different from the structures of the receptors used in the docking. Although it is now feasible to perform brute-force unbiased molecular dynamics simulations to dock a flexible compound to a flexible receptor [4, 5], such simulations are still prohibitively expensive for virtual screening in which a large number of compounds need to be evaluated. Ensemble docking has gained popularity in recent years because it is computationally less expensive and easier to use. Although this method is less rigorous, scientists have already found it useful to help select compounds from a chemical library that are more likely to show activity in experimental assays [6].

Ensemble docking [7–15] does not attempt to simulate directly the physical docking process, which involves the complex coupling between the structural changes of the two molecules during docking. Instead, it first generates an ensemble of the receptor structures without considering the ligands. It then docks ligands to this ensemble of receptor structures. The docking to each receptor structure simply calls for a rigid-receptor docking for which many useful programs have already been developed (e.g., [16–19]). This chapter introduces popular methods for generating structural ensembles and points out extra considerations in scoring and ranking compounds.

## 2    Generation of Receptor Structures for Ensemble Docking

### 2.1  From Experimental Structures

When many experimental structures of a receptor are available, one can construct a structural ensemble quickly [13, 20–22]. These structures might have different ligands bound, have different mutations made, be determined at different crystallization conditions, contain additional domains, or differ in some other ways. Together, they reflect the structural plasticity of the receptor.

Before these structures can be used for ensemble docking, they need to be processed to produce a consistent set of structures. These structures could have different residues missing, have different mutations made, or contain different number of residues. One can polish up these structures to include the same amino acid sequence and the same number of residues by using a structural modeling program such as MODELLER [23] to build the missing residues or make the necessary mutations.

### 2.2  From Homology Modeling

Sometimes no or only one or a few experimental structure(s) is (are) available for a receptor, but many experimental structures of one or more homologous proteins are available. In such cases, homology modeling provides a useful tool to build a structural ensemble for docking. In extreme cases when many structures of a family of proteins are available, large structural ensembles can be built for different members of the family. For example, because protein kinases have become popular targets for drug discovery, many experimental structures of protein kinases have been determined. Wong and Bairy [24, 25] leveraged this rich resource to build large structural ensembles for different protein kinases. They wrote a python wrapper around the MODELLER package to make it easier to build a large structural ensemble for a protein kinase and to refine the structural ensemble when new experimental structures become available.

### 2.3 From Conformational Transition Paths

When only a few experimental structures are available for a receptor, one could use a suitable method to generate conformational transition paths (e.g., [26–42]) and build a larger structural ensemble for docking by including structures along the paths. When the experimental structures are very different, such as between the closed and open forms of an enzyme, intermediate structures along minimum-energy paths connecting these structures could bind drastically different ligands from those accommodated by the experimental structures, thus increasing the diversity of the compounds identified as hits by a virtual screening through ensemble docking.

Wong [43] tested this idea by using proteins for which many experimental structures have been determined. He hypothesized that if the structures along conformational transition paths could accommodate known inhibitors, some of these structures might have already been determined for structurally well-studied proteins. This turned out to be the case for several protein kinases that have been studied extensively, including Bcr-Abl, the insulin receptor tyrosine kinase, the epidermal growth factor receptor, protein kinase A, and the Src kinase [43].

Methods for identifying conformational paths in proteins were introduced in the 1980s by Pratt [44] and Elber and Karplus [45]. Various similar approaches were added since then. A relatively simple one accessible by many users through the open-sourced software package MOIL [46] is introduced here. In particular, we focus on the chmin module in MOIL. It generates a conformational transition path between two structures by inserting a sequence of intermediate structures in between [45, 47–50]. It then refines this path by optimizing the function

$$
T\left(\vec{x}_2, \ldots, \vec{x}_{N-1} \middle| \vec{x}_1 \in \text{one end state}, \ \vec{x}_N \in \text{the other end state}\right)
= \sum_{i=2}^{N-1} U\left(\vec{x}_i\right) + C
\tag{1}
$$

where $U\left(\vec{x}_i\right)$ gives the potential energy of structure $i$, and the constraint function $C$ maintained roughly equal distances between adjacent structures along a path:

$$
C = \eta \sum_{i=1}^{N-1} \left(\Delta l_{i,i+1} - \langle \Delta l \rangle\right)^2 + \frac{\rho}{\lambda} \sum_{i=1}^{N-1} \exp\left(-\lambda \frac{\Delta l_{i,i+2}^2}{\langle \Delta l \rangle^2}\right)
\tag{2}
$$

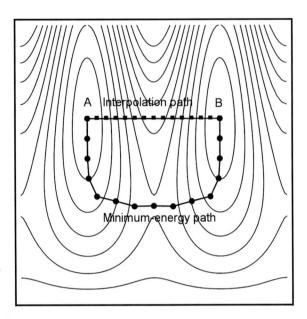

**Fig. 1** Schematic picture showing the refinement of an initial guess path, obtained by interpolation between structures A and B, to a minimum-energy path connecting the two structures (This figure was produced by modifying a Mathematica script made available in Professor Kristen Fichthorn's website.)

where

$$\langle \Delta l \rangle = \frac{1}{N-1} \sum_{i=1}^{N-1} \Delta l_{i,i+1} \tag{3}$$

Default values for the parameters $\eta$, $\rho$, and $\lambda$ controlling the strength of different factors in Eq. 2 can often be used.

Figure 1 illustrates schematically how this method works. One first guesses an initial path between structures A and B by interpolation between the two structures. This initial path may be rough in which many intermediate structures occupy high-energy regions of the potential energy surface. After optimization of the target function in Eq. 1, a minimum-energy path is generated. The two structures can interconvert more easily along this optimized path than the initial guess path. Inhibitors can bind to the intermediate structures just as transition-state analogues could bind to enzymes. Transition-state analogs have provided one strategy to develop drugs to inhibit enzymes [51].

Other methods have been developed to further refine this approach. For example, the nudged elastic band method [52] could produce smoother minimum-energy paths by including only the system force perpendicular to the paths and the constrain forces parallel to the paths. Variations to improve the location of the saddle points have also been introduced [32]. The string method was introduced later as another tool for obtaining smooth minimum-energy paths efficiently [53].

Normal mode analysis provides another fast technique to generate structural ensembles from one or a few experimental structures [11, 54, 55]. By assuming a harmonic potential near an experimental structure, the motion of the receptor can be described by a set of normal modes with a range of frequencies. The lowest frequency modes describe the largest amplitude motions of the receptor, and one can generate rather distinct structures of the receptor accessible at room or physiological temperatures by following these modes. In principle, one needs to diagonalize a Hessian matrix to obtain the normal modes. This is a $3N \times 3N$ matrix ($N$ = number of atoms in the receptor) containing the second derivatives of the potential energy with respect to often the Cartesian coordinates. As the computational time for diagonalizing this matrix grows as the cube of $3N$, it is common to use only the matrix elements corresponding to a subset of atoms, such as the alpha carbons of a protein, to perform normal mode analysis.

A normal mode analysis assumes that the potential energy behaves as a quadratic function around an energy minimum. Anharmonic effects can be accounted for approximately by using the quasi-harmonic model [56] in which one performs a molecular dynamics simulation to obtain the positional covariance matrix with each element calculated by

$$\langle (x_i - \langle x_i \rangle)(x_j - \langle x_j \rangle) \rangle \qquad (4)$$

in which $x_i$ is a coordinate of atom $i$, and $\langle y \rangle$ represents an ensemble average of the quantity $y$. Wong et al. [57] showed in the linear response limit that

$$\frac{\partial \langle x_i \rangle}{\partial f_j} = \frac{1}{k_B T} \langle (x_i - \langle x_i \rangle)(x_j - \langle x_j \rangle) \rangle \qquad (5)$$

where $f_j$ is a small force applied to atom $j$, $k_B$ is the Boltzmann constant, and $T$ is the absolute temperature. One can see that the inverse of $\frac{\partial \langle x_i \rangle}{\partial f_j}$ resembles an element of a Hessian matrix. This equation allows one to construct an effective Hessian matrix from the positional covariance matrix obtained from a molecular dynamics simulation to perform a quasi-harmonic analysis that can account for some anharmonic effects.

Although a normal mode analysis is usually carried out in vacuum or with an implicit-solvent model, the positional covariance matrix can be obtained from a molecular dynamics simulation using an explicit-solvent model so that solvation effects can be mimicked by a more realistic model.

Molecular dynamics simulation is most expensive among the methods described in this chapter, but it has been used for ensemble docking for a long time. For example, Pang and Kozikowski published a paper in 1994 using this approach in a docking model to predict how huperzine A bound to acetylcholinesterase [58]. The introduction of the relaxed complex scheme about 10 years later has made this approach popular [14, 59]. In this approach, one first performs a molecular dynamics simulation on the receptor, with or without ligand(s). One then docks different compounds to snapshots produced by the molecular dynamics simulation and uses the average docking energies to predict the binding strength of the compounds. Instead of using the docking energies from a docking program, one can also use the binding energies obtained from the more sophisticated molecular mechanics/Poisson-Boltzmann surface area (MM/PBSA) model [60–65] using the docked structures (e.g., [10]). In the MM/PBSA model, the electrostatics contributions were obtained by numerically solving the Poisson-Boltzmann equation taking into account the complex shape of the molecules, and the hydrophobic contributions were described by a term dependent on the surface area of the molecules.

**2.6   From Enhanced Sampling**

Molecular dynamics simulations at room or physiologically relevant temperatures suffer from slow sampling of conformational space. Various enhanced sampling techniques have been developed to alleviate this problem. Some of these techniques maintain rigorous thermodynamic ensembles so that various ensemble averages can be obtained from these structural ensembles. Relevant to this topic is the averaging of docking energies over the dynamics snapshots to provide a better estimation of the binding affinity between a compound and a receptor.

The replica-exchange method provides one popular example [42, 66–69]. Schematically shown in Fig. 2, this method not only run a molecular dynamics simulation on a system at a certain desired temperature, but also run many other simulations of the system at different higher temperatures. Structures of the simulations are allowed to exchange between adjacent temperature windows periodically according to the Metropolis criteria [70]. These higher temperature runs allow the system to explore a larger conformational space more easily. By exchanging structures between temperature windows, the sampling at the desired lower temperature is improved as well. Since the nonphysical structural exchanges between temperature windows disrupt the trajectories, one can no longer obtain dynamical information from these simulation trajectories. Nevertheless, structural exchanges according to the Metropolis criteria maintain rigorous thermodynamic ensembles at all the temperature windows so that proper thermodynamic averages can be obtained from the simulations. Similar averaging done in the relaxed complex scheme or in the MM/PBSA method described above can also be performed here after docking a ligand to the structures obtained from a replica-exchange simulation.

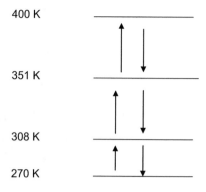

$$w(X_i \rightarrow X_j) = 1 \quad \text{for } \Delta \leq 0$$

$$= \exp(-\Delta) \quad \text{for } \Delta > 0$$

$$\text{where } \Delta = \left( \frac{1}{kT_j} - \frac{1}{kT_i} \right)(E_i - E_j)$$

**Fig. 2** Schematic representation of a replica-exchange simulation. Simulations are performed at multiple temperatures and structures are allowed to exchange between adjacent windows according to the Metropolis criteria [70] shown in the *bottom* of the figure. $w(X_i \leftrightarrow X_j)$ represents the probability of exchanging a structure $X_i$ at temperature $T_i$ with a structure $X_j$ at temperature $T_j$. $E_i$ represents the energy of structure $X_i$, and $k$ is the Boltzmann constant

Some methods enhance sampling by altering the potential energy surface rather than running simulations at many temperatures. Accelerated molecular dynamics [71–74] provides one example. It raises the energy near local energy minima so that a system does not spend as much time inside these energy wells. As a result, such a simulation samples a larger space than a regular molecular dynamics simulation does for the same amount of simulation time.

Some methods speed up sampling further by not requiring the simulation to maintain a rigorous thermodynamics ensemble. The simulated annealing cycling method represents one such approach, schematically shown in Fig. 3 [75–78]. It adopts the key idea of the replica-exchange method by running simulations at higher temperatures to improve sampling, but it does so by replacing simulations at multiple temperature windows with only one simulation spanning a range of temperatures. It implements this by introducing many successive simulated annealing cycles during a simulation. Each cycle begins with heating to a high temperature to encourage a system to move away from an energy well that it has already sampled. The system is then cooled down rapidly to 0 K in

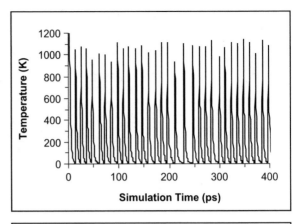

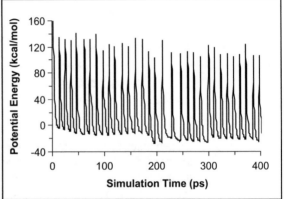

**Fig. 3** Schematic representation of the simulated annealing cycling approach. The *upper panel* shows that many simulated annealing cycles are introduced into a molecular dynamics simulation. A system is periodically heated up to a high temperature to encourage it to move away from a potential energy well that it has already sampled. The *bottom panel* shows that the system is moved into another energy well each time it is quenched to near 0 K after heating

the order of 10 ps to trap the system into a new energy well. This rapid cooling also prevents the biomolecular receptor from being unfolded or disintegrated. A trajectory repeats this cycle many times to speed up sampling. This approach was successfully applied to directly simulate a ligand-receptor docking process in which a flexible ligand was allowed to move inside a flexible receptor to find good docking poses [75–80]. One should be able to use this approach for the easier problem of generating the ensemble of a receptor structure for docking by only simulates the receptor without including its ligand. However, this approach does not maintain a system at a rigorous thermodynamic ensemble and thus one can no longer calculate an ensemble average simply by averaging a property over the structures obtained from the simulation.

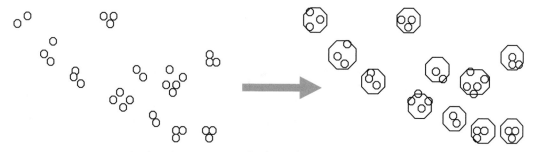

**Fig. 4** Schematic figure showing the clustering of similar structures into group

## 3  Clustering Structures to Reduce the Size of an Ensemble

Methods such as molecular dynamics simulations generate a large number of structures. Although the ensemble of structures generated conforms a thermodynamic ensemble and provides a means to calculate thermodynamic ensemble averages, docking a large number of compounds to a large number of structures is expensive. No large-scale screening efforts have yet used this method.

To reduce the costs of screening a large number of compounds in ensemble docking, an approximation of using only a small subset of structures and adopting a suitable ranking scheme is more practical with current computational capability. Clustering provides a popular method for reducing the large number of structures to a smaller subset for virtual screening (Fig. 4). Many clustering methods have been introduced. For an evaluation on different clustering methods applied to molecular dynamics trajectories, see [81]. As an example, clustering analysis by the GROMOS software package [82–84] uses the root-mean-square deviation (RMSD) between two structures as a measure of the distance between the two structures: The program first calculates the distance between any pairs of structures to be considered for clustering. It considers two structures as neighbors if their distance falls below a user-chosen cutoff. The structure that contains the largest neighbors is identified and the first cluster is then generated by including this structure and all its neighbors. Structures belonging to the first cluster are then removed and the same process is repeated for the remaining structures to obtain the next cluster. This process is repeated until no more structure is left. By choosing different cutoffs, a user can control the size and number of clusters being formed. The CHARMM software package [85], on the other hand, provides a self-organizing neural net approach for clustering [86–88]. This algorithm optimizes cluster assignment by minimizing the distance between members and the centroid structure within each cluster and by requiring this distance to be within a user-predefined cluster radius.

## 4    Extra Considerations in Ranking Compounds in Ensemble Docking

When docking compounds to a single receptor structure, one can simply use the docking scores, which reflects their binding strength, to rank the compounds for their potential to be actives. This is less straightforward in docking to multiple structures, especially when the structures are not generated according to a rigorous thermodynamic ensemble.

When using structures obtained from conventional molecular simulations (e.g., molecular dynamics and replica-exchange) that maintain rigorous thermodynamic ensembles, averaging the binding strength over all structures provides a reasonable approximation to the overall binding affinity between a ligand and a receptor. One can rationalize this by using the perturbation theory in free energy calculations [89–96]:

$$\Delta G(\text{binding}) = G\big((P:L) - G(P) - G(L)\big)$$

$$= -RT\ln \int e^{-\beta H(P:L)} d\vec{x}_P d\vec{x}_L + RT\ln \int e^{-\beta H(P)} d\vec{x}_P + RT\ln \int e^{-\beta H(L)} d\vec{x}_L$$

$$= RT\ln \frac{\int e^{-\beta H(P)} d\vec{x}_P \int e^{-\beta H(L)} d\vec{x}_L}{\int e^{-\beta H(P:L)} d\vec{x}_P d\vec{x}_L} = RT\ln \frac{\int e^{-\beta H(P)} e^{-\beta H(L)} d\vec{x}_P d\vec{x}_L}{\int e^{-\beta H(P:L)} d\vec{x}_P d\vec{x}_L}$$

$$= RT\ln \big\langle e^{-\beta H(P)} e^{-\beta H(L)} e^{\beta H(P:L)} \big\rangle_{P:L}$$

$$= RT\ln \big\langle e^{\beta \Delta H} \big\rangle_{P:L}$$

where $\Delta H = H(P:L) - H(P) - H(L)$

(6)

in which $H(P:L)$, $H(P)$, and $H(L)$ are the classical Hamiltonian of the complex, the receptor, and the ligand, respectively, $R$ is the gas constant, $T$ is the absolute temperature, and $\beta = RT$.

This formula is exact although not practical for calculating $\Delta G$ (binding) because the sampling favors that of the complex may not cover the important conformational space of the isolated protein and ligand well. However, it provides a formal theory to help understand the approximations introduced in different computational models. For example, simply averaging the binding affinity over all structure corresponds to making the approximation:

$\Delta G(\text{binding}) = RT\ln \big\langle e^{\beta \Delta H} \big\rangle_{P:L} \approx \langle \Delta H \rangle_{P:L}$    after expanding the exponential and logarithmic functions in Eq. 6 and keeping the lowest order term, and using energies from a docking program to estimate $\Delta H$. One can also see that the MM/PBSA model described above follows a similar approximation, but using a more sophisticated Poisson-Boltzmann surface area model to better account for solvation effects and reintroducing the entropic contributions using a harmonic approximation.

On the other hand, the ensemble average $\Delta H$ in Eq. 6 cannot be performed with structures that are not generated from a rigorous thermodynamic ensemble, such as those selected from a number of experimental structures or those from simulated annealing cycling molecular dynamics simulations as described above. Researchers have used less rigorous rules to select the best drug candidates when using these structures. Specific examples are given below.

## 5    Removing Non-productive Structures

Several studies reported that including more structures in an ensemble could decrease rather than increase the performance of a virtual screening [22, 97, 98]. If a structure could not bind any or many ligands properly, including such a structure could contaminate the overall ranking of the compounds, especially when one uses ranks rather than docking scores for compound prioritization. For example, including the top-ranked compounds from a "bad" structure could improperly overrate these compounds as good drug candidates.

One way to remove bad structures is to compare the docking scores of compounds throughout all structures. If most of the compounds do not give favorable docking scores for a structure, this structure is not or less useful to be included in ensemble docking. Huang and Wong [99] further quantitatively evaluated this strategy using available known active compounds. They first docked these actives to all the receptor structures in an ensemble and determined their binding scores. The averaged binding score was also calculated. They then ranked the structures for their usefulness in docking by the number of actives that docked with scores better than the averaged. They found this approach to identify good structures as well as more expensive methods that utilize not only actives but also a large number of decoys.

Besides allowing more actives to be identified from top-ranked compounds, removing "bad" structures could also reduce computational costs because one does not need to dock compounds to as many structures.

## 6    Metrics for Evaluating the Performance of a Virtual Screening Model

Various metrics have been introduced to measure the performance of a virtual screening. Two common and useful ones are discussed here.

Enrichment factor is used to measure how effective a screening model picks out actives from a chemical library. A screening model usually prioritizes the compounds in a library according to a ranking scheme. An effective model would have many actives among its top-ranked compounds. The enrichment factor quantifies this by using a random selection model as a reference. For example, assume that there are 100 active compounds in a library containing 10,000 compounds. A randomly picked 100 compounds from this library would find one active on average. However, a screening model might have prioritized the compounds in such a way that 30 actives are found within the first 100 compounds in its rank-ordered list. The enrichment factor for this model is then 30 because it finds 30 times more actives than a random model does. In a mathematic form, for a test library containing $N$ compounds, among which $n$ are actives, the enrichment factor EF for including $x$ % of compounds from the database is defined as

$$\mathrm{EF} = \frac{(n_s / N_s)}{(n / N)} \tag{7}$$

where $N_s$ is the number of compounds in the top $x$ % of the rank-ordered list and $n_s$ is the number of active compounds in this list.

However, the enrichment factor calculated this way cannot distinguish a case in which all the actives are piled up at the beginning of the top $x$ % of the rank-ordered list from the one in which the actives are positioned near the end of the list. The first case is more useful in practical drug discovery because if one were to start testing compounds from top-ranked compounds, one would identify all the actives earlier. Therefore, Truchon and Bayly introduced the Boltzmann-enhancement discrimination of receiver operating characteristics (BEDROC) to help distinguish these two situations [100]. Their paper provided a detailed description of the theory and concepts behind this method. Briefly, BEDROC scales the ranks of known actives according to a Boltzmann rather than a linear distribution so that a model that ranks actives earlier in an ordered list gives a significantly better performance score than one that ranks the actives later. In addition, a BEDROC score ranging between 0 and 1 is calculated for any screening model so that the performance of different models can be compared easily with 1 being the best score achievable by a model.

A practical consideration concerns the amount of time required to calculate the enrichment factor or BEDROC, both call for the docking of many actives along with an even larger number of decoys. This makes it computationally expensive to evaluate a screening model or to select the best receptor structures for docking, especially when many receptor structures need to be considered. Huang and Wong [99] introduced a cheaper solution to select the best receptor structures for ensemble docking by using only known actives without any decoy. They hypothesized that receptor structures capable of binding more known actives well were more likely to give favorable BEDROC scores. Indeed, they found that the structures that gave more actives with better docking scores than the average scores obtained over all structures also produced favorable BEDROC scores. This provides a computationally less expensive approach to help choose a smaller number of structures for ensemble docking: One could first dock the known actives to an initial ensemble of the receptor structures and calculates the average docking scores across all receptor structures. Then, for each receptor structure, find out the number of actives $P$ that have better docking scores than the average. Finally, select those structures that give the largest $P$ values.

# 7 Different Probabilities of Occurrence of Different Structures in an Ensemble

Methods that do not rely on rigorous calculations of thermodynamic ensemble averages but compare docking scores or ranks among different structures often ignore a factor that could deteriorate the performance of a screening campaign in picking out actives from a chemical library. This factor is the conformational energy of the receptor. A structure giving a favorable binding affinity for a compound could be one having a high energy and therefore lower probability of occurrence. This may overrate the importance of compounds showing good docking scores to this structure. A couple of studies have already suggested that including the conformational energy of the receptor could improve the performance of a screening campaign [98, 101]. However, these works only used crude models to estimate the conformational energies of the receptors. Further studies are needed to investigate more thoroughly how to reliably and practically include such effects to improve the compound ranking in ensemble docking.

# 8 Rescoring Could Improve the Performance of Virtual Screening

To speed up docking to facilitate the screening of a large number of compounds, simple energy models are often used. Using more sophisticated energy models to refine the docking poses and rescore them could improve the performance. For example, Degliesposti et al. [6] refined docking poses by performing energy minimization with programs designed for molecular mechanics and molecular dynamics simulations and rescored the new poses with the more sophisticated molecular mechanics/Poisson-Boltzmann surface area model or with its generalized Born counterparts. Using such a model, they were able to discover new inhibitors for plasmepsin II in plasmodium falciparum. Among the top 30 compounds they selected for experimental testing, 26 were found to be active with $IC_{50}$ values ranging from 4.3 nm to 1.8 μM.

## 9   Case Examples

### 9.1   Docking to Experimental Structures

It was reported over a decade ago that docking to several crystal structures could increase success rates of identifying bioactive compounds [20, 21]. Recently, Bottegoni et al. [97] performed a more detailed and systematic study. They used 36 systems and several modern metrics to compare the performance of the multiple-conformational model with those obtained from single-conformational models.

For each system, they docked both the actives and the decoys from the Directory of Useful Decoys (DUD) [102] to an ensemble of structures or an individual structure of the ensemble. Enrichment factor and BEDROC were two of the metrics that they used to evaluate the performance of the different docking models. They applied two different approaches to rank those compounds for their potential to be drug candidates based on their docking results to all the receptor structures. In one approach, they ranked the compounds based on the best docking score of each compound among all the structures (this involves only the comparison of the docking scores of each compound over all the receptor structures without considering the scores of the other compounds). In the other approach, they first used the best rank of each compound among all the receptors (in order to obtain the rank of a compound for each receptor structure, one needs to compare its docking score with those of the other compounds for this structure), but ended up with too many ties. To break the ties, the authors further used docking scores to rank the compounds.

In general, they found that docking to multiple conformations could identify more actives with more diverse chemical scaffolds. Their results also demonstrated the benefit of filtering out bad receptor structures. They found that removing the structures that gave unfavorable docking scores for most of the compounds gave better screening performance, according to metrics such as BEDROC. However, they were unable to conclude from this work which ranking approach, the one based on docking scores or the one based on ranking first, gave better screening performance.

### 9.2   Docking to Dynamics Snapshots

An extensive study performed recently by Ellingson et al. [103] provides a useful example here. They docked a much larger set of ligands than previous studies (e.g., [10, 14]). These ligands include known actives along with a large number of decoys. Their studies included four different receptors: β-lactamase, fibroblast growth factor receptor kinase, glucocorticoid receptor, and the tyrosine kinase Src. After running a 100 ns of molecular dynamics simulation for each receptor, they clustered the simulation generated structures to obtain a smaller number of receptor structures for docking using Autodock Vina [18]. Single crystal structures or dynamics snapshots were used to construct the single-conformational models. Using the enrichment factor as an indicator for performance, they found that the multiple-conformational model discovered more actives and identified more diverse compounds than the single-conformational models.

In selecting the top compounds from the docking results of a structural ensemble, Ellingson et al. first tried taking the top $x/N\%$ of compounds from each structure, where $N$ was the number of structures included in the structural ensemble to form the top overall $x\%$ of compounds. However, they found this method performed less well than the one that selected the top $x\%$ based on the best docking scores of the compounds among all the structures.

**9.3 Docking to Structures Obtained from Normal Mode Analysis**

Leis and Zacharias [54, 55] introduced an efficient approach to use a soft mode from a normal mode calculation to produce several structures surrounding an experimental structure for docking. In the more recent version, they modified the popular docking program Autodock [17] to perform this work. Autodock uses potential grid maps to speed up the calculations of the interactions between a ligand and its biological receptor. To incorporate protein flexibility in this representation, Leis and Zacharias created potential grid maps for each protein conformation generated by the normal mode calculation, and also allowed interpolation to obtain the grid maps of intermediate structures inserted between these structures. During docking using the Lamarckian genetic algorithm, they allowed an extra random variable to select a conformation or an interpolated conformation that the ligand could pair with. In a test case of docking three different ligands to protein kinase A, they found that incorporating protein flexibility this way had improved the placement of the ligands in the protein from over 2 Å from the experimental structures to a little over 1 Å. Particularly noteworthy in this approach is the interpolation representation that allows fewer structures to be explicitly included in the docking model. This idea could be applied to other methods of ensemble docking as well, not only those derived from normal mode analysis [104].

# 10 Summary

This chapter focuses on discussing ensemble docking as a method for incorporating receptor flexibility into virtual screening, a useful tool for structure-based drug discovery. This method is relatively inexpensive to use and could be used by many researchers in the near future. The simplicity lies in its ready use of programs that have already been developed for rigid-receptor docking. This chapter outlines different methods that have been used to produce structures for ensemble docking. It also discusses several different possible ways to rank the docking results to select compounds for experimental testing. In the case that the structures used for docking came from simulations that produce rigorous thermodynamic ensembles, averaging the binding affinities from all structures carries theoretical supports, even though some approximations still need to be made. One can use the averaged binding affinities of the compounds to rank their potential to become drug candidates. However, such averaging lacks theoretical rigor for structural ensembles not obtained from rigorous thermodynamic samplings. Some researchers take certain number of top-ranked compounds from each structure. Others use both the rank and the docking score/energy, which should be more informative. Another complication results from the different probabilities of finding different structures in an ensemble not generated by rigorous thermodynamic sampling. This factor was ignored in most ensemble docking. How to address this issue in an effective and a practical manner will need further research. With more scientists applying ensemble docking to more practical problems, it is conceivable that the performance of this approach will be evaluated more thoroughly and its shortcomings will be identified for further improvement.

## Acknowledgements

The author acknowledges his students and collaborators with whom some of the research discussed in this chapter was done. Dr. Zunnan Huang provided Fig. 3. The author also appreciates financial supports from the National Cancer Institute, the National Institute of Allergy and Infectious Diseases, the Research Board of the University of Missouri System, and the University of Missouri-St. Louis. The University of Missouri Bioinformatics Consortium has provided useful computational resources.

## References

1. Meng EC, Shoichet BK, Kuntz ID (1992) Automated docking with grid-based energy evaluation. J Comput Chem 13(4):505–524

2. Kuntz ID, Meng EC, Shoichet BK (1994) Structure-based molecular design. Acc Chem Res 27(5):117–123

3. Shoichet BK, Kuntz ID (1993) Matching chemistry and shape in molecular docking. Protein Eng 6(7):723–732

4. Shan Y, Kim ET, Eastwood MP, Dror RO, Seeliger MA, Shaw DE (2011) How does a drug molecule find its target binding site? J Am Chem Soc 133(24):9181–9183

5. Decherchi S, Berteotti A, Bottegoni G, Rocchia W, Cavalli A (2015) The ligand binding mechanism to purine nucleoside phosphorylase elucidated via molecular dynamics and machine learning. Nat Commun 6:6155

6. Degliesposti G, Kasam V, Da Costa A, Kang HK, Kim N, Kim DW, Breton V, Kim D, Rastelli G (2009) Design and discovery of plasmepsin II inhibitors using an automated workflow on large-scale grids. ChemMedChem 4(7):1164–1173

7. Sørensen J, Demir Ö, Swift RV, Feher VA, Amaro RE (2015) Molecular docking to flexible targets. Methods Mol Biol 1215:445–469

8. Osguthorpe DJ, Sherman W, Hagler AT (2012) Exploring protein flexibility: incorporating structural ensembles from crystal structures and simulation into virtual

screening protocols. J Phys Chem B 116 (23):6952–6959

9. Amaro RE, Li WW (2010) Emerging methods for ensemble-based virtual screening. Curr Top Med Chem 10(1):3–13

10. Wong CF, Kua J, Zhang Y, Straatsma TP, McCammon JA (2005) Molecular docking of balanol to dynamics snapshots of protein kinase A. Proteins 61(4):850–858

11. Cavasotto CN, Kovacs JA, Abagyan RA (2005) Representing receptor flexibility in ligand docking through relevant normal modes. J Am Chem Soc 127(26):9632–9640

12. Osterberg F, Morris GM, Sanner MF, Olson AJ, Goodsell DS (2002) Automated docking to multiple target structures: incorporation of protein mobility and structural water heterogeneity in AutoDock. Proteins 46(1):34–40

13. Knegtel RM, Kuntz ID, Oshiro CM (1997) Molecular docking to ensembles of protein structures. J Mol Biol 266(2):424–440

14. Lin JH, Perryman AL, Schames JR, McCammon JA (2002) Computational drug design accommodating receptor flexibility: the relaxed complex scheme. J Am Chem Soc 124(20):5632–5633

15. Lin JH, Baker NA, McCammon JA (2002) Bridging implicit and explicit solvent approaches for membrane electrostatics. Biophys J 83(3):1374–1379

16. Goodsell DS, Morris GM, Olson AJ (1996) Automated docking of flexible ligands: applications of AutoDock. J Mol Recognit 9 (1):1–5

17. Morris GM, Goodsell DS, Halliday RS, Huey R, Hart WE, Belew RK, Olson AJ (1998) Automated docking using a Lamarckian genetic algorithm and an empirical binding free energy function. J Comput Chem 19 (14):1639–1662

18. Trott O, Olson AJ (2010) Software news and update AutoDock Vina: improving the speed and accuracy of docking with a new scoring function, efficient optimization, and multi-threading. J Comput Chem 31(2):455–461

19. Kramer B, Rarey M, Lengauer T (1999) Evaluation of the FLEXX incremental construction algorithm for protein-ligand docking. Proteins 37(2):228–241

20. Cavasotto CN, Abagyan RA (2004) Protein flexibility in ligand docking and virtual screening to protein kinases. J Mol Biol 337 (1):209–225

21. Ferrari AM, Wei BQQ, Costantino L, Shoichet BK (2004) Soft docking and multiple receptor conformations in virtual screening. J Med Chem 47(21):5076–5084

22. Abagyan R, Rueda M, Bottegoni G (2010) Recipes for the selection of experimental protein conformations for virtual screening. J Chem Inf Model 50(1):186–193. doi:10.1021/ci9003943

23. Sali A, Blundell TL (1993) Comparative protein modelling by satisfaction of spatial restraints. J Mol Biol 234(3):779–815

24. Wong CF, Bairy S (2013) Rational drug design of inhibitors of protein kinases and phosphatases. Curr Pharm Des 19 (26):4739–4754

25. Bairy S (2011) Considering signaling pathway kinetics and protein flexibility in designing protein kinase inhibitors. University of Missouri-Saint Louis, Saint Louis

26. Pan AC, Sezer D, Roux B (2008) Finding transition pathways using the string method with swarms of trajectories. J Phys Chem B 112(11):3432–3440

27. Elber R (2007) A milestoning study of the kinetics of an allosteric transition: atomically detailed simulations of deoxy Scapharca hemoglobin. Biophys J 92(9):L85–L87

28. Hu J, Ma A, Dinner AR (2006) Bias annealing: a method for obtaining transition paths de novo. J Chem Phys 125(11):114101

29. Cardenas AE, Elber R (2003) Kinetics of cytochrome C folding: atomically detailed simulations. Proteins 51(2):245–257

30. Cardenas AE, Elber R (2003) Atomically detailed Simulations of helix formation with the stochastic difference equation. Biophys J 85(5):2919–2939

31. Bolhuis PG, Dellago C, Geissler PL, Chandler D (2000) Transition path sampling: throwing ropes over mountains in the dark. J Phys Condens Matter 12(8A):A147–A152

32. Henkelman G, Uberuaga BP, Jonsson H (2000) A climbing image nudged elastic band method for finding saddle points and minimum energy paths. J Chem Phys 113 (22):9901–9904

33. Chu JW, Trout BL, Brooks BR (2003) A super-linear minimization scheme for the nudged elastic band method. J Chem Phys 119(24):12708–12717

34. Fischer S, Karplus M (1992) Conjugate peak refinement—an algorithm for finding reaction paths and accurate transition-states in systems with many degrees of freedom. Chem Phys Lett 194(3):252–261

35. Ren W, Vanden-Eijnden E, Maragakis P, Weinan E (2005) Transition pathways in complex systems: application of the finite-temperature string method to the alanine dipeptide. J Chem Phys 123(13):1–12

36. Maragliano L, Vanden-Eijnden E (2007) On-the-fly string method for minimum free energy paths calculation. Chem Phys Lett 446(1–3):182–190

37. Peters B, Heyden A, Bell AT, Chakraborty A (2004) A growing string method for determining transition states: comparison to the nudged elastic band and string methods. J Chem Phys 120(17):7877–7886

38. Bowman GR, Beauchamp KA, Boxer G, Pande VS (2009) Progress and challenges in the automated construction of Markov state models for full protein systems. J Chem Phys 131(12)

39. Bowman GR, Huang X, Pande VS (2009) Using generalized ensemble simulations and Markov state models to identify conformational states. Methods 49(2):197–201

40. Donovan RM, Sedgewick AJ, Faeder JR, Zuckerman DM (2013) Efficient stochastic simulation of chemical kinetics networks using a weighted ensemble of trajectories. J Chem Phys 139(11):115105

41. Adelman JL, Grabe M (2013) Simulating rare events using a weighted ensemble-based string method. J Chem Phys 138(4):044105

42. Sugita Y, Okamoto Y (1999) Replica-exchange molecular dynamics method for protein folding. Chem Phys Lett 314 (1–2):141–151

43. Wong CF (2015) Conformational transition paths harbour structures useful for aiding drug discovery and understanding enzymatic mechanisms in protein kinases. Protein Sci. doi:10.1002/pro.2716

44. Pratt LR (1986) A statistical method for identifying transition states in high dimensional problems. J Chem Phys 85(9):5045–5048

45. Elber R, Karplus M (1987) A method for determining reaction paths in large molecules: application to myoglobin. Chem Phys Lett 139(5):375–380. doi:10.1016/0009-2614(87)80576-6

46. Elber R, Roitberg A, Simmerling C, Goldstein R, Li H, Verkhivker G, Keasar C, Zhang J, Ulitsky A (1995) MOIL: a program for simulations of macromolecules. Comput Phys Commun 91(1–3):159–189

47. Czerminski R, Elber R (1989) Reaction path study of conformational transitions and helix formation in a tetrapeptide. Proc Natl Acad Sci U S A 86:6963–6967

48. Choi C, Elber R (1991) Reaction path study of helix formation in tetrapeptides: effect of side chains. J Chem Phys 94(1):751–760

49. Czerminski R, Elber R (1990) Reaction path study of conformational transitions in flexible systems: applications to peptides. J Chem Phys 92(9):5580–5601

50. Nowak W, Czerminski R, Elber R (1991) Reaction path study of ligand diffusion in proteins: application of the self penalty walk (SPW) method to calculate reaction coordinates for the motion of CO through legheme-globin. J Am Chem Soc 113 (15):5627–5637

51. Schramm VL (2013) Transition states, analogues, and drug development. ACS Chem Biol 8(1):71–81

52. Henkelman G, Jonsson H (2000) Improved tangent estimate in the nudged elastic band method for finding minimum energy paths and saddle points. J Chem Phys 113 (22):9978–9985

53. Weinan E, Ren WQ, Vanden-Eijnden E (2002) String method for the study of rare events. Phys Rev B 66(5):052301

54. May A, Zacharias M (2008) Protein-ligand docking accounting for receptor side chain and global flexibility in normal modes: evaluation on kinase inhibitor cross docking. J Med Chem 51(12):3499–3506

55. Leis S, Zacharias M (2011) Efficient inclusion of receptor flexibility in grid-based protein-ligand docking. J Comput Chem 32 (16):3433–3439

56. Levy RM, Karplus M, Kushick J, Perahia D (1984) Evaluation of the configurational entropy for proteins: application to molecular dynamics simulations of an $\alpha$-helix. Macromolecules 17:1370

57. Wong CF, Zheng C, Shen J, McCammon JA, Wolynes PG (1993) Cytochrome c: a molecular proving ground for computer simulations. J Phys Chem 97(13):3100–3110

58. Pang YP, Kozikowski AP (1994) Prediction of the binding sites of huperzine A in acetylcholinesterase by docking studies. J Comput Aided Mol Des 8(6):669–681

59. Lin JH, Perryman A, Schames J, McCammon JA (2003) The relaxed complex method: accommodating receptor flexibility for drug design with an improved scoring scheme. Biopolymers 68:47–62

60. Kuhn B, Kollman PA (2000) A ligand that is predicted to bind better to avidin than biotin: insights from computational fluorine scanning. J Am Chem Soc 122(16):3909–3916

61. Kuhn B, Kollman PA (2000) Binding of a diverse set of ligands to avidin and streptavidin: an accurate quantitative prediction of their relative affinities by a combination of molecular mechanics and continuum solvent models. J Med Chem 43(20):3786–3791

62. Kollman PA, Massova I, Reyes C, Kuhn B, Huo S, Chong L, Lee M, Lee T, Duan Y, Wang W, Donini O, Cieplak P, Srinivasan J, Case DA, Cheatham TE III (2000) Calculating structures and free energies of complex molecules: combining molecular mechanics and continuum models. Acc Chem Res 33 (12):889–897

63. Massova I, Kollman PA (2000) Combined molecular mechanical and continuum solvent approach (MM-PBSA/GBSA) to predict ligand binding. Perspect Drug Discov Des 18:113–135

64. Lee MR, Duan Y, Kollman PA (2000) Use of MM-PB/SA in estimating the free energies of proteins: application to native, intermediates, and unfolded villin headpiece. Proteins 39 (4):309–316

65. Massova I, Kollman PA (1999) Computational alanine scanning to probe protein-protein interactions: a novel approach to evaluate binding free energies. J Am Chem Soc 121(36):8133–8143

66. Sugita Y, Okamoto Y (2000) Replica-exchange multicanonical algorithm and multicanonical replica-exchange method for simulating systems with rough energy landscape. Chem Phys Lett 329(3–4):261–270

67. Sugita Y, Kitao A, Okamoto Y (2000) Multi-dimensional replica-exchange method for free-energy calculations. J Chem Phys 113 (15):6042–6051

68. Mitsutake A, Sugita Y, Okamoto Y (2001) Generalized-ensemble algorithms for molecular simulations of biopolymers. Biopolymers 60(2):96–123

69. Sanbonmatsu KY, Garcia AE (2002) Structure of Met-enkephalin in explicit aqueous solution using replica exchange molecular dynamics. Proteins 46(2):225–234

70. Metropolis N, Rosenbluth AW, Rosenbluth MN, Teller AH, Teller E (1953) Equation of state calculations by fast computing machines. J Chem Phys 21:1087–1092

71. Voter A (1997) A method for accelerating the molecular dynamics simulation of infrequent events. J Chem Phys 106(11):4665–4677

72. Voter A (1997) Accelerating the dynamics of infrequent events. Abstr Pap Am Chem S 213:284-PHYS

73. Voter A (1997) Hyperdynamics: accelerated molecular dynamics of infrequent events. Phys Rev Lett 78(20):3908–3911

74. Hamelberg D, Mongan J, McCammon J (2004) Accelerated molecular dynamics: a promising and efficient simulation method for biomolecules. J Chem Phys 120 (24):11919–11929

75. Huang Z, Wong CF (2012) Simulation reveals two major docking pathways between the hexapeptide GDYMNM and the catalytic domain of the insulin receptor protein kinase. Proteins 80(9):2275–2286

76. Huang Z, Wong CF (2009) Docking flexible peptide to flexible protein by molecular dynamics using two implicit-solvent models: an evaluation in protein kinase and phosphatase systems. J Phys Chem B 113 (43):14343–14354

77. Huang Z, Wong CF (2009) Conformational selection of protein kinase A revealed by flexible-ligand flexible-protein docking. J Comput Chem 30(4):631–644

78. Huang Z, Wong CF, Wheeler RA (2008) Flexible protein-flexible ligand docking with disrupted velocity simulated annealing. Proteins 71(1):440–454

79. Huang Z, He Y, Zhang X, Gunawan A, Wu L, Zhang ZY, Wong CF (2010) Derivatives of salicylic acid as inhibitors of YopH in Yersinia pestis. Chem Biol Drug Des 76(2):85–99

80. Huang Z, Wong CF (2007) A mining minima approach to exploring the docking pathways of p-nitrocatechol sulfate to YopH. Biophys J 93(12):4141–4150

81. Shao JY, Tanner SW, Thompson N, Cheatham TE (2007) Clustering molecular dynamics trajectories: 1. Characterizing the performance of different clustering algorithms. J Chem Theory Comput 3 (6):2312–2334

82. Christen M, Hünenberger PH, Bakowies D, Baron R, Bürgi R, Geerke DP, Heinz TN, Kastenholz MA, Kräutler V, Oostenbrink C, Peter C, Trzesniak D, Van Gunsteren WF (2005) The GROMOS software for biomolecular simulation: GROMOS05. J Comput Chem 26(16):1719–1751

83. van Gunsteren WF, Berendsen HJC (1996) GROMOS. Biomos BV, Gronengen, The Netherlands

84. Daura X, Gademann K, Jaun B, Seebach D, Van Gunsteren WF, Mark AE (1999) Peptide folding: when simulation meets experiment. Angew Chem Int Ed 38(1–2):236–240

85. Brooks BR, Brooks CL III, Mackerell AD Jr, Nilsson L, Petrella RJ, Roux B, Won Y, Archontis G, Bartels C, Boresch S, Caflisch A, Caves L, Cui Q, Dinner AR, Feig M, Fischer S, Gao J, Hodoscek M, Im W, Kuczera K, Lazaridis T, Ma J, Ovchinnikov V, Paci E, Pastor RW, Post CB, Pu JZ, Schaefer

M, Tidor B, Venable RM, Woodcock HL, Wu X, Yang W, York DM, Karplus M (2009) CHARMM: the biomolecular simulation program. J Comput Chem 30 (10):1545–1614

86. Carpenter GA, Grossberg S (1987) ART 2: self-organization of stable category recognition codes for analog input patterns. Appl Optics 26:4919–4930

87. Feig M, Karanicolas J, Brooks CL III (2004) MMTSB Tool Set: enhanced sampling and multiscale modeling methods for applications in structural biology. J Mol Graph Model 22 (5):377–395

88. Karpen ME, Tobias DJ, Brooks CL III (1993) Statistical clustering techniques for the analysis of long molecular dynamics trajectories: analysis of 2.2-ns trajectories of YPGDV. Biochemistry (Mosc) 32(2):412–420

89. Zwanzig RW (1954) High-temperature equation of state by perturbation method. I. Nonpolar gases. J Chem Phys 22:1420–1426

90. Tembe BL, McCammon JA (1984) Ligand-receptor interactions. Comput Chem 8:281

91. Wong CF, McCammon JA (1986) Dynamics and design of enzymes and inhibitors. J Am Chem Soc 108(13):3830–3832

92. Wong CF, McCammon JA (1986) Computer simulation and the design of new biological molecules. Isr J Chem 27:211–215

93. Mezei M, Beveridge DL (1986) Free energy simulations. Ann N Y Acad Sci 482:1–23

94. Bash PA, Singh UC, Langridge R, Kollman PA (1987) Free energy calculation by computer simulation. Science 236:564–568

95. Jorgensen WL (1989) Free energy calculations: a breakthrough for modeling organic chemistry in solution. Acc Chem Res 22 (5):184–189

96. Beveridge DL, DiCapua FM (1989) Free energy via molecular simulation: applications to chemical and biomolecular systems. Annu Rev Biophys Biophys Chem 18:431–492

97. Bottegoni G, Rocchia W, Rueda M, Abagyan R, Cavalli A (2011) Systematic exploitation of multiple receptor conformations for virtual ligand screening. PLoS One 6(5):e18845

98. Barril X, Morley SD (2005) Unveiling the full potential of flexible receptor docking using multiple crystallographic structures. J Med Chem 48(13):4432–4443

99. Huang Z, Wong CF. An Inexpensive Method for Selecting Receptor Structures for Virtual Screening. submitted

100. Truchon JF, Bayly CI (2007) Evaluating virtual screening methods: good and bad metrics for the "early recognition" problem. J Chem Inf Model 47(2):488–508. doi:10.1021/ci600426e

101. Wei BQ, Weaver LH, Ferrari AM, Matthews BW, Shoichet BK (2004) Testing a flexible-receptor docking algorithm in a model binding site. J Mol Biol 337(5):1161–1182

102. Huang N, Shoichet BK, Irwin JJ (2006) Benchmarking sets for molecular docking. J Med Chem 49(23):6789–6801

103. Ellingson SR, Miao Y, Baudry J, Smith JC (2015) Multi-conformer ensemble docking to difficult protein targets. J Phys Chem B 119(3):1026–1034

104. Leis S, Zacharias M (2012) ReFlexIn: a flexible receptor protein-ligand docking scheme evaluated on HIV-1 protease. PLoS One 7 (10):e48008

Methods in Pharmacology and Toxicology (2016): 85–110
DOI 10.1007/7653_2015_58
© Springer Science+Business Media New York 2015
Published online: 10 February 2016

# Understanding Water and Its Many Roles in Biological Structure: Ways to Exploit a Resource for Drug Discovery

Mostafa H. Ahmed, Alessio Amadasi, Alexander S. Bayden,
Derek J. Cashman, Pietro Cozzini, Chenxiao Da, Deliang L. Chen,
Micaela Fornabaio, Vishal N. Koparde, Andrea Mozzarelli,
Hardik I. Parikh, Aurijit Sarkar, J. Neel Scarsdale, Francesca Spyrakis,
J. Andrew Surface, Ashutosh Tripathi, Saheem A. Zaidi, and
Glen E. Kellogg

## Abstract

The importance of water molecules in biological interactions is not debatable, but the various diverse and specific roles that water can play are not as well understood on a molecular scale. In this methods report, the theoretical basis for a computational framework that focuses on water is described. The framework is HINT (for Hydropathic INTeractions) and is a related series of algorithms and methods for probing and modeling the hydrophobic effect, solvation and desolvation, ionization of acids and bases, and tautomerism. HINT is derived from the experimental measurement of the partition coefficient for solute transfer between water and 1-octanol, stylized as log $P_{o/w}$, which is a free energy term. Discussion of computational approaches to quantitating the hydrophobic effect, scoring biological associations with a free energy force field, evaluating the conservation of water molecules in complexes, modeling ionization state ensembles in complex environments, enumerating putative small-molecule tautomers in complexes, and predicting the location of important bridging waters are provided. These factors are summarized in terms of their potential effects on drug discovery projects.

Keywords: Hydrophobic effect, Hydropathic interactions, HINT, Log $P_{o/w}$, Free energy of association, Computational titration, Structure-based drug discovery, Bridging water molecules

## 1 Introduction

Water is ubiquitous in the biological milieu, not just for the obvious macroscale, but also for the micro- and nanoscales. The simple and often repeated statement "Water is Life" could not be more true. The roles that water molecules play in biological structure and function are broad and amazingly varied. To truly understand biological action on an atomic scale almost always involves assessing the actions of the molecules of water—or the lack thereof, which is itself interesting—surrounding the action. Intimately related to water are the acidic and basic properties of molecules. While Lewis acids and bases are occasionally required to understand biological reactions, far more often the Brønsted-Lowry model applies and water molecules have critical roles as both donors and acceptors of protons. Finally, the tautomerism of organic molecules is also dependent on the presence of water acting as an acid and/or a base.

The energetics of water molecules in biological systems is also interesting and has received much scrutiny over the years. Clearly, each water molecule, as it possesses two hydrogen bond acceptor and two hydrogen bond donor loci, is a potent interacting species with other molecules. This is tempered somewhat by the fact that water also likes to interact with other waters. Intra-water interactions are perhaps the most interesting water property because the enthalpic driving force that "structures," i.e., locks together, collections of water molecules also tends to exclude or encage nonpolar moieties, yielding what is called "the hydrophobic effect." Because water molecules have such a strong compulsion to self-associate or interact with other hydrogen bond donor or acceptor functional groups, unwelcome nonpolar compounds or molecular fragments *appear* to associate amongst themselves, giving rise to the misnomer hydrophobic "bonding." This is also a multi-scale phenomenon: the macro observation that "oil and water don't mix" is rooted in these molecular scale principles. Interestingly, although the root cause of the hydrophobic effect is clearly the enthalpic interactions between water molecules, the manifestation of it is entropic! When a *structured* water molecule is displaced to "bulk," e.g., squeezed out by the interaction of two biological molecules, that produces an increase of degrees of freedom and thus entropy. Therefore, the importance of evaluating the many contributions of water molecules to biological systems should not be underestimated, especially in the context of drug discovery.

## 1.1 Modeling of Water

Experimental measurements of these effects are difficult to impossible, particularly for biologically relevant systems, so computational simulations are applied in attempts to unravel the various energetic contributions to free energy of association between molecules. Molecular dynamics simulations of model small-molecule systems have appeared to support the conventional understanding of the hydrophobic effect [1], but large-scale, **all**-atom, constraint-free simulations wherein the modeled system (including the water molecules) self-assembles in the expected manner have been extremely rare [2, 3]. Thus, while protein folding can be simulated for small "toy" proteins with current computational assets, most impressively with the D.E. Shaw specialty supercomputer called Anton [4], the obvious problem is time scale—the cumulative set of translations, reorientations, and interactions, resulting in a folded protein, bound ligand, subunit association, etc., *and* driven by the actual first-principle forces involving discrete water molecules, are clearly very long time-scale phenomena. Desolvation and related phenomena are clearly vital barriers during molecular associations, as was demonstrated in long-term simulations [2, 3]. This level of computation is all but inaccessible for the larger proteins of interest in drug discovery. It is important to reiterate that, beyond the van der Waals attractions felt by *all* pairs of atoms, there is **not** a hydrophobic attraction between nonpolar atoms or molecules: it is an emergent property of the entire ensemble, *especially* the water. Thus, simpler models have been applied to understanding the hydrophobic effect. A relatively simple observation that is easy to model is the hydrophobic surface contact area between molecules (or within a folded biomolecule). Modeling this area is a way of recognizing that the larger the area, the more water molecules that must have been displaced. Empirical terms representing this effect can be found in a variety of free energy scoring functions, but such an approach is obviously a quite crude oversimplification of a complex phenomenon. Other approaches have involved various constructs where properties are assigned to pseudo-atoms representing water, e.g., in cellular automata models [5], or in statistical mechanics models [6].

We have taken a more holistic approach to treating and modeling the hydrophobic effect. Our models were developed *based on the hydrophobic effect*, i.e., the experimental measurements of the partitioning of a solute between two solvents—water and 1-octanol. There has been a rich collection of such data, going back many decades, because it has been known since the late 1800s that the activity of drugs is strongly related to their ability to pass through biological membranes, e.g., pass through the

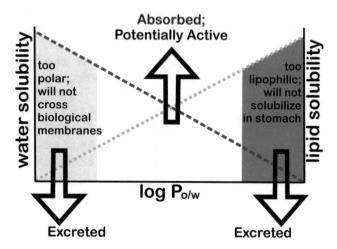

**Fig. 1** Water solubility and lipid solubility as a function of log $P_{o/w}$. Compounds either too hydrophobic or too polar will be excreted without being therapeutically beneficial. Compounds with intermediate hydrophobicities will cross biological membranes and will be potentially active

stomach wall or the blood-brain barrier (*see* Fig. 1). Only molecules balancing two competing effects, water solubility and lipid solubility, can be orally active. Equally important is that many computational algorithms have been developed to predict this partitioning, which is usually reported as **log $P_{o/w}$**. The C-LOGP method by Hansch, Leo, and Weininger [7] is typical. It is also very important to recognize that the measurement of log $P_{o/w}$ is probing a free energy process, and in fact log $P_{o/w}$ is a $\Delta G$ for solute transfer between the two solvents. We have named our model HINT (for Hydropathic INTeractions) and have applied it over the past 2+ decades to a wide variety of biological chemistry problems.

As we have explored these biological systems, involving proteins, small molecules, and polynucleotides, alone and in just about every combination, we have found the pervasive influence of water—usually playing multiple roles—the key to understanding structure and function. Concomitantly, we developed several new and novel computational tools to help us in these studies. Thus, the focus of this chapter is on our set of computational tools for evaluating and predicting the roles of water in biological systems. As our tools were developed over an extended period of time, we have not previously described them together in a single focused contribution. Also, we discuss a few strategies for drug discovery that exploit water as a "natural resource."

## 2   Understanding the Hydrophobic Effect

As we alluded to above, modeling the hydrophobic effect in a de novo sense has been quite impractical to date as part of drug discovery studies because of the complexity of such systems and the time scales required. The oversimplification of the phenomenon by calculation of buried surface area is a useful approximation, but is also clearly flawed. We have instead built a model wherein the properties of atoms were derived from their propensity to associate with water (polar, hydrophilic) or "associate" with lipids, e.g., 1-octanol (hydrophobic, lipophilic). These propensities are atomistic deconstructions of log $P_{o/w}$ [8] guided by principles and data used in the C-LOGP empirical algorithm for prediction of log $P_{o/w}$ [9, 10], which itself has roots in a fragmental approach proposed by Rekker [11]. Thus, instead of carrying atomic charges, the atoms in our model carry atomic hydrophobicities ($a_i$), where $a_i > 0$ is found on a hydrophobic atom, $a_i < 0$ is found on a polar atom, and

$$\sum a_i = \log P_{o/w}.$$

Our atoms also carry a second descriptor, $S_i$, which represents their relative solvent-accessible surface area, or degree of exposure to solvent, which is, of course, water.

The HINT model was a unique idea that Don Abraham had a long-standing interest in developing. It was his notion that the same forces that "partitioned" a small molecule between two solvents are found in all biomolecular interactions in water. That is, hydrogen bonding, Coulombic interactions, acid-base interactions, hydrophobic interactions, and solvation/desolvation are found both in the "shake flask" and in protein-protein and protein-ligand interactions. Furthermore, many of the effects of entropy are encoded simply because log $P_{o/w}$ is itself a free energy.

**2.1 The HINT Algorithm**

The HINT algorithm simply calculates a "score" between each interacting pair of atoms, e.g.:

$$b_{ij} = a_i S_i a_j S_j T_{ij} \exp(-r) + L_{ij},$$

where $r$ is the distance between the atoms $i$ and $j$ in Å, $T_{ij}$ is a logic function described previously [12] that assigns acid-base character to polar atoms, and $L_{ij}$ is an implementation of the Lennard-Jones function based on the models of Levitt and Perutz [13, 14]. The sum over all $i$–$j$ pairs within a single molecule or between two molecules, i.e.,

$$H_{\text{TOTAL}} = \sum \sum b_{ij},$$

represents the total interaction.

Figure 2 illustrates the behavior of the logic function for the interaction between atoms $i$ and $j$ that have the characters shown. Recall that hydrophobic atoms have $a > 0$ and polar atoms (regardless if acid or base) have $a < 0$. Thus, all favorable atom-atom interactions will have $b_{ij} > 0$ and unfavorable interactions will have

|  | hydro-phobic | polar (acid) | polar (base) |
|---|---|---|---|
| hydro-phobic | +1 | +1 | +1 |
| polar (acid) | +1 | −1 | +1 |
| polar (base) | +1 | +1 | −1 |

**Fig. 2** Values of $T_{ij}$ for combinations of atomic hydropathic properties. Color coding of matrix cells: *blue*, favorable polar-polar and hydrogen bond; *red*, unfavorable polar-polar; *green*, favorable hydrophobic-hydrophobic; *purple*, hydrophobic-polar (desolvation). Since hydrophobic atoms have $a > 0$ and polar atoms have $a < 0$, the $T_{ij}$ values in the cells yield the convention that favorable atom-atom interactions have $b_{ij} > 0$

$b_{ij} < 0$. $H_{TOTAL}$ should, in principle, be similarly positive for a molecule-molecule or related interaction with a favorable $\Delta G$. However, being a state function like Gibb's free energy, the difference in $H_{TOTAL}$ holds more information than just its absolute value. $H_{TOTAL}$ can be correlated with the free energy of association: fairly extensive examination of protein-protein associations in wild-type and mutant hemoglobins [15–17] and a variety of protein-ligand systems [18–20] defined $\Delta\Delta G$ as ~500 HINT units/kcal mol$^{-1}$.

*Polar-Polar Interactions.* Because the most polar (hydrophilic) functional groups (or atoms) tend to possess higher (more positive *or* more negative) partial charges, or even formal charges, it is not surprising that there is a fairly good correlation between $|a_i|$ and partial charge [12]. Thus, electrostatic effects are inherently included in the HINT interaction formalism, although clearly not as accurately as with explicit use of Coulomb's law and the Poisson-Boltzmann equation [21], and with using higher level theory to estimate partial atomic charges.

Hydrogen bonding is, in the HINT formalism, a special case of polar-polar interactions, i.e., when the interacting atoms are within defined distances of each other and are of appropriate character (an H-bond donor **and** an acceptor). HINT scores, i.e., $b_{ij}$s, for well-formed hydrogen bonds range up to around 700, which corresponds to about $-1.4$ kcal mol$^{-1}$ [16, 18, 19].

*Hydrophobic-Hydrophobic Interactions.* Hydrophobic interactions are a ubiquitous force in biological systems, but their contribution is hard to assess or model. First, as described above, the hydrophobic effect is an emergent property. Second, simple molecular mechanics force fields have an inherent bias against favorable hydrophobic interactions because the partial charges of hydrophobic groups like methyls, which are usually treated as united atom $CH_3$ constructs, are usually $>0$. Thus, application of the Coulombic term suggests that the interaction, for example, between two methyls would be repulsive. Fortunately, the van der Waals (London) forces as modeled by the Lennard-Jones equation do partially compensate. In HINT, each hydrophobic interaction contributes relatively little energetically to a system, typically with $b_{ij}$ values ranging between 25 and 75 (0.05–0.15 kcal mol$^{-1}$), but there can be many such interactions in a system. Consider a stacked pair of aromatic rings, where there are 36 C–H to C–H interactions, some obviously weaker than others. In our early studies of the subunit interfaces within hemoglobin, we found that interfaces with little discernable movement like $\alpha_1\beta_1$ have more hydrophobic interactions than the more fluid $\alpha_1\beta_2$ interface, which changes dramatically between the tense and relaxed states [22]. The number of polar interactions in these two pairs of interfaces is similar. Overall, we have found that about 1/3 of a total interaction is attributable to hydrophobic terms as calculated by HINT on many systems.

*Hydrophobic-Polar Interactions.* This HINT interaction type is the most intriguing. Similar to most hydrophobic-hydrophobic interactions, some hydrophobic-polar interactions could be mischaracterized based on simple electrostatics: e.g., oxygens of a carboxylate or carbonyl will have negative partial charges, which would indicate an attractive interaction with (positively charged) hydrophobic atoms—the opposite of what we expect hydropathically. Based on our macro view of the hydrophobic effect and many high-resolution crystal structures of biological systems, we would like to observe a different response when modeling such structures with Newtonian force field methods.

While hydrophobic-hydrophobic and polar-polar interactions are relatively simple, obvious, and intuitive, the hydrophobic-polar interaction is not. To appreciate it, we must first separate and isolate the interacting molecular species. Here, all polar atoms will be surrounded by water molecules that complete their "hydropathic valence" [23], i.e., acting as complementary donors to the molecule's acceptors and vice versa. Exposed hydrophobic atoms or groups will have no such partners, but may be in some cases encaged by sets of structured water molecules that are being careful not to get too close. With this in mind, we bring the two species together again: (1) where two polar atoms interact favorably, there is no solvation-related energetic difference from their point of view between the before and after cases—the polar atoms still have partners and the previously associated waters engage with other waters; (2) where two polar atoms interact unfavorably, except in rare cases, a water molecule will be retained to mitigate the repulsion; otherwise, from their point of view, there is no energetic difference between before and after; (3) where two hydrophobic atoms interact, they were not solvated before the association and are still not solvated; but lastly, (4) in a hydrophobic-polar interaction, the polar atom has *lost* its solvation without reprisal from another atom—and this is the energy cost of **desolvation**. In all cases, HINT inherently accounts for costs and gains of desolvation because entropy and solvation/desolvation effects are implicitly encoded in the log $P_{o/w}$ measurements.

**2.2 Interpretation of HINT Score**

As mentioned above, we showed that the total HINT score for an interaction correlated with its free energy of association in many studies. In particular, we looked at $\Delta G = f(H_{TOTAL})$. We constructed a simple equation that could predict $\Delta G$ from $H_{TOTAL}$ with a standard error of about 2.5 kcal mol$^{-1}$ for an arbitrary protein-ligand system [18, 19]. Interestingly, when specific molecular systems were studied, i.e., a single protein with multiple putative ligands, the slopes of those $\Delta G$ vs. $H_{TOTAL}$ lines were surprisingly consistent with each other and with the "all systems" correlations. The differences were largely in the "$y$-intercept" portion of the correlation equation, which can be attributed to internal energetic effects such as conformation entropy that are not accounted for in the pairwise sums of $b_{ij}$. This led us to advocate [24] that the best scoring function for a molecular system is one that is constructed from known data for that system—rather than one purported to be universal for all systems. It is also significant that nearly all "universal" scoring functions are optimized based on recreating poses seen in the corresponding X-ray crystal structures. We chose to optimize our scoring functions with respect to free energy of binding [24]. *See* Fig. 3, where docking results for 19 proteins using three algorithms and scoring functions (AutoDock, GOLD, and FlexX) were compared to the results from HINT scoring functions customized for each protein/ligand set. While the experimental pose should correspond to the most energetically

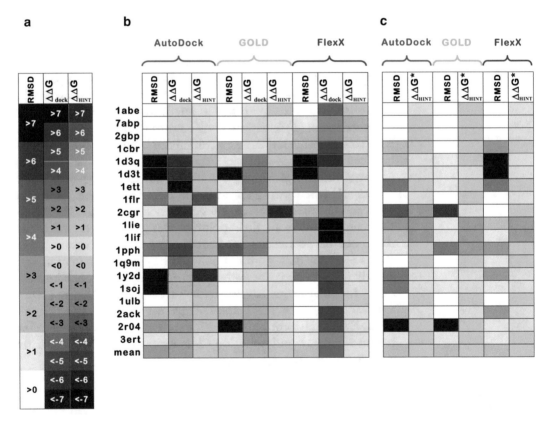

**Fig. 3** Representation of the results of 19 protein-ligand docking experiments using AutoDock, GOLD, and FlexX with color-temperature scale. (**a**) Color temperature coding: first column, root mean square deviation (RMSD) between docking and crystal poses (Å); second column, $\Delta\Delta G_{dock}$—difference between free energy calculated by internal scoring function (and/or published calibration) of the docking program and experimental free energy of binding (kcal mol$^{-1}$); third column, $\Delta\Delta G_{HINT}$—difference between free energy calculated by HINT ($\Delta G_{binding} = -0.001079 H_{TOTAL} - 8.08$, calibrated for this particular dataset) and experimental free energy of binding (kcal mol$^{-1}$). (**b**) Results for best-scoring conformers as chosen by internal scoring functions of AutoDock, GOLD, and FlexX docking programs. (**c**) Results for best-scoring conformers chosen by HINT from poses generated by AutoDock, GOLD, and FlexX. Figure adapted from reference 24

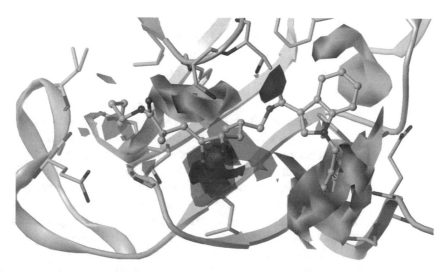

**Fig. 4** HINT interaction maps illustrating the binding between a novel nonpeptide orally active inhibitor of human renin for treatment of hypertension (PDB ID: 2V11). *Green* contours correspond to regions where hydrophobic-hydrophobic binding is dominant; *blue* contours correspond to regions dominated by favorable polar interactions, such as hydrogen bonding; *red* contours correspond to regions dominated by unfavorable polar-polar interactions; and *purple* contours correspond to regions where the dominant interactions are hydrophobic-polar. Close examination of these maps can provide a rational basis for compound design, e.g., by reducing the unfavorable polar-polar interactions and hydrophobic-polar interactions

favorable conformation, our work showed that this is not always the case.

The overall HINT score for a biomolecular association is a useful metric of the quality of the interaction, but since HINT is based on pairwise summations, careful examination of the individual interaction types and scores reveals much more detailed information. In fact, this information was so revealing of drug discovery and design/optimization information that we developed a novel visualization tool—HINT interaction maps that color code and quantify the types and strengths of interactions between two interacting molecules. Figure 4 shows an example of this type of map. By creating these maps we unleashed a tool that guides molecular design by clearly highlighting regions (atom-atom interactions) that are suboptimal.

## 3 Water Makes It Wetter

Truth be told, there are many thousands of water molecules in a biological system comprised of a protein, cofactors, and a potential ligand. Clearly most of them are solely engaged with other water molecules, a smaller fraction of them serve to anchor the collection to the protein in uninteresting places, and just a relative few of them engage the molecules of interest in ways that overtly effect the system's energetics. In fact, only a small handful of water molecules are seen to interact with **both** the protein **and** ligand in a binding pocket [25, 26] and less than one-fourth of water molecules found at protein-protein interfaces make favorable interactions with both proteins [27, 28].

One interesting question that makes modeling the biological environment difficult is which water molecules does one consider as "bulk" and which ones should be considered explicitly. A practitioner of molecular dynamics would, of course, argue that all waters could be included in simulations by application of periodic boundary conditions and other mathematical constructs. Many such studies have been performed at a cost of millions of CPU hours. The counterargument is that explicitly simulating all water molecules makes it difficult to see the trees because such a view of the entire forest all but obscures what we are interested in about a few key water molecules. Poisson-Boltzmann approaches [29] simulate the presence of water with different dielectric constants for outside and inside the macromolecule, which is adequate for treating electrostatics, but still ignores the issue of which water molecules in a solvated macromolecular ensemble should be treated explicitly.

We had considered this problem extensively, and felt that the HINT model, because of its genesis in solvation phenomena, could provide a rational framework for exploring water. First, in the model described above, the HINT scores surely encode some of the apparently invisible transfers and rearrangements of water structure represented and recorded in free energies of association and underlying biomolecular associations. However, water molecules found in binding sites, etc. are more persistent and must be treated explicitly.

### 3.1 Water Rank

Partly because 15 years ago we did not have the resources (or patience) to perform molecular dynamics on entire solvated proteins just to optimize a water network; we were interested in alternative approaches. We recognized that steepest descent molecular mechanics energy minimization tools have limitations—especially in terms of reaching (false) local minima, even in terms of optimizing something as simple as water molecules. It is easy to envision situations where a water molecule is not optimally oriented because other species blocks its ability to explore full rotation. With this in mind, we developed a very simple computational tool that *exhaustively* rotates a water completely through all axes and optimizes its HINT score with respect to the species in its immediate environment [30]. Similarly, the torsion angles of –OH, –SH, –NH$_2$, etc. groups in protein side chains or within ligands could be optimized to maximize hydrogen bonding with maximal HINT score.

A conundrum was thus created: Which water in a collection should be optimized first? The optimization of one water's orientation would profoundly impact the orientations of its neighbors, and so forth. Our solution was to assume that the water capable of making the best set of hydrogen bonds should be the "seed" and that all other water molecules would be optimized in "rank" order. Thus was created the Rank descriptor:

$$\text{Rank} = \sum \left\{ (2.80 \, \text{Å}/r_n) + \left[ \sum \cos(\theta_{\text{Td}} - \theta_{nm}) \right]/6 \right\},$$

where $r_n$ is the distance between the water oxygen atom and the target heavy atom $n$ ($n$ is the number of valid targets or a maximum of 4). This is scaled relative to 2.8 Å, which is presumed to be the ideal hydrogen bond length. $\theta_{\text{Td}}$ is the ideal tetrahedral angle (109.5°) and $\theta_{nm}$ is the angle between targets $n$ and $m$ ($m = n$ to number of valid targets). This allows for a maximum of 4 targets ($\leq 2$ donors and $\leq 2$ acceptors). Lastly, to properly weight the geometrical quality of hydrogen bonds, any $\theta_{nm}$ angle less than 60° is rejected along with its associated target [30]. Practically, each water molecule, which is in reality only known as the coordinates of the central O unless the structure is of exceptionally high resolution, is analyzed with an environmental survey of the closest H-bond donors or acceptors, and these positions are used to calculate its Rank.

Using our exhaustive algorithm, the highest Rank water molecule can then be optimized with respect to its "receptor," which is all other non-water atoms in the system. The optimized water is then added as a member of the receptor, and the second highest Rank water is optimized. This continues until all water molecules in the system are optimized. With this approach, we are able to create very plausible water networks in a short amount of time compared to stochastic techniques such as molecular dynamics. Our use of the term "plausible" is not an accident: it is impossible, even with high-resolution X-ray crystallographic models, to definitively determine the hydrogen bonding patterns within even a modest size water network. In fact, even neutron diffraction may not locate all hydrogens in a protein structure, while the number of water molecules actually observed in either X-ray or neutron diffraction patterns or reported in the resulting models is highly variable, but correlatable with resolution—i.e., higher resolution structures usually report more water positions.

Nonetheless, the Rank algorithm has been applied successfully in a number of computational chemistry problems. In one study from our group [25], we manually evaluated the role played by water molecules in a set of protein-ligand structures, which we classified as second shell, first shell, active site, cavity, or buried $H_2Os$. Rank was able to differentiate among these various roles somewhat more convincingly than the water's HINT score. We also showed, in that work, the disposition of water molecules between un-liganded proteins and their resulting liganded analogues; water molecules were shown to be displaced for either functional or steric reasons, while others were simply missing. In other work, Kuhn et al. [31] used an adaptation of the Rank algorithm to discriminate waters that have a role in binding from waters that can be ignored in their derivation of their empirical ScorpionScore. Much like our goal for the HINT model, they demonstrated the value of intuitive visualization of key intermolecular interactions, interaction networks, and binding hot-spots in rationalizing ligand binding.

### 3.2 Water Relevance

A common view in medicinal chemistry is that, based on thermodynamics, the more tightly bound a water molecule is, the more energy that might be gained by replicating its interactions in a designed ligand. This design approach was demonstrated with the second-generation HIV-1 protease inhibitors (cyclic ureidic and cyclic sulfamide derivatives) that displaced the water ("301") found between Ile 150α and Ile 150β in the un-liganded structure and retained in all previous HIV-1 protease-ligand structures [32, 33]. We showed, later, that HINT quantitatively mapped the contribution of individual structural waters to binding energy and that the contributions of structural water molecules should be included for reliable free energy predictions, with the caveat that *only* water molecules that **add** information value should be included [26].

At a first pass, water molecules that interact with atoms in both the receptor and ligand should meet the criterion of adding information value, but we felt that a more precise definition or metric would be valuable. Since both the HINT score for a water—with respect to its environment or "pseudo-receptor"—and Rank were revealing of the water's role in structure, and yet were not highly correlated [25], we hypothesized that the combination of these metrics might yield a more powerful predictive tool [26]. The goal was, based on its properties in a un-liganded protein structure, to determine the conservation of a water molecule with respect to ligand binding. In other words, can the water molecules most likely to be displaced be predicted a priori? Clearly, such data may provide important drug design clues. Another parameter previously proposed to be indicative of water conservation is the water's crystallographic B-factor [34–36], which indicates the magnitude of oscillation of an atom due to temperature, disorder, or other factors; thus, we also included this as a potentially useful descriptor in our study. Other studies have focused on the dynamical nature of the biological environment [37] or as part of a docking-like investigation [38] to estimate water binding.

To construct a training set, we used 125 discrete waters in 13 proteins for which high-resolution structures were available in both un-liganded and liganded forms. In training, water molecules conserved between the two forms were assigned target values of "1," while non-conserved water molecules were assigned target values of "0." With this data set, we built a heuristic model combining Rank and HINT score such that

$$P_A = \frac{P_R \left( |W_R| + 1 \right)^2 + P_H \left( |W_H| + 1 \right)^2}{\left( |W_R| + 1 \right)^2 + \left( |W_H| + 1 \right)^2}$$

where $P_A$ is the overall probability of the entire system and $P_R$ and $P_H$ are the percent probabilities for conservation based on Rank and HINT score, respectively, while $W_R$ and $W_H$ are the weights of those terms [26]. The original paper provides further explanation of $P_R$, $P_H$, $W_R$, and $W_H$. We termed $P_A$ water Relevance; that is, the more conserved a water is, the more *relevant* it is structurally. Applying this model to a test set of an additional 68 water molecules, again in proteins for which high-resolution structures were available in both un-liganded and liganded forms, yielded a success rate of 87 % correct rate of conserved vs. displaced. Significantly, when the training and test sets were restricted to higher resolution structures, the success rate improved. Using the B-factor alone, or in combination with one or both of our parameters, yielded inferior models, i.e., 66 % success for B-factor alone.

There are a few water displacement caveats, however: compounds interacting through tightly bound bridging waters can be as potent as those interacting directly with the binding site. Direct-binding ligands are generally bulkier, more hydrophobic and complex, and often more difficult to develop. In contrast, water-mediated ligands are often smaller, less hydrophobic, and more flexible, and have better ligand efficiencies [39]. In effect, water can act as a glue or a third partner, contributing to the specificity of interaction and the ligand's pharmacodynamic properties and retaining the correct water molecule in a binding site can be a very successful design strategy [40]. Also, notable recent work by the AstraZeneca group [41] using SZMAP (OpenEye Scientific Software, Santa Fe, NM) shows that the changes in rotational entropy of a water molecule due to charge interactions are good indications of conservation in *holo* protein-ligand complexes. The more rotational entropy the water loses due to charge-charge interactions, the harder it is to displace with ligand groups. We observed a similar phenomenon when examining the water molecules of HIV-1 protease in 2004 [42]—while displacing water 301 did gain binding energy for the cyclic ligands [32, 33]—that gain appeared to be largely attributable to the binding energy of the water; that is, these ligands made the same interactions that the water did.

### 3.3 Prediction of Water Positions

Peter Goodford's 1985 GRID program [43] uses finely tuned potential energy functions to evaluate potential sites for the binding of various functional groups, and especially water. For example, Wallnoefer et al. recently showed that water networks generated using GRID could be used to stabilize molecular dynamics simulations [45]. However, while GRID is still being used, it is being succeeded by WaterFLAP, based on FLAP [44]. Also in current use are WaterMap [46], which uses cluster analysis of molecular dynamics trajectories to determine water network geometry and thermodynamics; AQUARIUS [47], which is a knowledge-based approach that identifies water sites from experimental electron density maps; CS-Map [48], which predicts favorable binding position for water molecules using an interaction potential accounting for van der Waals, electrostatic, and solvation contributions; and Fold-X [49], which predicts bound water positions from interaction sites that would involve two or more polar atoms.

Nevertheless, Relevance provided us with a novel, interesting, and highly "relevant" target variable for a water prediction algorithm. Our algorithm functions in a manner somewhat similar to GRID, except that the result is a set of positionally and rotationally optimized water molecules rather than a 3D map of energetically favorable positions [50]. See Fig. 5 for an operational view of the algorithm. The user simply sets the "Relevance level" for insertion of new water molecules and the algorithm can fill a pocket, solvate an interface, or water-mediate a protein-ligand interaction with water molecules with Relevance at or above that level.

It is interesting, however, that a water molecule does not have to be in the same exact position to perform the same role. For example, a water molecule acting as a H-bond donor to two other atoms that would nominally be repelled by each other could sit in a multitude of positions. In other words, it is entirely possible that energetically plausible water placement might not correspond to experimental structural data.

## 4    Protons? What Protons?

With the exception of a few neutron diffraction structures for proteins and a small number of X-ray diffraction studies at extraordinarily high resolution, experimentally determined structure models do not have explicit protons. For hydrogen atoms that are covalently bonded to carbon atoms, whether aliphatic or aromatic, their positions can be assumed without error from known and virtually invariant bond lengths and geometries. However, for only a few of the hydrogens that are covalently bonded to polar atoms, the same is true. In the remainder of cases, there can be free rotation, i.e., as around the R–OH or R–NH$_2$ dihedrals (*vide supra*), the possibility of ionization, i.e., as between R–C(=O)OH and R–CO$_2^-$ or R–NH$_2$ and R–NH$_3^+$, or tautomerization, i.e., enol to keto or lactam to lactim. Since protons cannot normally be resolved in most biomolecular structural data, a variety of inferences or assumptions are made to build molecular models from these data. For example (1) since bond lengths generally reflect bond order, it might be possible to distinguish between tautomeric forms; (2) since distances between heavy-atom H-bond donors and

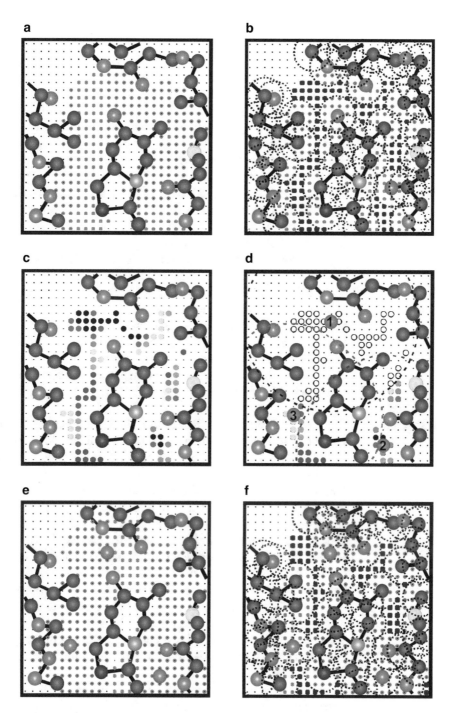

**Fig. 5** The algorithm employed in Relevance-based water prediction. (**a**) Grid points within a specified distance (related to the radius of water) from atoms in **both** the ligand and protein are marked in *green*; (**b**) the remaining grid points after those too close to existing atoms are marked in *purple*; (**c**) HINT scores for putative waters, optimized for orientation, at each of these grid points are indicated by the color spectrum from *blue*—most favorable to *red*—least favorable; (**d**) the highest scoring water (*red circle 1*) is placed and all grid points within a "knockout" distance are disabled, followed by the placement of additional waters (*red circles 2* and *3*) in a similar manner; (**e**) when all grid points are assigned as water molecules or disabled, the next cycle includes these new water molecules as part of the defined molecule; and (**f**) grid points too close to existing atoms (including those from new waters) are eliminated. Figure adapted from reference 50

their partner acceptors should be shorter than uninvolved atom pairs, it might be possible to "find" hydrogens that way; or (3) since we know that in solution at pH 7 (or whatever) carboxylic acids are in their carboxylate forms and amines are protonated, the same must be always true even in proteins. Unfortunately, however, there are at least three undermining and confounding factors: (1) the resolution in these structures is really not good enough to resolve differences in bond order distances, which are typically on the order of 0.1–0.2 Å; (2) many of these are situations that are in equilibrium with potentially small energetic differences between species; and (3) the local pH within a protein can be very different from that of the overall solution.

We proposed a term to describe such cases—isocrystallographic [51]. A structure model is to be considered isocrystallographic with another if both structure models would fit within the same experimental electron density envelopes. This is, of course, resolution dependent. Higher resolution structures will have better defined envelopes and thus lower structural uncertainty [52]. Simply in terms of protons, whether related to rotation, ionization, or tautomerization, there are often *many* structure models that can be constructed for evaluation.

## 4.1 Computational Titration

We first considered the ionization state problem to be one of sampling, much like that in systematic conformational search. If we calculated the energy for all models, then we should be able to identify the lowest energy and therefore "correct" structure model. Figure 6 illustrates a typical case: a carboxylic acid, an amine, and a single water molecule. There are a total of six models that can be constructed by placing zero (Fig. 6a), one (Fig. 6b–d), or two (Fig. 6e, f) protons at the carboxylate/carboxylic acid and/or amine/ammonium cation. Each of the six models, including their waters, is optimized and scored as described above. The model with the highest HINT score would presumably be the lowest energy structure. As this approach is somewhat analogous to a titration where a basic solution is neutralized by stepwise addition of an acidic titrant, we have called our algorithm **Computational Titration** because we are simulating the stepwise addition of *protons*— one at a time.

For relatively small systems, e.g., a protein with one or two ionizable residues (mostly Asp, Glu, and His, possibly Lys and Arg, and less likely Cys and Tyr) and one or two ionizable functional groups on the ligand, there will be a manageable number of ensemble states and their energies will likely be spread out over a fairly wide range. However, with increasing numbers of ionizable groups

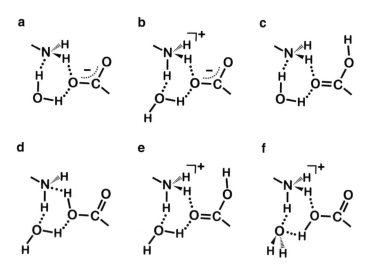

**Fig. 6** Ionization state ensemble from Computational Titration models of amine, carboxylic acid, and water. (**a**) Zero added protons—amine is in unionized state, acid in ionized carboxylate form, water acts as two proton donor; (**b**) one added proton—amine is protonated, acid in ionized carboxylate form, water donates one proton and accepts one proton; (**c**) one added proton—amine is in unionized state, acid in protonated neutral form, water acts as two proton donor; (**d**) one added proton—amine is in unionized state, acid in protonated neutral form (alternate oxygen), water donates one proton and accepts one proton; (**e**) two added protons—amine is protonated, acid in protonated neutral form, water donates one proton and accepts one proton; and (**f**) two added protons—amine is protonated, acid in protonated neutral form (alternate oxygen), water acts as two proton acceptor

in the system, the number of potentially accessible states ($N$) increases dramatically, as

$$N = (3)^{n1} \cdot (2)^{n2},$$

where $n1$ is the total number of carboxylates (where the three possible states are as shown in Fig. 7a–c) and guanidines (where the three possible states are as shown in Fig. 7d–f), and $n2$ is the number of amines (where the two states are $R–NX_2$ and $R–NX_2H^+$), phenols (where the two possible states are $Ar–OH$ and $Ar–O^-$), and thiols (where the two possible states are $R–SH$ and $R–S^-$). In a system with four carboxylates (from Asp, Glu, or the ligand), two amines (from Lys or the ligand), and a single phenol (from Tyr or the ligand), $N = 512$. We found that with such systems, the differences in HINT scores could be very small, especially amongst the protonation models contending for lowest energy. This near-degeneracy may be partly due to summing the more subtle HINT score terms that tend to mediate and compensate for the more dramatic electrostatic-like terms.

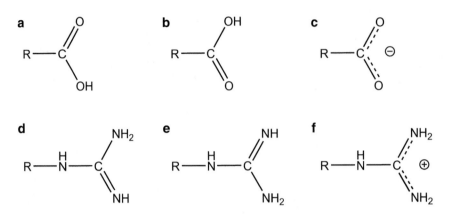

**Fig. 7** Ionization state options for carboxylic acid and guanidine. (**a–c**) Three isocrystallographic forms for carboxylic acid/carboxylate; (**d–f**) three isocrystallographic forms for guanidine/guanidinium

This led us to question the prevailing wisdom that there was only one "true" model for a biomolecular system. Obviously, simultaneously dealing with a few hundred molecular models to describe a protein-ligand interaction is not practical, but applying statistical thermodynamics principles to the collection of ensemble states and their HINT scores, i.e., as

$$E = -RT\log\left\{\left[\sum e^{-\frac{E_H}{RT}}\right]/n\right\}$$

where $E_H$ is the total HINT score ($H_{\text{TOTAL}}$) for a model translated to free energy by a previous correlation fit and $n$ is the number of states in the collection, appears to reveal an energetically reasonable estimate of interaction energy. While this is a useful equation and can be used in other situations, e.g., calculating binding energy from multiple docking solutions, the salient point is that, within the framework of isocrystallographic models, one cannot know which model is true because many models are contributing similarly to the overall energetics. This is an especially significant point because crystallography is generally performed at low temperatures—approaching liquid $N_2$, while chemistry and biology occur at or above room temperature where exchange of protons and flexibility are much more prevalent.

A few points are worth mentioning here about Computational Titration. First, the goal in CT is practical and rational model building, not in estimating pH or $pK_a$, which are very well performed by other methods such as finite difference Poisson-Boltzmann [53–56] and molecular dynamics [57–59] or with empirical models such as PROPKA [60]. Second, the water/polar network is responsive to changes in ionization state: any neighboring water molecules need to be optimized for each of the models conceived during a CT run. Third, while the protocol we described here and elsewhere [42, 61–63] is based on the HINT force field, the concepts and strategy could be simply translated to another paradigm.

**4.2  Tautomers**

There are a handful of well-documented cases where a tautomeric rearrangement of a small-molecule ligand—in contrast to its expected form—was necessary to model that ligand's binding. Such cases are also isocrystallographic as there is little or no data in the crystallographic data to place the telling protons or definitively assign bond orders. Yvonne Martin emphasized the importance of tautomerization by stating that about 25 % of drug-like molecules existing as more than one form [64]. These few cases are not the problem; it is the fact that virtual screening tools often ignore the possibility that alternate tautomers can exist and/or fail to consider the energetic consequences of such. Clearly, energetically accessible molecules that could fit very well in a database screen should be considered.

Tautomer analysis remains a work in progress in our laboratory, but the similarity of this problem to Computational Titration is striking. In effect, it is "simply" a matter of adding another combinatorial layer to the number of models to be examined in the analysis. In the example above, assuming that the tautomer set is independent of the acids and bases of the ligand, which it should normally be, a tautomeric functional group with four states would increase the number of models to be evaluated fourfold, to 2048. The more difficult-to-implement issues are the organization of a database encoding such groups, designing algorithms that build in situ the tautomeric isomers, and collecting/validating reasonable penalty/reward values for scoring. Again, a change in tautomer may require a re-optimization of members in the water network surrounding the ligand.

# 5  Hydropathic Valence "Bond" Theory

Much like an atom may have unpaired electrons in orbitals that need to be fulfilled by bonding with other atoms in the same predicament, each amino acid residue and, for that matter all molecules in the biological environment, also have what can be thought of as a valence. This valence, however, possesses the hydropathic character of the molecule or residue and can only be satisfied by associating non-covalently with other species (or intramolecularly) providing complementary character. Simply, where the target species possesses a hydrogen bond donor, its complement should be an acceptor, or where the target is hydrophobic, its complement is likewise hydrophobic. This "theory" is, of course, an expression of a well-known and accepted dogma. However, with our unique HINT computational framework we have a powerful set of tools to systematize, tally, and visualize all such interactions.

**5.1  Conformation and Folding**

In a protein or other complex biomolecule, fulfillment of the hydropathic valence of each residue or distinct domain may be wholly or partially reached by the molecule's adaptation of alternate conformations wherein complementary groups within the molecule are paired. Thus, the folding of proteins to "bury" their hydrophobic portions as much as possible, the formation of salt bridges and other hydrogen bonds, and the notably higher population of the most polar residues on the surface of a protein can be explained. We recently showed that even the specific conformations that a residue adopts, i.e., its sidechain rotameric state as expressed by the $\chi$ dihedrals, are responsive to this principle [23]. At least for tyrosine [23], the small set of experimentally observed side-chain conformations are associated with a limited number of 3D hydropathic environments, which provide different approaches to satisfy tyrosine's hydropathic valence. We are continuing to document this phenomenon with other residue types. Also, we are exploring extensions of the principle to protein backbone angles, which represent the local secondary structure.

## 5.2 Solvation

In the context of hydropathic valence, solvation is just a consequence of fulfilling the valence needs of the polar portion of a molecule. Within a protein, water molecules are found in locations that meet both the hydropathic valence needs of the location *and* have adequate space for it. The large majority of waters are thus found in locations accessible to the surface and bulk solvent, i.e., in pockets, crevices, and cavities. Water molecules on a protein surface that are structurally conserved are often most strongly associated with the most polar protein side chains such as Asp, Glu, Lys, or Arg. Other water molecules found on the surface are, in turn, associated with these. As a specific example, while tyrosine does not carry a strongly polar side chain, the phenolic –OH can act as either or both a hydrogen bond acceptor and donor. Also, the phenyl ring can potentially act as an acceptor from a water molecule although this is rarely observed in crystal structures. Our analysis of tyrosine environments [23] clearly indicated that water molecules played hydropathic roles in fulfilling valence that were indistinguishable to the tyrosine from those played by other polar atoms on amino acid residues.

## 5.3 Docking

Docking two molecules together is in practice an attempt to computationally satisfy—optimally—both of the molecules' hydropathic valences. However, as seen above, there are many easy-to-ignore factors at play, like ionization state, tautomerization, and especially water. Nowhere have these blind spots been more obvious than in protein-protein docking. Only in the last 2–3 years have protein-protein docking algorithms even started to incorporate water in their methodologies [65–68], although a number of programs and protocols have been available for ligand-protein docking with water for a number of years: the genetic-algorithm GOLD [69] suite has an option for one-by-one toggling of known crystallographic waters [69]. Similarly, Flex-X [70], AutoDock [71], and

GLIDE [72, 73] have shown significant improvements in docking performance with algorithms to simulate contributions of interfacial waters. Lastly, full-scale molecular dynamics run post-docking in explicit solvent [74, 75] has shown some success but at much higher computational cost. Such explicit water methods have been developed to estimate ligand-binding free energy with thermodynamic integration, free energy perturbation theory, and linear interaction energy (LIE) models [76–78].

We were specifically interested in the roles that water molecules play at protein-protein interfaces, as PPI inhibitors are an emerging area for drug discovery research [79]. A huge obstacle is that there is seldom a well-defined binding pocket for small molecules. Instead, areas at PPIs with high energy must be identified as potential sites for ligand binding, and interfacial water molecules are obvious targets [27, 28, 80]. We performed two exhaustive studies of these complexes [27, 28]. Among the several key conclusions of this work, two stand out: (1) water-mediated protein-protein interactions are more pH change resistant than direct interactions because the "bridging" water can easily adapt donating two protons to donating one and accepting one to accepting two protons, and (2) there are more water molecules apparently "trapped" (~26 %) between the two proteins and not making favorable interactions with either than there are water molecules "bridging" (~21 %) between the two. These two observations highlight the crucial importance of explicitly including water in modeling of interactions and the inherent difficulty of doing so: If over one-fourth of all water molecules at a protein-protein interface are seemingly unfavorable energetically, how can such water molecules be predicted?

# 6  Conclusions

Although water molecules are ubiquitous in the biological milieu, they are often ignored or poorly represented in many computational studies. Many of the methods and algorithms described above for dealing with water are not very computationally sophisticated and are not CPU intensive. They are, however, intuitive, which is, in our view, *very* important. Also, because of their basis in an experimental measurement of a thermodynamic property, the technologies that we have provided are also inherently inclusive of thermodynamic properties.

There are many moving parts in real molecular associations such as a small-molecule binding to a protein to elicit a biological activity. The two isolated molecules are at first solvated and as they come together the water–molecule interactions are mostly replaced by molecule–molecule and water–water interactions, although some of the water molecules may be retained to fill voids or to form bridging molecule–water–molecule interactions. De-structuring a water molecule by sending it to the bulk is an entropic effect. Conformational adjustments are made by both molecules, if doing so gains more free energy of binding than is expended for adopting a higher energy conformation. Ionization states of acidic or basic moieties may be changed or alternate tautomeric forms may be adopted—again if that is energetically worthwhile. Of course, this is all proceeding in a concerted manner. Some of these events are amenable to quantum mechanical methods, others are amenable to molecular dynamics simulations, but still others are more phenomenological in nature and cannot be expressed with first principle physics.

So, how can we use the knowledge of water and its many roles for drug discovery and design? First, pay attention to hydrophobic interactions and recognize that, in water, they are more than just London force interactions and contribute one-third or more of the binding free energy. Also, the presence of hydrophobic-polar inter-actions often indicates good possibilities for chemical modification that yields improved binding. Second, be guarded in acceptance of water molecules reported in crystal structures because (a) they could actually be an ion or other species and/or (b) the set may be incomplete—the number of waters reported correlates strongly with structure resolution. Third, carefully evaluate the ionization states of key residues in the target site and putative ligands. There is some good news here: because the two prototypical interactions depicted in Fig. 8a, b are not too energetically dissimilar, it may be possible to perform virtual screening, etc. by enumerating only the target's ionization state options in multiple runs (i.e., not enumer-ating every potential ligand state). Fourth, Rank or other simple metrics of water conservation can provide design clues, but the more conserved a water appears to be, the more tenacious it will

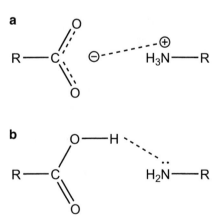

**Fig. 8** Two interaction models for amine interacting with carboxylic acid. (**a**) Carboxylate with ammonium; (**b**) carboxylic acid with amine

be. However, there may not be the substantive gain in energy expected by displacing such a water molecule as it may not actually be a large gain in entropy, and constrained bridging water molecules can be equally effective and, in fact, make the complex more resistant to pH changes [28].

## Acknowledgements

Dedicated to Donald J. Abraham for his many contributions to the development of structure-based drug discovery, to understanding of the hydrophobic effect, and to the conception of HINT.

## References

1. Jensen MØ, Mouritsen OG, Peters GH (2004) The hydrophobic effect: molecular dynamics simulations of water confined between extended hydrophobic and hydrophilic surfaces. J Chem Phys 120(20):9729–9744

2. Shan Y, Kim ET, Eastwood MP, Dror RO, Seeliger MA, Shaw DE (2011) How does a drug molecule find its target binding site? J Am Chem Soc 133(24):9181–9183

3. Dror RO, Pan AC, Arlow DH, Borhani DW, Maragakis P, Shan Y, Xu H, Shaw DE (2011) Pathway and mechanism of drug binding to G-protein-coupled receptors. Proc Natl Acad Sci U S A 108(32):13118–13123

4. Lindorff-Larsen K, Piana S, Dror RO, Shaw DE (2011) How fast-folding proteins fold. Science 334(6055):517–520

5. Kier LB, Tombes R, Hall LH, Cheng C-K (2013) A cellular automata model of proton hopping down a channel. Chem Biodivers 10(3):338–342

6. Mobley DL, Dumont E, Chodera JD, Dill KA (2007) Comparison of charge models for fixed-charge force fields: small-molecule hydration free energies in explicit solvent. J Phys Chem B 111(9):2242–2254

7. Hansch C, Hoekman D, Leo A, Weininger D, Selassie CD (2002) Chem-bioinformatics: comparative QSAR at the interface between chemistry and biology. Chem Rev 102(3):783–812

8. Kellogg GE, Joshi GS, Abraham DJ (1992) New tools for modeling and understanding hydrophobicity and hydrophobic interactions. Med Chem Res 1:444–453

9. Hansch C, Leo A (1979) Substituent constants for correlation analysis in chemistry and biology. Wiley, New York

10. Abraham DJ, Leo AJ (1987) Extension of the fragment method to calculate amino acid zwitterion and side chain partition coefficients. Proteins 2(2):130–152

11. Nys G, Rekker R (1974) The concept of hydrophobic fragmental constants (f-values). II Extension of its applicability to the calculation of lipophilicities of aromatic and heteroaromatic structures. Chem Ther 9(4):361–374

12. Kellogg GE, Abraham DJ (2000) Hydrophobicity: is $LogP_{o/w}$ more than the sum of its parts? Eur J Med Chem 35(7):651–661

13. Levitt M (1983) Molecular dynamics of native protein. I Computer simulation of trajectories. J Mol Biol 168(3):595–617

14. Levitt M, Perutz MF (1988) Aromatic rings act as hydrogen bond acceptors. J Mol Biol 201(4):751–754

15. Burnett JC, Kellogg GE, Abraham DJ (2000) Computational methodology for estimating changes in free energies of biomolecular association upon mutation. The importance of bound water in dimer-tetramer assembly for beta 37 mutant hemoglobins. Biochemistry 39(7):1622–1633

16. Burnett JC, Botti P, Abraham DJ, Kellogg GE (2001) Computationally accessible method for estimating free energy changes resulting from site-specific mutations of biomolecules: systematic model building and structural/hydropathic analysis of deoxy and oxy hemoglobins. Proteins 42(3):355–377

17. Kellogg GE, Burnett JC, Abraham DJ (2001) Very empirical treatment of solvation and entropy: a force field derived from log $P_{o/w}$. J Comput-Aided Mol Des 15(4):381–393

18. Cozzini P, Fornabaio M, Marabotti A, Abraham DJ, Kellogg GE, Mozzarelli A (2004)

Free energy of ligand binding to protein: evaluation of the contribution of water molecules by computational methods. Curr Med Chem 11(23):3093–3118

19. Cozzini P, Fornabaio M, Marabotti A, Abraham DJ, Kellogg GE, Mozzarelli A (2002) Simple, intuitive calculations of free energy of binding for protein-ligand complexes. 1. Models without explicit constrained water. J Med Chem 45(12):2469–2483

20. Fornabaio M, Cozzini P, Mozzarelli A, Abraham DJ, Kellogg GE (2003) Simple, intuitive calculations of free energy of binding for protein-ligand complexes. 2. Computational titration and pH effects in molecular models of neuraminidase-inhibitor complexes. J Med Chem 46(21):4487–4500

21. Honig B, Nicholls A (1995) Classical electrostatics in biology and chemistry. Science 268 (5214):1144–1149

22. Abraham DJ, Kellogg GE, Holt JM, Ackers GK (1997) Hydropathic analysis of the noncovalent interactions between molecular subunits of structurally characterized hemoglobins. J Mol Biol 272(4):613–632

23. Ahmed MH, Koparde VN, Safo MK, Neel Scarsdale J, Kellogg GE (2015) 3D interaction homology: the structurally known rotamers of tyrosine derive from a surprisingly limited set of information-rich hydropathic interaction environments described by maps. Proteins 83 (6):1118–1136

24. Spyrakis F, Amadasi A, Fornabaio M, Abraham DJ, Mozzarelli A, Kellogg GE, Cozzini P (2007) The consequences of scoring docked ligand conformations using free energy correlations. Eur J Med Chem 42(7):921–933

25. Amadasi A, Spyrakis F, Cozzini P, Abraham DJ, Kellogg GE, Mozzarelli A (2006) Mapping the energetics of water-protein and water-ligand interactions with the "natural" HINT forcefield: predictive tools for characterizing the roles of water in biomolecules. J Mol Biol 358 (1):289–309

26. Amadasi A, Surface JA, Spyrakis F, Cozzini P, Mozzarelli A, Kellogg GE (2008) Robust classification of "relevant" water molecules in putative protein binding sites. J Med Chem 51(4):1063–1067

27. Ahmed MH, Habtemariam M, Safo MK, Scarsdale JN, Spyrakis F, Cozzini P, Mozzarelli A, Kellogg GE (2013) Unintended consequences? Water molecules at biological and crystallographic protein-protein interfaces. Comput Biol Chem 47:126–141

28. Ahmed MH, Spyrakis F, Cozzini P, Tripathi PK, Mozzarelli A, Scarsdale JN, Safo MA,

Kellogg GE (2011) Bound water at protein-protein interfaces: partners, roles and hydrophobic bubbles as a conserved motif. PLoS One 6:e24712

29. Grochowski P, Trylska J (2008) Continuum molecular electrostatics, salt effects, and counterion binding—a review of the Poisson-Boltzmann theory and its modifications. Biopolymers 89(2):93–113

30. Kellogg GE, Chen DL (2004) The importance of being exhaustive. Optimization of bridging structural water molecules and water networks in models of biological systems. Chem Biodivers 1(1):98–105

31. Kuhn B, Fuchs JE, Reutlinger M, Stahl M, Taylor NR (2011) Rationalizing tight ligand binding through cooperative interaction networks. J Chem Inf Model 51(12):3180–3198

32. Schaal W, Karlsson A, Ahlsén G, Lindberg J, Andersson HO, Danielson UH, Classon B, Unge T, Samuelsson B, Hultén J, Hallberg A, Karlén A (2001) Synthesis and comparative molecular field analysis (CoMFA) of symmetric and nonsymmetric cyclic sulfamide HIV-1 protease inhibitors. J Med Chem 44(2):155–169

33. Lam PY, Jadhav PK, Eyermann CJ, Hodge CN, Ru Y, Bacheler LT, Meek JL, Otto MJ, Rayner MM, Wong YN (1994) Rational design of potent, bioavailable, nonpeptide cyclic ureas as HIV protease inhibitors. Science 263 (5145):380–384

34. García-Sosa AT, Mancera RL, Dean PM (2003) WaterScore: a novel method for distinguishing between bound and displaceable water molecules in the crystal structure of the binding site of protein-ligand complexes. J Mol Model 9(3):172–182

35. Lu Y, Wang R, Yang C-Y, Wang S (2007) Analysis of ligand-bound water molecules in high-resolution crystal structures of protein-ligand complexes. J Chem Inf Model 47 (2):668–675

36. Raymer ML, Sanschagrin PC, Punch WF, Venkataraman S, Goodman ED, Kuhn LA (1997) Predicting conserved water-mediated and polar ligand interactions in proteins using a K-nearest-neighbors genetic algorithm. J Mol Biol 265(4):445–464

37. Barillari C, Taylor J, Viner R, Essex JW (2007) Classification of water molecules in protein binding sites. J Am Chem Soc 129 (9):2577–2587

38. Trott O, Olson AJ (2010) AutoDock Vina: improving the speed and accuracy of docking with a new scoring function, efficient optimization, and multithreading. J Comput Chem 31 (2):455–461

39. Spyrakis F, Cavasotto CN (2015) Open challenges in structure-based virtual screening: receptor modeling, target flexibility consideration and active site water molecules description. Arch Biochem Biophys 583:105–119

40. Alphey MS, Pirrie L, Torrie LS, Boulkeroua WA, Gardiner M, Sarkar A, Maringer M, Oehlmann W, Brenk R, Scherman MS, McNeil M, Rejzek M, Field RA, Singh M, Gray D, Westwood NJ, Naismith JH (2013) Allosteric competitive inhibitors of the glucose-1-phosphate thymidylyltransferase (RmlA) from Pseudomonas aeruginosa. ACS Chem Biol 8(2):387–396

41. Bayden AS, Moustakas DT, Joseph-McCarthy D, Lamb ML (2015) Evaluating free energies of binding and conservation of crystallographic waters using SZMAP. J Chem Inf Model 55 (8):1552–1565

42. Fornabaio M, Spyrakis F, Mozzarelli A, Cozzini P, Abraham DJ, Kellogg GE (2004) Simple, intuitive calculations of free energy of binding for protein-ligand complexes. 3. The free energy contribution of structural water molecules in HIV-1 protease complexes. J Med Chem 47(18):4507–4516

43. Goodford PJ (1985) A computational procedure for determining energetically favorable binding sites on biologically important macromolecules. J Med Chem 28(7):849–857

44. Cross S, Baroni M, Carosati E, Benedetti P, Clementi S (2010) FLAP: GRID molecular interaction fields in virtual screening. Validation using the DUD data set. J Chem Inf Model 50(8):1442–1450

45. Wallnoefer HG, Liedl KR, Fox T (2011) A GRID-derived water network stabilizes molecular dynamics computer simulations of a protease. J Chem Inf Model 51(11):2860–2867

46. Yang Y, Lightstone FC, Wong SE (2013) Approaches to efficiently estimate solvation and explicit water energetics in ligand binding: the use of WaterMap. Expert Opin Drug Discov 8(3):277–287

47. Pitt WR, Goodfellow JM (1991) Modelling of solvent positions around polar groups in proteins. Protein Eng 4(5):531–537

48. Kortvelyesi T, Dennis S, Silberstein M, Brown L, Vajda S (2003) Algorithms for computational solvent mapping of proteins. Proteins 51(3):340–351

49. Schymkowitz JWH, Rousseau F, Martins IC, Ferkinghoff-Borg J, Stricher F, Serrano L (2005) Prediction of water and metal binding sites and their affinities by using the Fold-X force field. Proc Natl Acad Sci U S A 102 (29):10147–10152

50. Kellogg GE, Fornabaio M, Chen DL, Abraham DJ (2005) New application design for a 3D hydropathic map-based search for potential water molecules bridging between protein and ligand. Internet Electron J Mol Des 4:194–209

51. Spyrakis F, Fornabaio M, Cozzini P, Mozzarelli A, Abraham DJ, Kellogg GE (2004) Computational titration analysis of a multiprotic HIV-1 protease-ligand complex. J Am Chem Soc 126(38):11764–11765

52. Koparde VN, Scarsdale JN, Kellogg GE (2011) Applying an empirical hydropathic forcefield in refinement may improve low-resolution protein X-ray crystal structures. PLoS One 6: e15920

53. Ullmann GM, Kloppmann E, Essigke T, Krammer E-M, Klingen AR, Becker T, Bombarda E (2008) Investigating the mechanisms of photosynthetic proteins using continuum electrostatics. Photosynth Res 97(1):33–53

54. Antosiewicz JM, Shugar D (2011) Poisson–Boltzmann continuum-solvation models: applications to pH-dependent properties of biomolecules. Mol Biosyst 7(11):2923–2949

55. Bashford D (2004) Macroscopic electrostatic models for protonation states in proteins. Front Biosci J Virtual Libr 9:1082–1099

56. Gunner MR, Mao J, Song Y, Kim J (2006) Factors influencing the energetics of electron and proton transfers in proteins. What can be learned from calculations. Biochim Biophys Acta Bioenerget 1757:942–968

57. Goh GB, Knight JL, Brooks CL 3rd (2012) Constant pH molecular dynamics simulations of nucleic acids in explicit solvent. J Chem Theor Comput 8(1):36–46

58. Wallace JA, Shen JK (2011) Continuous constant pH molecular dynamics in explicit solvent with pH-based replica exchange. J Chem Theor Comput 7(8):2617–2629

59. Donnini S, Tegeler F, Groenhof G, Grubmüller H (2011) Constant pH molecular dynamics in explicit solvent with $\lambda$-dynamics. J Chem Theor Comput 7(6):1962–1978

60. Li H, Robertson AD, Jensen JH (2005) Very fast empirical prediction and rationalization of protein $pK_a$ values. Proteins 61(4):704–721

61. Bayden AS, Fornabaio M, Scarsdale JN, Kellogg GE (2009) Web application for studying the free energy of binding and protonation states of protein-ligand complexes based on HINT. J Comput Mol Des 23(9):621–632

62. Tripathi A, Fornabaio M, Spyrakis F, Mozzarelli A, Cozzini P, Kellogg GE (2007) Complexity in modeling and understanding

protonation states: computational titration of HIV-1-protease-inhibitor complexes. Chem Biodivers 4(11):2564–2577

63. Kellogg GE, Fornabaio M, Chen DL, Abraham DJ, Spyrakis F, Cozzini P, Mozzarelli A (2006) Tools for building a comprehensive modeling system for virtual screening under real biological conditions: the computational titration algorithm. J Mol Graph Model 24 (6):434–439

64. Martin YC (2009) Let's not forget tautomers, J Comput Mol Des 23(10):693–704

65. Chen J, Brooks CL III, Khandogin J (2008) Recent advances in implicit solvent-based methods for biomolecular simulations. Curr Opin Struct Biol 18(2):140–148

66. Kastritis PL, van Dijk ADJ, Bonvin AMJJ (2012) Explicit treatment of water molecules in data-driven protein-protein docking: the solvated HADDOCKing approach. Methods Mol Biol 819:355–374

67. Van Dijk ADJ, Bonvin AMJJ (2006) Solvated docking: introducing water into the modelling of biomolecular complexes. Bioinformatics 22 (19):2340–2347

68. Parikh HI, Kellogg GE (2014) Intuitive, but not simple: including explicit water molecules in protein-protein docking simulations improves model quality. Proteins 82 (6):916–932

69. Verdonk ML, Chessari G, Cole JC, Hartshorn MJ, Murray CW, Nissink JWM, Taylor RD, Taylor R (2005) Modeling water molecules in protein-ligand docking using GOLD. J Med Chem 48(20):6504–6515

70. Kramer B, Rarey M, Lengauer T (1999) Evaluation of the FLEXX incremental construction algorithm for protein-ligand docking. Proteins 37(2):228–241

71. Morris GM, Huey R, Lindstrom W, Sanner MF, Belew RK, Goodsell DS, Olson AJ (2009) AutoDock4 and AutoDockTools4:

automated docking with selective receptor flexibility. J Comput Chem 30(16):2785–2791

72. Friesner RA, Banks JL, Murphy RB, Halgren TA, Klicic JJ, Mainz DT, Repasky MP, Knoll EH, Shelley M, Perry JK, Shaw DE, Francis P, Shenkin PS (2004) Glide: a new approach for rapid, accurate docking and scoring. 1. Method and assessment of docking accuracy. J Med Chem 47(7):1739–1749

73. Halgren TA, Murphy RB, Friesner RA, Beard HS, Frye LL, Pollard WT, Banks JL (2004) Glide: a new approach for rapid, accurate docking and scoring. 2. Enrichment factors in database screening. J Med Chem 47(7):1750–1759

74. Jorgensen WL, Chandrasekhar J, Madura JD, Impey RW, Klein ML (1983) Comparison of simple potential functions for simulating liquid water. J Chem Phys 79(2):926–935

75. Toukan K, Rahman A (1985) Molecular-dynamics study of atomic motions in water. Phys Rev B Condens Matter 31(5):2643–2648

76. Kästner J, Senn HM, Thiel S, Otte N, Thiel W (2006) QM/MM free-energy perturbation compared to thermodynamic integration and umbrella sampling: application to an enzymatic reaction. J Chem Theory Comput 2 (2):452–461

77. Gutiérrez-de-Terán H, Aqvist J (2012) Linear interaction energy: method and applications in drug design. Methods Mol Biol 819:305–323

78. Abel R, Young T, Farid R, Berne BJ, Friesner RA (2008) Role of the active-site solvent in the thermodynamics of factor Xa ligand binding. J Am Chem Soc 130(9):2817–2831

79. Wells JA, McClendon CL (2007) Reaching for high-hanging fruit in drug discovery at protein-protein interfaces. Nature 450 (7172):1001–1009

80. Guo W, Wisniewski JA, Ji H (2014) Hot spot-based design of small-molecule inhibitors for protein-protein interactions. Bioorg Med Chem Lett 24(11):2546–2554

Methods in Pharmacology and Toxicology (2016): 111–132
DOI 10.1007/7653_2015_45
© Springer Science+Business Media New York 2015
Published online: 12 August 2015

# CAVITY: Mapping the Druggable Binding Site

## Weilin Zhang, Yaxia Yuan, Jianfeng Pei, and Luhua Lai

## Abstract

Identifying reliable binding sites based on three-dimensional structures of proteins and other macromolecules is a key step in drug discovery. A good definition of known binding site and the detection of a novel site can provide valuable information for drug design efforts. CAVITY is developed for the detection and analysis of ligand-binding site(s). It has the capability of detecting potential binding site as well as estimating both the ligandabilities and druggabilites of the detected binding sites. CAVITY has been successfully applied in many research projects as a stand-alone program or combined with other drug discovery software. In this chapter, we introduce the computational methods and protocols used in CAVITY, and use examples to further illustrate the detailed procedures of how to apply this computational software.

**Keywords:** Druggability, Ligandability, Binding site detection, CavityScore, CavityDrugScore

## 1 Introduction

Protein-ligand (macromolecule-ligand) interactions are involved in many essential biological processes. Experimental techniques such as X-ray crystallography, nuclear magnetic resonance (NMR), as well as cryo-EM have been used to obtain a large amount of 3D structural data, which provide enriched resources for structure-based drug design. For a certain protein structure, evaluation of whether it might be a potential drug target is important. Such an assessment could help the researchers avoid intractable targets and focus their efforts on the target sites with better prospective. Suitable geometry and physical-chemistry properties of a binding site are essential for potent ligand binding. In this sense, many detailed aspects are considered at molecular level to estimate the feasibility of drug discovery on a certain target. For example, both NMR fragment-based and virtual screening-based approaches have suggested that favorable druggability is highly correlated with pocket hydrophobicity and shape [1, 2].

Many computational structure-based methods have been developed for the detection of binding sites in the past years [3]. Geometry-based, energy-based, and geometry-energy hybrid schemes [4–6] are the most commonly used strategies. The major properties adopted in these methods include volume, hydrophobicity, hydrogen bonding, potential energy, solvent accessibility, desolvation energy, and residue propensities depending on the individual algorithm. The geometry-based methods usually use geometric criteria generated by first making a regular 3D grid embracing the protein and then moving a small-molecule probe around the grid to check for positions that are accessible and inaccessible, or energetically favorable and unfavorable, based on the distance and/or relatively simple interaction energy equations. Energy-based methods adopt similar gridding procedure, but apply certain particular strategies to compute the interaction energy between protein atoms and small-molecule probes. For most of the cases, both geometry-based and energy-based methods perform well. As demonstrated by different studies, over 95 % of the known binding sites could be retrieved within the top five ranked pockets detected by such programs [7, 8]. In general, geometry-based algorithms are relatively faster and more robust in the case of structural variations, while the energy-based methods tend to have better accuracy in sub-pocket predictions. We will use CAVITY as an example to show how such a program could help researchers in their studies.

CAVITY is a structural geometry-based ligand-binding site detection program with the capability of predicting both the ligandabilities and druggabilites of the detected binding sites [8]. CAVITY was originally used in the de novo drug design tool Ligbuilder 2.0 [9] to accurately reflect the key interactions within a binding site as well as to confine the ligand growth within a reasonable region; it was later developed into a stand-alone program for binding site detection and analysis. The CAVITY approach generates clear and accurate information about the shapes and boundaries of the ligand-binding sites, which provide helpful information for drug discovery studies: (1) For cases where a protein-ligand complex of the target protein is available, CAVITY can be used to detect the binding site regions which are not covered by the known ligand(s) and provide clues for the improvement of ligand-binding affinity. In addition, the predicted ligandability and druggability of the binding site would tell the researchers whether further improvement of the known ligand is promising. (2) For cases where ligands are known, but the structural information of ligand-target interactions is not available, CAVITY can be used to detect the binding site and the binding mode of the known ligands could be predicted by using molecular docking technique. (3) For cases with no reported ligand, CAVITY can not only be used to detect potential binding sites, but also to provide qualitative estimations of ligandability and druggability for potential binding sites on the target protein, which is very important for making an early-stage decision about whether the protein is a promising target for a drug discovery project. CAVITY has been used in many different projects to help generate such information and clues [10–15].

## 2   Computational Methods Used in CAVITY

### 2.1 Binding Site Detection

CAVITY is a geometry-based method. The binding site detection process includes six steps (Fig. 1).

1. A large 3D grid is made first to embrace the protein.

2. A spherical probe is used to roll around the surface of a protein to erase the far-away grid positions and leave the occupied

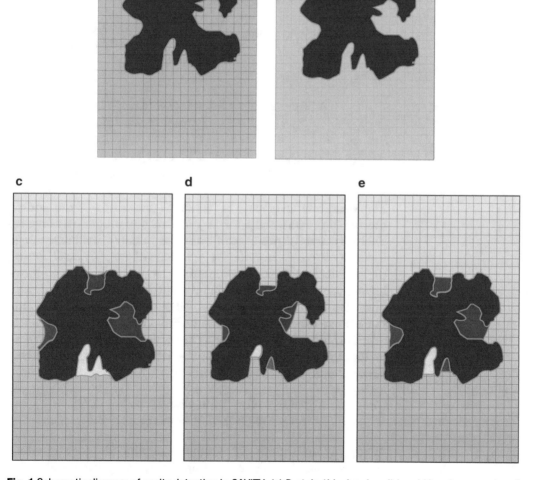

**Fig. 1** Schematic diagram of cavity detection in CAVITY. (**a**) Protein (*black colored*) in grid box (*green colored*). (**b**) Using the eraser ball to remove grid points outside protein. (**c**) "Vacant" grid points after erasing. Four cavities were shown in different colors. (**d**) Shrink each cavity until the depth reaches the minimal depth. (**e**) Recover cavities to obtain the final result

positions by protein atoms and vacant positions on the protein surface.

3. Continuous pockets are split into separated cavities based on the decrease of "layer depth."

4. The sizes of the cavities are recovered to their original size after shrinking separation process by increase of the "layer depth."

5. Detected cavities are sorted according to CavityScore value.

6. Druggability of the detected cavities is characterized by Cavity-DrugScore value.

**2.2 Binding Site Analysis**

CAVITY uses CavityScore and CavityDrugScore [8] to make quantitative and qualitative predictions for the ligandability and druggability of a binding site, respectively. Ligandability is defined as the chance of finding a small molecule binds to a certain target; druggability is the chance of being a good target for drug discovery.

The Cavity Score is defined as

$$\text{Cavity Score} = \frac{\text{Volume} - \text{Adjust volume}}{\text{Surface area} - \text{Adjust surface area}}$$

where

$$\text{Adjust volume} = \text{Boundary volume (2 layers)} - \text{Hydrophobic volume}$$

$$\text{Adjust surface area} = \text{Hydrogen bond donor surface area} + \text{Hydrogen bond acceptor surface area}$$

The value of CavityScore is related to the depth of the pocket, the size of the pocket lip, the physicochemical properties of hydrophobicity, and the presence of hydrogen bond(s). Generally, a high CavityScore comes from (1) large vacant volume, (2) small lip size, (3) large hydrophobic volume, and (4) large hydrogen-bond-forming surface. By using the training sets from PDBBIND [16, 17], both the maximal experimental binding affinity $pK_d(\text{Max})$ and the average experimental binding affinity $pK_d(\text{Ave})$ showed linear relationship with CavityScore. Therefore, CavityScore is used to predict the maximal and the average $pK_d$ of the binding site by a linear equation [8, 18] (*see* **Note 1**):

$$pK_d(\text{Max}) = 1.80 \times \text{CavityScore} + 2.7$$
$$pK_d(\text{Ave}) = 0.62 \times \text{CavityScore} + 3.6$$

"Druggability" stands for a more complicated property which could be related to higher level properties of ligands (ADME/T) as well as the role of the macromolecules act in cellular pathways [19]. Sometimes marketing factors are also involved. Considering the complexity of "druggability," many researchers have applied machine learning algorithms to make a qualitative prediction, where the descriptors related to more detailed and local specific characteristics such as curvature, lipophilic surface, enclosure, and polar interactions [20, 21]. For such approaches, a better training set could improve the performance of the generated models [22–25].

The Cavity Drug Sore is defined as

$$\text{Cavity Drug Score} = \frac{N_b \times N_h}{N_v} - 6000 \times \text{Enclosure}$$

where:

$$\text{Enclosure} = \frac{N_s}{N_v}$$

$N_b$ is the number of the hydrophobic and hydrogen-bonding grid points inside the cavity; $N_h$ is the number of hydrophobic grid points; $N_v$ is the total number of grid points inside the cavity; and $N_s$ is the number of grid points in the lip layers of the cavity. These descriptors were trained and validated by NRDLD data set [25] which contains crystal structures of 71 druggable and 44 less druggable proteins from literatures. The main cutoff value between druggable and less druggable proteins is −180. If a CavityDrugSore value is lower than −180, the Druggability category will be labeled as "Undruggable" which means that it may not be a good targeting site. If a CavityDrugSore value is larger than −180 but less than 600, the Druggability category will be labeled as "Hard" which means that it may be relatively difficult to find a druggable small molecule by targeting this site than a Druggable cavity. If the CavityDrugSore value is larger than 600, the Druggability category will be labeled as "Druggable."

## 2.3   Availability of CAVITY

CAVITY can be used on LINUX platforms. The binary files of CAVITY are freely available to academic users at the website http://www.ligbuilder.org.

An online computation server was also established at http://www.ligbuilder.org/cavity/home.php

To install CAVITY, first uncompress the downloaded CAVITY package:

tar -zxf cavity.tar.gz

The software package contains the following directories and files:

| example/ | Example file directory |
|---|---|
| default/ | Default and preset input parameters |
| parameter/ | Necessary structure parameters |
| cavity32 | 32-bit program |
| cavity64 | 64-bit program |
| cavity.input | An input file template |
| whole.input | An input file template for whole protein mode |
| ligand.input | An input file template for ligand-guided detecting mode |
| area.input | An input file template for area mode |

The default executable file was compiled under 32-bit system (cavity32) and 64-bit system (cavity64).

## 3 Procedure of Using CAVITY

For simplicity, we will use a protein-ligand complex as a starting point to demonstrate the procedure of CAVITY. The protein we choose is secretory phospholipase A2 (sPLA2). sPLA2 hydrolyzes the acyl ester bond of phosphoglycerides at its sn-2 position and liberates free fatty acids. It has been considered as a key enzyme of inflammation [26] and many crystal structures of protein-ligand complexes were reported [27–29].

A practical CAVITY process includes three major steps: (1) prepare structure files (Section 3.1), (2) prepare CAVITY input file for different running mode and run the program (Sections 3.2–3.4), and (3) analyze the results (Section 3.7). Because CAVITY is a geometry-based method, it could also be used for detecting pockets on DNA/RNAs (Section 3.5). Besides normal parameters in the template input files, other parameters could also be adjusted to satisfy more specific jobs for the advanced users (Section 3.6). A server mode is also presented as the last part of this section.

### 3.1 Preprocess Protein Structures as Input Data

A 3D-protein structure file in the Protein Data Bank (PDB) format is required as input for CAVITY. Such a structure file could be downloaded from PDB and preprocessed by visualization software such as PyMOL [30] or generated by using other computational modeling tools in PDB format [31]. If the "ligand-guided detecting" mode is chosen, a ligand file must also be provided in Tripos Mol2 file format [32].

The structure file of the example protein, human secretory phospholipase A2 (PDB ID: 1DB4), could be downloaded from http://www.rcsb.org/pdb/files/1db4.pdb.

The PDB files will be preprocessed first. With the help of visualization modeling tools, we can easily remove the unwanted molecules such as waters and ions. It is also important to examine the structure for missing residues. In the following, we illustrate the procedure of using the PyMOL program for protein structure preparation. Other visualization tools can be used similarly (*see* **Notes 2** and **3**).

1. Make a directory under the CAVITY directory and put the downloaded PDB file here:

   mkdir 1db4

   cp 1DB4.pdb 1db4/.

2. Load original protein file with PyMOL, and open the downloaded PDB file 1DB4.pdb by File -> Open or

   load 1DB4.pdb

3. Extract ligands if exists:

   (a) Open the sequence viewer in the PyMOL viewer by

   - Choose "Display" in the Menu and then choose "sequence" or
   - Click the small "S" button on the lower left panel.

   (b) Select the ligand residue as indicated in Fig. 2 and a "(sele)" item will be generated on the left panel.

   (c) Click the small "A" button just behind (sele).

   (d) From the prompt out menu, choose "extract object" and then a new object "obj01" will be generated.

4. Remove water molecules:

   Remove all the water molecules by:
      remove resn HOH

5. Remove ion atoms:

   Because the calcium atom is essential here for the binding site. We will keep it in this example. If they are not necessary we could remove them using similar command as we remove water molecules (*see* **Note 4**).

6. Save input files:

   Save the protein into file 1db4_protein.pdb. Save the ligand into file 1db4_ligand.mol2 for later usage.

*3.2 Binding Site Detection: The Whole Protein Detection Mode*

The whole protein detection mode is usually used when there is no ligand reported for a target protein. CAVITY will search the entire protein surface for all potential pockets as illustrated in Fig. 1. This mode is the most time-consuming mode. Depending on the

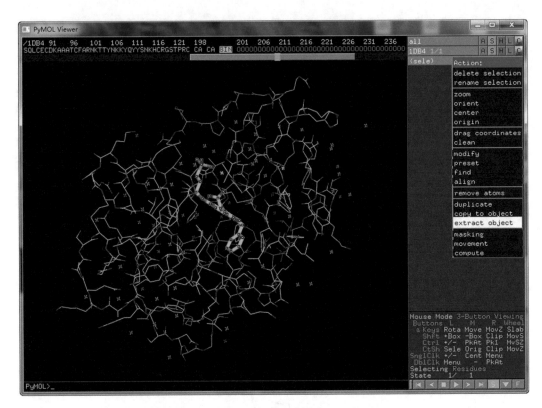

**Fig. 2** Extract ligand from protein-ligand complex in PDB format using PyMOL

size of the target and the speed of the hardware, one computation may take about 1 min to half an hour. Besides detecting potential binding sites, CAVITY can also be used to provide a qualitative estimation of ligandability and druggability for potential binding site in the target protein, which would be important for early-stage judgment of whether this target is promising for drug discovery. In this part, we only use the 1db4_protein.pdb file.

1. Create an input file from template input file "whole.input" by:
   cp whole.input cavity_1db4.input

2. Edit the input file with a text editor (vi, gedit, etc.).
   Change the following lines of cavity_1db4.input:
   RECEPTOR_FILE example/AA/1db4.pdb

   to

   RECEPTOR_FILE 1db4_protein/1db4_protein.pdb

   Save this file.

3. Run CAVITY program:
   cavity64 cavity_1db4.input

It will take 1–2 min for CAVITY to finish the calculation.

**3.3 Binding Site Detection: The Ligand-Guided Detection Mode**

When a protein-ligand complex of the target protein is available, CAVITY can be used to detect the binding site regions that are not covered by the known ligand and provide clues for the improvement of ligand-binding affinity. With a prepositioned ligand in the target protein, CAVITY is guided to define a detection boundary much narrower than the whole protein mode, which is still larger enough for the indicated local area. Therefore it will be ideal if the size, shape, and location of the ligand are proper. To use this mode, a ligand file in Mol2 format is required (*see* **Note 5**). In most of the cases, a ligand extracted directly from the complex structure will be just fine. In this part, we use both 1db4_protein.pdb and 1db4_ligand.mol2 files.

1. Create a new directory "1db4_ligand" and copy the receptor and ligand file to this directory:

   mkdir 1db4_ligand

   cp 1db4/* 1db4_ligand/.

2. Create an input file from template input file "cavity.input" by:

   cp ligand.input cavity_1db4_ligand.input

   Then edit the input file with a text editor. Change the following lines to user-defined receptor and ligand file names ("1db4_protein.pdb" and "1db4_ligand.mol2" respectively):

   | RECEPTOR_FILE | example/AA/1db4.pdb |
   |---|---|
   | LIGAND_FILE | example/AA/1db4.mol2 |

   to

   | RECEPTOR_FILE | 1db4_ligand/1db4_protein.pdb |
   |---|---|
   | LIGAND_FILE | 1db4_ligand/1db4_ligand.mol2 |

3. Run CAVITY program:

   cavity64 cavity_1db4_ligand.input

   It will take 1–2 min for CAVITY to finish the calculation.

**3.4 Binding Site Detection: The Area Mode**

In some cases, we may be only interested in certain part of the protein, but do not have a protein-ligand complex structure available to use the ligand-guided detection mode. Manually assigning the detection boundary will be a solution for such cases. In the "Area mode," a detection boundary is defined by the minimum and maximum 3D dimensional coordinates. Therefore, the region could be adjusted to various volumes and positions.

1. Open the 1db4_protein.pdb file in PyMOL.

   (a) Open the sequence viewer as we did in Section 3.1.

(b) Select HIS47.

(c) In the lower command line type:

get_extent sele

(d) The minimum and maximum *XYZ* coordinates of this selection will be returned as an array:

cmd.extent: min: [56.222, 26.532, 37.984]

cmd.extent: max: [61.443, 29.846, 41.611]

Here, we define the Area mode detection region by subtracting and adding 16 to the minimum and the maximum coordinates, respectively. The values are as follows:

min: [40.222, 10.532, 21.984]

max: [77.443, 45.846, 57.611]

We will put these values into the input file later.

2. Create a new directory "1db4_ligand" and copy the receptor file to this directory:

mkdir 1db4_area

cp 1db4/1db4_protein.pdb 1db4_area/

3. Create an input file from template input file "cavity.input" by:
cp area.input cavity_1db4_area.input

Then edit the input file by a text editor to define the region for CAVITY to search. As we already have the values in **step 1**, change the following lines:

| RECEPTOR_FILE | example/AA/1db4.pdb |
|---|---|
| MIN_X | XX.XX |
| MAX_X | XX.XX |
| MIN_Y | XX.XX |
| MAX_Y | XX.XX |
| MIN_Z | XX.XX |
| MAX_Z | XX.XX |

To

| RECEPTOR_FILE | example/AA/1db4.pdb |
|---|---|
| MIN_X | 40.22 |
| MAX_X | 77.44 |
| MIN_Y | 10.53 |
| MAX_Y | 45.85 |
| MIN_Z | 21.98 |
| MAX_Z | 57.61 |

4. Run CAVITY program:

cavity64 cavity_1db4_area.input

It will take 1–2 min for CAVITY to finish this calculation.

**3.5 DNA/RNA**

With the force field parameters for DNA and RNA, CAVITY can also be used to detect potential pockets on DNA and RNA segments. In the example directory, a brief example is provided using a DNA double-helix fragment (4AH1).

1. Create a new directory DNA_test and copy the input pdb file to this directory:

cp example/DNA/4AH1 DNA_test/.

2. Create an input file from template input file cavity.input by:

cp whole.input cavity_DNA_test.input

Then edit the input file with a text editor to assign the receptor's file name. Change the following lines:

RECEPTOR_FILE example/AA/1db4.pdb

to

RECEPTOR_FILE DNA_test/4AH1.pdb

Because the cavities in DNA/RNA system are relatively larger compared to protein-ligand system, we will use a specialized input parameter set contained in file "large.input" instead of standard input by commenting out the line:

INCLUDE ./default/standard.input

By adding a "#" at the beginning of the line. Then deleting "#" at the beginning of this line:

#INCLUDE ./default/large.input

To

INCLUDE ./default/large.input

Save this file.

3. Run CAVITY program:

cavity64 cavity_DNA_test.input

It will take 1–2 min for CAVITY to finish the calculation.

### 3.6 Result Analysis

The names of the output files resulted from CAVITY will be pre-fixed with the name indicated by RECEPTOR_FILE and the binding-site index number. For the example (1db4) described above, the following files will be generated in the same directory as indicated in the RECEPTOR_FILE parameter's value:

1db4_protein_summary.txt

1db4_protein_surface.pdb

1db4_protein_vacant.pdb

1db4_protein_surface_1.pdb

1db4_protein_vacant_1.pdb

1db4_protein_pharmacophore_1.pdb

1db4_protein_pharmacophore_1.txt

. . .

### 3.6.1 View the Summary and Estimate the Ligandability and Druggability

Name_summary.txt(1db4_protein_summary.txt): This file contains the main characteristics to describe the potential pockets, including CavityScore, $pK_d$(Max), $pK_d$(Ave), Vacant volume, Surface, DrugScore, and Druggability Category. Some of these descriptors are also included in the visualization files. User can view this file with a plain text editor.

Example:

1db4_protein/1db4_protein_surface_1.pdb

| REMARK | 5 Predicted Maximal pKd: 10.61 |
| --- | --- |
| REMARK | 5 Predicted Average pKd: 6.26 |
| REMARK | 6 DrugScore: 567.00 |
| REMARK | 6 Druggability: Hard |

The $pK_d$(Max) and $pK_d$(Ave) indicate the ligandability of the binding site in a more intuitive way. The $pK_d$(Max) suggests the upper limit of binding affinity for compound optimization; the $pK_d$(Ave) suggests the most possible average $K_d$ values for the ligands in this pocket. If these values especially the $pK_d$(Max) are less than 6.0 (equivalent to $K_d = 1$ μM), this binding site may not be a suitable drug design target [8, 18].

"ligandability" is only part of the "druggability" that reflects the possibility of finding small active ligands. To have a better discrimination between druggable binding sites and undruggable binding site, druggability category derived from CavityDrugScore is used to give a more readable version. If the cavity's druggability category is labeled as "Undruggable," it may not be a good position for the binding of druggable small molecules. If the cavity's Druggability category is labeled as "Hard," it may take much more efforts to find a druggable small molecule. If the Druggability category is "Druggable," it is possible to find a high affinity as well as druggable small molecule.

Besides these properties, Vacant volume is another important geometrical descriptor. If it is less than 200 $Å^3$, it will be difficult for a small molecule to bind to this cavity.

*3.6.2 Graphic Visualization of the CAVITY Result*

CAVITY will also output the following visual files for a graphic view of the detection results.

NAME_surface.pdb: This output file stores the surface shape of the binding site and CavityScore. By using molecular modeling software like PyMOL (*see* **Note 6**), users could view this file and obtain an insight into the geometrical shape of the binding site.

NAME_vacant.pdb: This output file stores the volume shape of the binding site. By using molecular modeling software, user could view this file, obtain an insight into the geometrical shape of the binding site, and evaluate the size of small molecules that may bind to this site.

NAME_cavity.pdb: This output file stores the protein atoms forming the binding site. By using molecular modeling software, user could view this file and obtain an insight into the residues that constitute the binding site.

NAME_pharmacophore.pdb: This output file stores the pharmacophore model derived from key interaction grid site inside the binding site [33]. It is in the PDB file format, in which nitrogen atoms represent hydrogen-bond donor sites; oxygen atoms represent hydrogen-bond acceptor sites; and carbon atoms represent hydrophobic sites. By using molecular modeling software, user could view this file and obtain an insight into the key pharmacophore features of the binding site.

NAME_pharmacophore.txt: This output file stores the information of the derived pharmacophore model. It lists the pharmacophore features and the internal distances between them. It also ranks all the features according to their binding scores. It is the text version of the corresponding NAME _pharmacophore. pdb. It can be used as input for other software.

**3.7  Input Parameters**

There are several other input parameters besides the input parameters that we modified in the template files above. We put several critical parameters in the predefined input parameter files which can be used for different types of systems (Section 3.7.1). For advanced users, more detailed descriptions of important parameters are provided in Section 3.7.2.

For convenience, we provided default running parameter sets to adapt different tasks. Predefined critical parameters for pocket detection, such as SEPARATE_MIN_DEPTH, are included in such parameter sets. Users may simply load them into input parameter file by using the keyword INCLUDE. These predefined files are under the path cavity/default/:

Overall default set:

default.input: The overall default parameter set of CAVITY.

Detection mode set:

standard.input: For common binding site, default.

peptide.input: For shallow cavity, e.g., peptide-protein and protein-protein interface.

large.input: For large and complex cavity, e.g., large protein-protein interface, multi-function cavity, multi-substrate cavity, channel, and nucleic acid site.

super.input: For super-sized cavity, e.g., large channel and large polymer interface.

Users can manipulate individual parameters for their own purpose. Such parameter assignment should be declared in the top input parameter file (such as cavity_1db4_protein.input). The values assigned here will override the values in those predefined parameter set files. The declaration could be commented out by adding # at the beginning of the line. Below are detailed descriptions of the important files and parameters for running CAVITY.

RECEPTOR_FILE: The PDB file presenting the target protein. This file is required for running CAVITY.

DETECT_MODE: Detect mode of CAVITY.

0: Whole protein mode: CAVITY will detect the whole protein to find all potential binding sites, and this is the default mode.

1: Ligand mode: CAVITY will detect around the ligand-binding region indicated by a given Mol2 file. It helps the program to locate the interested binding site. However in most cases, CAVITY could locate the binding site without a given ligand's coordinates. Users may try this mode if not satisfied with the result from using the whole protein mode and only interested in the known ligand-binding region.

LIGAND_FILE parameter is required for this mode.

2: Area mode: CAVITY will detect the specific space area assigned by user. X_MIN, X_MAX, Y_MIN, Y_MAX, Z_MIN, and Z_MAX are the minimum and maximum coordinates in 3D space of the detection region. These parameters are required for this mode.

LIGAND_FILE: This Mol2 file presenting a ligand of the target protein (needed if DETECT_MODE is 1). It guides CAVITY to define detection boundary; therefore it will be ideal if the size, shape, and location of the ligand are properly set. A ligand extracted directly from the complex structure will be just fine. Below are some advanced parameters:

*For input section*:

PARAMETER_DIRECTORY: The path of the directory "parameter" where the force field parameters used by Cavity are located.

HETMETAL: Determine whether metal irons are considered when detecting the cavities. Default: Yes.

YES: Metal irons in the protein will be considered.

NO: Metal irons in the protein will not be considered.

HETWATER: Determine whether water molecules are considered when detecting the cavities. Default: No.

YES: Water in the protein will be considered.

NO: Water in the protein will not be considered.

*For output section*:

OUTPUT_RANK: This is a user-defined CavityScore cutoff. CAVITY will only output detected binding sites whose CavityScore is greater than OUTPUT_RANK. User may increase this value to prevent CAVITY outputting useless results.

*For cavity detection process*:

RADIUS_LENTH: The radius of eraser ball (unit: 0.5 Å). User may increase this radius to detect plane and shallow binding site, e.g., peptide-binding site and protein-protein interface. Default: 10.

SEPARATE_MIN_DEPTH: Default minimal depth of binding site. When linkage between sub-cavities does not reach this value, the sub-cavities will be split.

MAX_ABSTRACT_DEPTH: Default abstract depth. Increase this value if the real binding site is much larger than the detection result, and vice versa.

MAX_ABSTRACT_LIMIT_V: Default abstract volume. Increase this value if the real binding site is much larger than the detection result, and vice versa.

SEPARATE_MAX_LIMIT_V: Default max limit volume. Increase this value if the real binding site is much larger than the detection result, and vice versa.

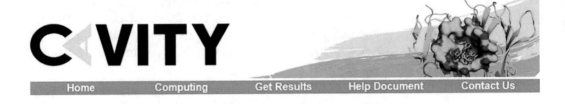

| | |
|---|---|
| MODE | Whole Receptor Mode ▼ |
| Receptor File | 浏览… 未选择文件。<br>PDB file is allowed! |
| Ligand File | 浏览… 未选择文件。<br>mol2 file is allowed! |
| SEPARATE_MIN_DEPTH | 8    Angstrom |
| MAX_ABSTRACT_LIMIT | 1500    Square Angstrom |
| SEPARATE_MAX_LIMIT | 6000    Square Angstrom |
| MIN_ABSTRACT_DEPTH | 2    Angstrom |
| RULER_1 | 100    0.125 Cubic Angstrom |
| OUTPUT_RANK | 1.5 |
| Email | |

Submit    Reset

**Fig. 3** The interface of the CAVITY web server

**3.8 The CAVITY Online Server**

In case the user does not want to use the command line version of CAVITY, an online CAVITY server is also available (*see* Fig. 3). The url is

http://www.ligbuilder.org/cavity/home.php

Below are the procedures of binding site mapping using the CAVITY server:

1. Preprocess protein file as in Section 3.2.
2. Upload the protein PDB file and a ligand file if your want to use ligand-guided detecting mode. Set advanced parameters if necessary.
3. Provide an e-mail address to receive the notification when job is finished.
4. Submit.
5. When the job is finished, the server will send an e-mail to the user with a link to a result page that contains all the result files for download.

## 4    Case Study

In this section, we use a practical example to illustrate the use of CAVITY for the detection of novel druggable binding site.

D-3-Phosphoglycerate dehydrogenase (PGDH) from *Escherichia coli* catalyzes the first critical step in serine biosynthesis, and can be allosterically inhibited by serine (*see* Fig. 4). PGDH contains three distinctive domains: the substrate-binding domain, the nucleotide-binding domain, and the regulatory domain, and it forms a tetramer composed of four identical subunits. The overall structure of the PGDH tetramer could be described as a dimer of dimers [34]. Each fundamental dimer is stabilized by a contact of the nucleotide-binding domain, further dimerized through contacts of the regulatory domains. L-Serine binds to the two adjacent regulatory domains by forming a hydrogen bond network [35].

Structure-based drug design has been applied mainly on the discovery of small molecules directly targeting the sites of known ligands. As most of the known ligands bind to the substrate-binding sites, the biological effects of these ligands are based on the direct inhibition of certain target's function. Recognition of

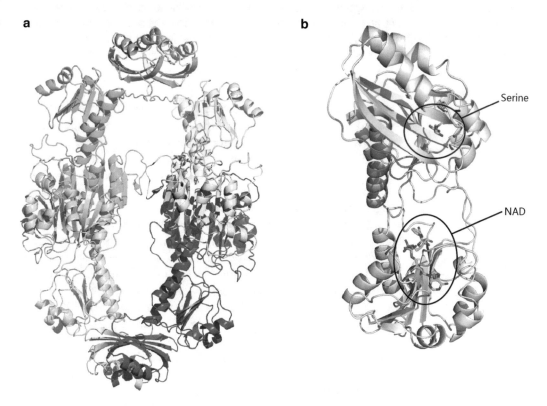

**Fig. 4** The structure of PGDH (PDB ID: 1PSD). (**a**) The PGDH Tetramer with each monomer showed in a different color. (**b**) Binding sites of NAD and L-serine on a PGDH monomer. Pictures were generated using PyMOL

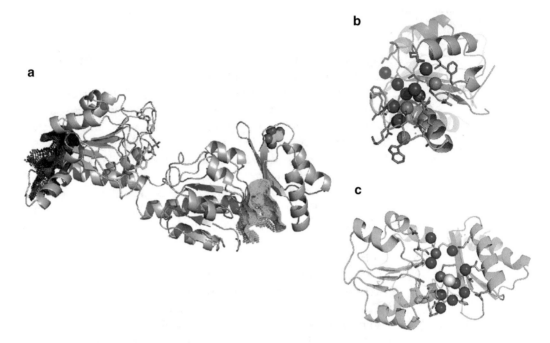

**Fig. 5** The CAVITY predicted binding pockets of PGDH. (**a**) Three binding pockets of PGDH using the inactive conformation were detected by program CAVITY. The NAD-binding position is denoted by the ligand NAD. The site I (in *red brown*) locates at the opposite side of the NAD-binding site. The site II (in *cyan*) locates near the L-serine-binding site. (**b**) Residues and key interaction sites in site I. (**c**) Residues and key interaction sites in site II. These figures are generated based on the residue files and pharmacophore files. This picture was generated using PyMOL

allosteric sites as potential targeting sites presents an entirely new way to design diverse effectors [36]. However, it is challenging to directly find a ligand for a potential site with unknown functions. Although high-throughput screening (HTS) with carefully designed bioassay could be a solution [37, 38], a well-developed computational method for allosteric site detection is also an attracting strategy for such problem.

For the PGDH project, it is interesting to know whether there are other sites, besides the L-serine-binding site, for small molecule binding and enzyme activity regulation. To this end, we first identified potential ligand-binding sites of PGDH using CAVITY [39]. In addition to the known substrate-binding site and L-serine-binding site, more than ten sites were detected by CAVITY in each monomer. Five to six sites with high CavityScores were then evaluated using the two-state Go model-based allosteric site prediction method [11, 14]. Sites I and II (Fig. 5) were predicted as potential allosteric sites, which were then used to virtually screen for binding molecules using molecular docking [15].

Below we described the process of identifying potential binding sites using CAVITY. By examining the potential sites' Druggability, the potential allosteric sites could be distinguished from other undruggable sites for further computational/biological verifications.

Files of this case study could be downloaded from http://www.ligbuider.org/cavity/1YAB_protein.tar.gz

**4.1 About the Input PDB Files**

This compressed downloadable package contains two directories: the "inactive" and the "active," for the two conformational studies presented below.

The "inactive" directory contains the bound conformation denoted in [11]. The X-ray structure of inactive conformation of PGDH (PDB ID: 1PSD) contains both NAD and serine bound at their corresponding binding sites. The "active" directory contains the bound conformation denoted in [11]. The X-ray structure of the active conformation PGDH (PDB ID: 1YAB) contains NAD at its binding site.

**4.2 Preprocess and Computation**

For computational efficiency, only a monomer (chain A) is extracted from the PDB file without small molecules for the study of the inactive conformation (1PSD). For the active conformation (1YAB), one further step was conducted to mutate the MSE residue to Met due to the lack of force field for the MSE residue (*see* **Note 7**). After the extraction of monomers, the whole protein mode mentioned in Section 3.2 was used to detect the potential cavities.

**4.3 Result Analysis and Discussion**

In both the active and inactive PGDH conformations, the NAD-binding site was ranked No. 1. For the inactive conformation, site I was ranked No. 2 with a predicted average $pK_d$ of 6.96 and volume of 1012 $\text{Å}^3$. Site II was ranked No. 4 with a predicted average $pK_d$ 6.57 and volume 1201 $\text{Å}^3$. Both of their druggabilities were categorized as "HARD."

For the active conformation, site I was ranked No. 4 with a predicted average $pK_d$ 6.08 and volume 955 $\text{Å}^3$. Site II was ranked No. 3 with a predicted average $pK_d$ 6.49 and volume 954 $\text{Å}^3$. Here, the druggability of site I was categorized as "HARD" while site II was categorized as "Undruggable" with a DrugScore very close to the cutoff value.

The differences in the rank and category were due to the variation of the PGDH conformations. Although ranked differently, both allosteric binding sites could be discriminated from other "undruggable" sites. These results illustrated the robustness of CAVITY for different conformations.

In our PGDH project, a two-state Go model-based allosteric site prediction algorithm was applied to distinguish these two potential allosteric sites from other detected sites. These two sites were then used for virtual screen to identify potential allosteric effectors. For site II, three inhibitors with the lowest $IC_{50}$ 21.6 μM were found [11]. For site I, two compounds demonstrated low-concentration activation and high-concentration inhibition phenomenon in enzymatic bioassay. One compound exhibited an $AC_{50}$ value of 34.7 nM and $IC_{50}$ of 34.8 μM [15]. The discovered novel allosteric sites of PGDH were substrate independent and different from the known L-serine-binding site.

This example demonstrates that CAVITY can be used in the identification of novel binding site(s), which is particularly useful in locating potential allosteric sites for proteins and other macromolecules.

## 5    Notes

1. The linear equations of $pK_d$(Max) and $pK_d$(Ave) have been modified to current form in the updated version of CAVITY.

2. When the structural information of certain part of the target macromolecule was not available (such as flexible loop regions), CAVITY will continue its detection on the rest part of the target. Therefore if the missing residues are far away from the true binding sites, the overall result of identified cavities will not be affected too much. But if that missing part is at an essential region, then reconstruction by certain computational modeling approaches [40, 41] may be needed.

3. Currently, CAVITY will process PDB files with one model. For NMR structure file which usually contains multiple models, user may split them into multiple files and use CAVITY to calculate each of them.

4. If certain water molecule is considered to be important, user may keep that water molecule(s) and remove other water molecules in the preprocess step. Then declare "HETWATER YES" in the main input parameter file.

5. According to our experience, sometimes the mol2 file generated by PyMOL [30] is not in good quality. In such a situation, user may first save the ligand structure into PDB format, and then use Open Babel [42] or ChemAxon Standardizer [43] to generate the mol2 file.

6. PyMOL is recommended for graphic visualization. The residue PDB files and pharmacophore PDB files could be displayed correctly in most of the molecular modeling software. Because we use condensed atom points to represent the surface and vacant, some molecular modeling software may not display these files correctly. Please try different software if you cannot view these files.

7. For advanced user, it is possible to add a custom-defined residue in the file parameter/RESIDUE_DEF. The format is in an Amber [44] like style.

# Acknowledgments

This work was supported in part by the Ministry of Science and Technology of China (grant numbers: 2012AA020308, 2012AA020301) and the National Natural Science Foundation of China (grant numbers: 81273436, 91313302).

# References

1. Hajduk PJ, Huth JR, Fesik SW (2005) Druggability indices for protein targets derived from NMR-based screening data. J Med Chem 48 (7):2518–2525

2. Huang N, Jacobson MP (2010) Binding-site assessment by virtual fragment screening. PLoS One 5(4)

3. Villoutreix BO, Lagorce D, Labbe CM, Sperandio O, Miteva MA (2013) One hundred thousand mouse clicks down the road: selected online resources supporting drug discovery collected over a decade. Drug Discov Today 18(21–22):1081–1089

4. Laurie ATR, Jackson RM (2006) Methods for the prediction of protein-ligand binding sites for structure-based drug design and virtual ligand screening. Curr Protein Pept Sci 7 (5):395–406

5. Henrich S et al (2010) Computational approaches to identifying and characterizing protein binding sites for ligand design. J Mol Recognit 23(2):209–219

6. Leis S, Schneider S, Zacharias M (2010) In silico prediction of binding sites on proteins. Curr Med Chem 17(15):1550–1562

7. Schmidtke P, Souaille C, Estienne F, Baurin N, Kroemer RT (2010) Large-scale comparison of four binding site detection algorithms. J Chem Inf Model 50(12):2191–2200

8. Yuan Y, Pei J, Lai L (2013) Binding site detection and druggability prediction of protein targets for structure-based drug design. Curr Pharm Des 19(12):2326–2333

9. Yuan Y, Pei J, Lai L (2011) LigBuilder 2: a practical de novo drug design approach. J Chem Inf Model 51(5):1083–1091

10. Chen H, Van Duyne R, Zhang N, Kashanchi F, Zeng C (2009) A novel binding pocket of cyclin-dependent kinase 2. Proteins 74 (1):122–132

11. Qi Y, Wang Q, Tang B, Lai L (2012) Identifying allosteric binding sites in proteins with a two-state Go model for novel allosteric effector discovery. J Chem Theory Comput 8 (8):2962–2971

12. Wu Y et al (2012) Dynamic modeling of human 5-lipoxygenase–inhibitor interactions helps to discover novel inhibitors. J Med Chem 55(6):2597–2605

13. Chen J, Ma XM, Yuan YX, Pei JF, Lai LH (2014) Protein-protein interface analysis and hot spots identification for chemical ligand design. Curr Pharm Des 20(8):1192–1200

14. Ma X, Qi Y, Lai L (2014) Allosteric sites can be identified based on the residue-residue interaction energy difference. Proteins. doi:10.1002/prot.24681

15. Wang Q, Qi Y, Yin N, Lai L (2014) Discovery of novel allosteric effectors based on the predicted allosteric sites for Escherichia coli D-3-phosphoglycerate dehydrogenase. PLoS One 9 (4):e94829

16. Wang RX, Fang XL, Lu YP, Wang SM (2004) The PDBbind database: collection of binding affinities for protein-ligand complexes with known three-dimensional structures. J Med Chem 47(12):2977–2980

17. Wang RX, Fang XL, Lu YP, Yang CY, Wang SM (2005) The PDBbind database: methodologies and updates. J Med Chem 48 (12):4111–4119

18. Yuan Y (2012) An integrated system for de novo drug design. Ph.D., Peking University, Beijing

19. Pei JF, Yin N, Ma XM, Lai LH (2014) Systems biology brings new dimensions for structure-based drug design. J Am Chem Soc 136 (33):11556–11565

20. Nayal M, Honig B (2006) On the nature of cavities on protein surfaces: application to the identification of drug-binding sites. Proteins 63(4):892–906

21. Halgren TA (2009) Identifying and characterizing binding sites and assessing druggability. J Chem Inf Model 49(2):377–389

22. Cheng AC et al (2007) Structure-based maximal affinity model predicts small-molecule druggability. Nat Biotechnol 25(1):71–75

23. Schmidtke P, Barril X (2010) Understanding and predicting druggability. A high-throughput

method for detection of drug binding sites. J Med Chem 53(15):5858–5867

24. Sheridan RP, Maiorov VN, Holloway MK, Cornell WD, Gao Y-D (2010) Drug-like density: a method of quantifying the "bindability" of a protein target based on a very large set of pockets and drug-like ligands from the protein data bank. J Chem Inf Model 50 (11):2029–2040

25. Krasowski A, Muthas D, Sarkar A, Schmitt S, Brenk R (2011) DrugPred: a structure-based approach to predict protein druggability developed using an extensive nonredundant data set. J Chem Inf Model 51(11):2829–2842

26. Nevalainen TJ (1993) Serum phospholipases A2 in inflammatory diseases. Clin Chem 39 (12):2453–2459

27. Schevitz RW et al (1995) Structure-based design of the first potent and selective inhibitor of human nonpancreatic secretory phospholipase-A(2). Nat Struct Biol 2(6):458–465

28. Hansford KA et al (2003) D-Tyrosine as a chiral precursor to potent inhibitors of human nonpancreatic secretory phospholipase A2 (IIa) with antiinflammatory activity. ChemBioChem 4(2–3):181–185

29. Lee LK et al (2013) Selective inhibition of human group IIA-secreted phospholipase A (2) (hGIIA) signaling reveals arachidonic acid metabolism is associated with colocalization of hGIIA to vimentin in rheumatoid synoviocytes. J Biol Chem 288(21):15269–15279

30. Schrodinger, LLC (2010) The PyMOL molecular graphics system, Version 1.3r1

31. Bernstein FC et al (1977) The protein data bank. Eur J Biochem 80(2):319–324

32. Tripos Mol2 File Format documentation. http://www.tripos.com/tripos_resources/fileroot/pdfs/mol2_format.pdf

33. Chen J, Lai L (2006) Pocket v. 2: further developments on receptor-based pharmacophore modeling. J Chem Inf Model 46 (6):2684–2691

34. Schuller DJ, Grant GA, Banaszak LJ (1995) The allosteric ligand site in the Vmax-type cooperative enzyme phosphoglycerate dehydrogenase. Nat Struct Mol Biol 2(1):69–76

35. Sugimoto E, Pizer LI (1968) The mechanism of end product inhibition of serine biosynthesis I. Purification and kinetics of phosphoglycerate dehydrogenase. J Biol Chem 243 (9):2081–2089

36. Merdanovic M, Mönig T, Ehrmann M, Kaiser M (2013) Diversity of allosteric regulation in proteases. ACS Chem Biol 8(1):19–26

37. Wolan DW, Zorn JA, Gray DC, Wells JA (2009) Small-molecule activators of a proenzyme. Science 326(5954):853–858

38. Hardy JA, Lam J, Nguyen JT, O'Brien T, Wells JA (2004) Discovery of an allosteric site in the caspases. Proc Natl Acad Sci U S A 101 (34):12461–12466

39. Qi Y (2012) Molecular dynamics simulation of protein folding, dynamics and function. Ph.D. Thesis, Peking University, Beijing

40. Fiser A, Do RKG, Sali A (2000) Modeling of loops in protein structures. Protein Sci 9 (9):1753–1773

41. Carlsson J et al (2011) Ligand discovery from a dopamine D-3 receptor homology model and crystal structure. Nat Chem Biol 7 (11):769–778

42. O'Boyle N et al (2011) Open Babel: an open chemical toolbox. J Cheminform 3(1):33

43. ChemAxon (2012) Standardizer 6.1.0

44. Case DA, Babin V, Berryman JT, Betz RM, Cai Q, Cerutti DS, Cheatham TE III, Darden TA, Duke RE, Gohlke H, Goetz AW, Gusarov S, Homeyer N, Janowski P, Kaus J, Kolossváry I, Kovalenko A, Lee TS, LeGrand S, Luchko T, Luo R, Madej B, Merz KM, Paesani F, Roe DR, Roitberg A, Sagui C, Salomon-Ferrer R, Seabra G, Simmerling CL, Smith W, Swails J, Walker RC, Wang J, Wolf RM, Wu X, Kollman PA (2014) AMBER 14, University of California, San Francisco

Methods in Pharmacology and Toxicology (2016): 133–151
DOI 10.1007/7653_2015_48
© Springer Science+Business Media New York 2015
Published online: 12 August 2015

# Methods for Detecting Protein Binding Interfaces

## Nurit Haspel

## Abstract

Protein molecules often come together in complexes in order to achieve their biological functions in the living cell. Since the three-dimensional structure and the functionality of proteins are closely related to each other, characterizing the structural and dynamical properties of protein complexes through experiments or computational modeling is important for understanding their roles in the basic biology of organisms. Certain specific regions of a protein may play a critical role in its structural, dynamical, and functional properties. A protein molecule binds to another protein or to a drug molecule through a specific site on its surface, which is commonly known as the binding interface. Prediction of binding interfaces can assist in drug design, protein engineering, protein function elucidation, molecular docking, and analyzing the networks of protein-protein interactions. Experimental detection of binding interfaces can provide a wealth of information, but is time consuming and sometimes inaccurate. Computational methods can validate and complement experimental studies in a cost-efficient way. In this chapter we present a short survey of computational methods that have been suggested over the past two decades for the detection of protein-protein and protein-drug binding interfaces, focusing on methods that use specific amino acids as determinants of binding interfaces. Later, we describe our work in using evolutionary conservation and structural features to detect binding interfaces in proteins and guide protein-protein docking.

Keywords: Docking, Evolutionary conservation, Machine learning, Protein binding interfaces, Protein-protein interaction

## 1 Introduction

Protein complexes play a central role in cellular organization and functions, including ion transport and regulation, signal transduction, protein degradation, and transcriptional regulation [1–3]. Since the three-dimensional structure and the functionality of proteins are closely related to each other, analyzing protein complexes and their structures is crucial for understanding the roles of protein complexes in the basic biology of organisms. Such structural information is also essential for drug discovery. Proteins usually bind to drug molecules or to other proteins through a specific site on their surfaces; residues of such sites tend to be evolutionarily conserved. Below we review some of the recent methods for the detection of binding interfaces through sequence conservation and the characteristics of protein surfaces.

## 1.1 Detecting Binding Interfaces Through Amino Acid Conservation

The amino acids on protein binding interfaces are evolutionarily highly conserved due to their importance to protein functions. Different approaches have been developed to detect the specific amino acids that contribute to the specificity and strength of protein interactions. Studies have shown that protein binding interfaces are often hydrophobic [4]. Hydrophobic residues interact with each other through van der Waals (VdW) interactions. Electrostatic interactions and hydrogen bonds also contribute to protein interaction with other molecules [5]. Binding interfaces can be detected experimentally through mass spectrometry, crystallographic structures of protein complexes, thermodynamic studies, alanine-scanning mutagenesis for hotspot detection [5–7], and yeast-two-hybrid (Y2H) [8] among others. The subject has been reviewed in [9].

Experimental methods are often costly and sometimes inaccurate. To this end, computational methods can complement and aid experimental techniques. Many computational methods focus on finding the so-called hotspots, which are residues on protein surfaces that are involved in binding by forming energetically favorable interactions. Hotspot residues are normally clustered on the protein surface rather than randomly distributed [10]. Those computational methods detect binding interfaces using sequence information [11], structural information [5], as well as physicochemical properties of binding interfaces [12]. For example, the evolutionary trace (ET) method [13, 14] extracts sequence conservation information from families of homologous proteins and ranks the amino acids according to their conservation. The sequence conservation patterns are then mapped onto the protein surface to generate clusters and identify functional interfaces. Figure 1 shows an example of a protein complex with the conserved residues obtained by the ET server highlighted [14]. The SiteLight method [15] uses phage display libraries, which can be tested for binding to target molecules by means of binding affinity-based selection: It maps the peptide library onto a protein surface. Given a collection of sequences derived from biopanning against the target molecule, the binding interface between the template and the target can be predicted. This method is applicable to any types of complexes made up of a protein template and a target molecule. The joint evolutionary trees (JET) method [16] is a more recent method based on the ET method described above. In this method, Gibbs-like sampling of distance trees is used to analyze homologous sequences to reduce the effects of erroneous multiple alignment and weak homologues on distance tree construction. Sequence analysis using the JET method is sensitive to the effect of individual residues and avoids the overrepresentation of highly homologous sequences. Patches of protein surfaces are predicted to be binding sites through clustering, which takes into account both physicochemical properties and sequence conservation.

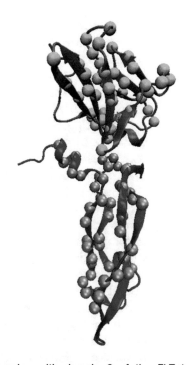

**Fig. 1** VEGF in complex with domain 2 of the FLT-1 receptor (PDB:1flt). Conserved residues are *highlighted* as *spheres*. The conservation information is taken from the Evolutionary Trace (ET) server [14]

*1.2 Detecting Protein Complexes Through Docking*

Protein docking is the computational modeling of the binding of two or more proteins or a protein and a smaller ligand, often a drug candidate, into a complex. It is a challenging problem [17–20] because docking two protein molecules involves searching for low-energy complexes in a space of $N \times M + 6$ dimensions, where $N$ and $M$ are the total number of $(x, y, z)$ coordinates that are employed to represent each one of the unbound protein structures. For a protein containing $m$ atoms, its total number of coordinates equals $m \times 3$. The extra six degrees of freedom is the number of translation and rotation parameters that correspond to the different placements of one monomer onto another. The large number of parameters results in a high-dimensional search space. As a result, most protein-protein docking methods focus on rigid-body docking, where the monomeric structures are considered rigid. In this way, the focus is on finding the placements that result in low-energy dimeric structures. Protein-drug docking involves the docking of a small molecule onto a protein, and flexibility can often be introduced at the ligand level, with limited flexibility at the receptor level [21]. Due to the size of small molecules, docking can be performed as part of virtual screening of large databases.

The geometric search of protein docking is followed by a ranking stage, where the docking candidates from the search stage are ranked by a scoring function that takes into account geometric and physicochemical factors. Computational docking methods often produce, in addition to near-native but slightly incorrect complexes, a large number of low-energy false-positive complexes, where the two proteins are bound on the wrong interface. Scoring functions are used to distinguish the near-native complexes from the false positives.

Detecting the correct interaction interface is a fundamental challenge in molecular docking. Studies have demonstrated that such interfaces exhibit a higher degree of evolutionary conservation than other regions on the molecular surface [13, 16]. However, conserved residues may form a small part of interaction interfaces for various reasons [22]. These findings suggest that ranking of amino acids by evolutionary conservation is a reasonable approach to locate the interaction interface, even if partially. The extent to which binding interfaces contain evolutionary-conserved amino acids has been employed as a scoring function to rank computed bound configurations [23]. Some methods have incorporated knowledge of the location of conserved residues to guide the search for bound configurations. For instance, the energy function employed for minimization can include terms that reward matching of surface regions with high conservation [24].

In the next section we describe our work in detecting binding interfaces through geometry, biophysics, and evolutionary conservation. First, we describe a method for protein-protein docking and refinement guided by geometry and detection of clusters of conserved residues. Next, we describe a method that combines evolutionary conservation, rigidity analysis, and machine learning to detect critically important regions in proteins, including binding interfaces. It should be noted that while our work focuses on protein-protein binding, the methods described here can be readily applied to protein-ligand binding and incorporated into drug design and virtual screening.

## 2    Methods

### 2.1    Using Evolutionary Conservation to Guide Protein Docking

In our earlier work [25, 26] we suggested a docking approach followed by complex refinement. This is a geometry-guided method, which considers transformations that match complementary regions on the protein surfaces. The search and refinement are guided by geometry, and by finding clusters of conserved residues on the protein surface. This allowed us to narrow the search space to find near-native docking candidates. Based on findings that evolutionary conserved regions are good indicators of functional interfaces [16], the search was limited to evolutionarily conserved regions. This greatly reduced the number of considered transformation. The JET method mentioned above [16] was used by the docking method to rank amino acids according to their evolutionary conservation. This information was then used to filter geometrically complementary surface regions on the input proteins. Matching geometrically complementary and evolutionary conserved regions resulted in rigid transformations that produce putative docking results. In what follows we describe the docking and refinement methods in detail.

*Molecular Surface Representation and Critical Points:* Docking algorithms aim to find the best match between the binding surfaces of two molecules. Therefore, the molecular surface of the input protein(s) is first represented by solvent-accessible surface area (SASA) which is calculated by computing the Connolly surface [27]. This is a dense representation that maintains the 3D coordinate, the normal mode, and a numerical value to indicate the type of the surface—convex, saddle, or concave. A sparse, simpler representation is then calculated [28]. This representation retains critical points, which are projections of the center of gravity of a Connolly face on the molecular surface. Critical points are denoted caps, pits, or belts that correspond to convex, concave, or saddle faces, respectively. The critical points cover key locations on the molecular surface and represent the shape of a molecule. Every critical point inherits the conservation score of its closest amino acid on the molecular surface.

*Active Triangles:* The JET score for each amino acid ranges from 0.0, least conserved, to 1.0, most conserved. An iterative version, iJET, repeats the analysis 50 times to obtain an average score for each amino acid. Amino acids with at least 50 % surface accessibility and JET score above a predefined threshold are denoted "active" and assumed to participate in the interaction interface. The rest of the amino acids are treated as "passive". Lower threshold leads to larger surface area and more rigid-body transformations to be considered. Higher threshold leads to smaller surface area and more targeted docking process. Our experiments [25] suggest that thresholds of 0.25–0.75 do not affect the accuracy of the method in reproducing the native assembly. The active/passive designation is inspired by [29].

We define active triangles using critical points. A critical point p1 with conservation score above a predefined threshold (we used 0.5 in [25]) is selected first. Two more critical points, p2 and p3 (not necessarily conserved), are then selected from the molecular surface according to angle and distance constraints: We make sure that the points are not collinear, and that p2 and p3 lie no closer than 2 Å and no further than 5 Å from p1. The minimum and maximum distances ensure that no two points are on the same VdW sphere of an amino acid, and that no triangle covers large parts of the molecular surface. The angle and distance parameters were taken from [30]. See Fig. 2a. We use active triangles to limit the number of tested transformations. We then sort the triangle's

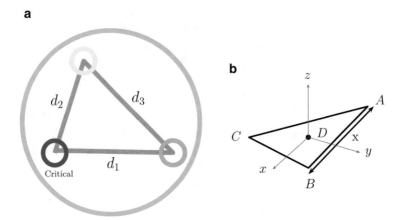

**Fig. 2** (**a**) An illustration of an active *triangle*. The *triangle* has three non-collinear surface points, at least one of which must be critical. The distances between the points are between 2 and 5 Å. (**b**) A reference frame (coordinate system) defined by three non-collinear points

vertices by lexicographic order. Since triangles capture a small surface area, two triangles that share the first vertex in the lexicographic ordering usually represent the same region in the molecular surface. For this reason, no two triangles are allowed to share the first vertex in the lexicographic ordering. Triangles are hashed by their center of mass to further reduce the number of unique active triangles. Given $n$ critical points, the above constraints result in fewer than $n$ active triangles.

*Rigid Body Transformations*: To calculate a rigid-body transformation we define a local coordinate frame for each monomer. Active triangles are employed for this purpose. First, one of the monomers, denoted as A, is arbitrarily selected as the "base" monomer. The other "moving monomer" is referred to as B. For each active triangle selected from A, a matching active triangle is selected from B. We only consider geometry at this stage, as in [31]. These two triangles define two local coordinate frames. The rigid-body transformation aligns the frames by superimposing their origins and rotating B to be congruent with A (see Fig. 2b).

**2.2 Docking Refinement Using Evolutionary Traces**

The protein-protein interfaces predicted by computational docking methods are often not accurate and need to be further refined. We devised a docking refinement method using geometry and evolutionary conservation to improve the interface packing [26]. The input to the refinement process is a protein complex structure generated by a docking method. The refinement proceeds in cycles—each cycle seeks to improve the conformation of one unit with respect to the other one (a unit corresponds to a monomer of the complex). Application of this method is not limited to dimers, as done in this paper. It can be extended to complexes with multiple chains [32]. The refinements are done through small-scale rigid-body rotations focusing on the vicinity of the input structure in order to reduce the computation time and avoid large changes to the protein structure. Monomers are rotated by a random angle within a predefined range around an arbitrary axis passing through the centroid of the unit (see below). Each rotation results in a new complex conformation, which is ranked by an ET- and biophysics-based scoring function for the interface. This process is repeated several times to further improve the results. During each cycle, only K top-scoring conformations are selected for the next iteration to avoid exponential growth of the search space. After the new top scoring conformations are obtained for the selected pair of units, the results are energy minimized for 200 steps using NAMD [33] at the end of each cycle. A small number of minimization steps were applied to relax the local structure near the interface without affecting the overall protein structures. The output structures are the minimized top K conformations generated at the last cycle, which are the refined versions of the input structure.

*Creating Random Conformations with Uniform Distribution*: A probabilistic approach is used to expand the search space. For each input docked conformation, 100 random conformations are generated by rotations around an arbitrary axis [34] passing through the centroid of the monomer. Both the rotation angle and the rotation axis are selected randomly from a uniformly distributed set. As the input docked conformations are supposed to be rather close to the native conformation, large-scale changes to the protein structures need to be avoided. Therefore, ±5° is considered a reasonable range for small-scale rotations. The arbitrary rotation axis is selected from the set of all unit vectors in a unit sphere centered at the centroid of the chain (see details below). A 3D vector $V$ is represented by two angles: the angle between $V$- and $X$-axis ($\alpha$) and the angle between $V$- and $Z$-axis ($\beta$). Then the $x$, $y$, and $z$ components of $V$ can be expressed as follows:

$$V_x = \cos(\alpha); V_y = \sin(\alpha); V_z = \cos(\beta)$$

The arbitrary rotation axis is selected out of the $360 \times 360$ three-dimensional unit vectors by randomly selecting $\alpha$ and $\beta$ values between 1 and 360°. This approach allows a wide conformational search space.

*Scoring Function*: The scoring function we aim to optimize is computed for the interface atoms, which are defined for each chain as the atoms within at most 6 Å to the adjacent chain atoms. In our previous work [35], the scoring function consisted of effective distance restraints [29] and surface complementarity [24] based on evolutionary conservation of residues, as well as VdW and electrostatic terms taken from the AMBER ff03 force field [36]. In the work described here [26], we calculated the interface conservation based on the ET scores of each interface residue, as described below. The scoring function contains a conservation component, based on the assumption that the functionally important surfaces of proteins should consist of clusters of highly conserved residues [13]. We experimented with native structures of different proteins and observed that indeed such clusters are created (see Fig. 1). It should be noted that clusters of conserved residues appear in other parts of the protein as well, possibly due to protein allostery and the fact that many proteins have multiple interaction sites. The ET rank files for every protein are taken from the Evolutionary Trace Server [13, 37]. For each interface atom, we define the evolutionary conservation value as in the equation below:

$$c_i = (\mu - \text{residueRank})/\sigma$$

where residueRank is the ET rank value of the residue that the atom belongs to, $\mu$ is the mean of ET rank values of residues in the chain, and $\sigma$ is the standard deviation of ET rank values of residues in the chain. It is easy to see that for lower ET rank values, which represent lower mutation rates, conservation values will be higher. Similarly, ET rank values larger than the mean will have negative conservation values. Atoms with positive conservation values are considered conserved. We found that the conservation values significantly correlate with lRMSD (least root mean square deviation) values between the refined complexes and the native structures.

The conservation term of our interface scoring function is then defined as

$$E_{\text{conservation}} = \sum_{i,\, j} f(i, j)$$

where $f$, the conservation value for the interface atom pair $i$ and $j$, is defined as

$$f(i, j) = \begin{cases} -c_i \times c_j & \text{if } c_i < 0 \text{ and } c_j < 0 \\ c_i \times c_j & \text{otherwise} \end{cases}$$

Each interface atom $i$ on one monomer and interface atom $j$ on the other monomer are considered in computing the conservation term. We should make sure that $E_{\text{conservation}}$ is not biased towards larger interfaces. For example, given two conformations—one with an interface of 1000 atoms where 300 of them are conserved, and the other with an interface of 300 atoms where 200 of them are conserved. In this case, the former interface should not be preferred over the latter by only counting the number of conserved atoms on the interface. For this reason, non-conserved atoms (i.e., atoms with negative conservation values) also have negative impact on the calculation. It should be noted that the VdW term used for the refinement had the more permissive 9–6 terms, to allow soft clashes.

*2.2.1 Case Study: Complex of Eglin with Subtilisin Carlsberg*

We docked several complexes produced by the method described above and subsequently refined them. The refinement is performed iteratively in two steps. In the first step, 100 conformations are generated as described above and are ranked using our scoring function. The 10 conformations with lowest interface energies are fed into the second step for further refinement. In the second step, 100 new conformations are generated for each of the 10 conformations produced in the first step. The resulting 1000 new conformations are ranked by the scoring function and the 10 lowest energy conformations are returned. We found that further iterations do not significantly improve the results. We show here an example of the results obtained for one protein-protein system—the complex formed by eglin with subtilisin Carlsberg (PDB: 1CSE). In this case, the refinement improved the lRMSD values up to 23 % and all 10 solutions are better than the input docked structure. Table 1 shows the results for the top five solutions. Figure 3 shows the native, docked

**Table 1**
**Refinement results**

| Conformation | Docked | Sol. 1 | Sol. 2 | Sol. 3 | Sol. 4 | Sol. 5 |
|---|---|---|---|---|---|---|
| lRMSD | 3.35 | 2.58 | 2.58 | 2.64 | 2.56 | 2.67 |
| Total interface size | 879 | 709 | 725 | 744 | 722 | 735 |
| Conserved interface size | 530 | 450 | 467 | 482 | 466 | 476 |

lRMSD values in Å with respect to the native structure, number of interface atoms, and number of conserved interface atoms are shown for the initial docked structures and the top five refinement solutions for 1CSE

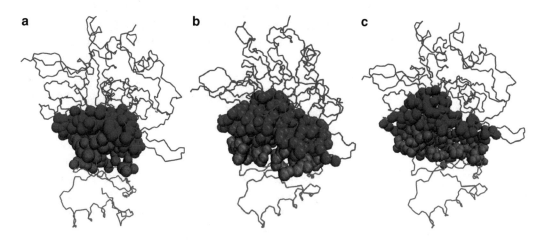

**Fig. 3** Illustration of the 1CSE complex: (**a**) Native complex. (**b**) Input docked complex. (**c**) Refined complex

and refined complex with the interface atoms highlighted as spheres. The correlation coefficient between the lRMSD values and the VdW, electrostatic, and conservation terms were $-0.56, -0.11$, and $-0.57$, respectively, which shows the relative contribution of the conservation term to the refinement.

**2.3 Detecting Critical Regions in Proteins**

Functionally important amino acids are not limited to the binding interface. Other regions in a protein, such as flexible hinges, also play an important role in protein structure and function. Detecting various critical regions in proteins facilitates the analysis and simulation of protein rigidity and conformational changes, and aids in characterizing protein-protein binding. We developed a machine-learning-based method to analyze and predict critical residues in proteins [38, 39]. We combined residue-specific information and data obtained by two complementary methods: KINARI-Mutagen [40], which performs graph-based analysis to find rigid clusters of amino acids in a protein, and combining evolutionary conservation scores to find functional interfaces in proteins, similar to the docking refinement work discussed above. We devised a machine learning model that combined both methods and other features including amino acid type and SASA. We applied the method to a dataset of proteins with experimentally known critical residues, and were able to achieve over 77 % prediction rate, more than either of the methods separately. The ET Server [17] provided the residue rank files for a large number of proteins. The range of rank values in ET files vary from protein to protein, which makes it a difficult task to evaluate the relative conservation of a residue in one protein chain with respect to another. We used the normalized score devised in [26] and described above: $c_i = (\mu - \text{residueRank})/\sigma$, where residueRank is the ET rank value of the residue, $\mu$ is the mean of ET rank values of residues in the chain, and $\sigma$ is the standard deviation of ET rank values of residues in the chain. Lower ET rank values represent lower mutation rates and higher conservation rates. Similarly, Larger ET rank values will have negative conservation values. Atoms with positive conservation values are considered critical.

*Rigidity Analysis and KINARI*: Rigidity analysis [41, 42] is a graph-based method that detects rigid and flexible regions in proteins. A mechanical model of the molecule is built based on covalent bonds as hinges and other interactions, like hydrogen bonds and hydrophobic interactions, are represented as hinges or bars. A graph is constructed from the mechanical model such that each body is associated to a node, a hinge between two bodies is associated to five edges between two nodes, and a bar is associated to an edge. Efficient algorithms based on the pebble game paradigm [43, 44] are used to analyze the rigidity of the graph and infer the rigid and flexible regions of the mechanical model and the protein.

KINARI-Web [45] is a web server for rigidity analysis of molecular structures. KINARI-Mutagen [40] is a tool that relies on a rigidity-theoretical approach that evaluates the effects of mutations that may not be easy to perform in vitro. It relies on the loss of hydrogen bonds and hydrophobic interactions upon a residue's change to glycine, to predict the effects of a mutation. It simulates mutating a residue to glycine by removing its side-chain hydrogen bonds and hydrophobic interactions from the molecular model. It identifies critical residues based on the degree to which an in silico mutation to glycine affects the protein's rigidity. Because there are more experimental data on alanine mutations than glycine, another feature, which allows the mutation of residues to alanine, was added to KINARI-Mutagen.

*Towards a Combined Approach*: While evolutionary conservation and rigidity analysis use different approaches that measure different properties, they have one important thing in common—both aim to discover highly important residues in proteins. Therefore, combining them can provide richer, more accurate information about the relative importance of residues in a protein. Therefore, in [38] we applied the evolutionary conservation-based score and KINARI-Mutagen to a large dataset of proteins to test whether a combination of these methods can provide more information about the importance of residues than any of the methods separately. Our aim was to use machine learning to smoothly integrate the two approaches into a combined method that can provide more accurate and robust prediction of the importance of residues in proteins. We tested our data against the Protherm dataset [46] that contains information about single-point mutations, and a dataset of interaction partners, PiSite [47]. PiSite searches the PDB for different protein complexes that include the same protein, and returns information about that protein's interaction sites and partners, at the residue level.

*Classification Using Machine Learning*: Machine learning is a branch of artificial intelligence, which aims to classify, group, and learn from data. The classification generally contains the following stages: (1) Representing a set of known data points (training data) as a set of feature vectors labeled by classes. Often there are two classes—positive and negative, but there can be more than two; (2) training the set to construct a model that best explains the data, and (3) using the model to classify a set of unknown data points (test data). Support Vector Machines (SVM) [48] are a type of machine learning model which constructs a high-dimensional hyperplane that best separates the two classes of data and defines a kernel function to map the data onto the plane. There are many different types of kernels, and the most popular ones are linear, polynomial, radial basis function (RBF), or sigmoid. Many machine learning and statistical methods have been developed to help predict the effects of mutations and to infer which residues are critical [49–52].

*Extraction of Experimental Data*: We searched the Protherm Database [46] for single point mutations to Glycine or Alanine with known $\Delta\Delta G$ values. $\Delta\Delta G$ is the change to the protein's free energy value ($\Delta G$) following the mutation. A negative value means that the mutation has a destabilizing effect on the protein.

*Feature Selection*: We used an SVM library, libsvm [48], to train and test our data. The features we selected were:

1. Amino acid type: Charged (D,E,K,R), polar (N,Q,S,T), aromatic (F,H,W,Y), or hydrophobic (A,C,G,I,L,M,P,V).

2. Evolutionary Trace score, normalized according to the equation above.

3. Rigidity score, expressed as the size of the largest rigid cluster obtained by KINARI Mutagen.

4. SASA of the residue.

The feature vectors were labeled as +1 (destabilizing mutation according to Protherm) or $-1$ (not destabilizing). Our threshold for destabilization was a $\Delta\Delta G$ value of $-0.5$ or less. We conducted a threefold cross-validation by conducting three tests where the roles of the test and training set rotated between three equal sized, randomly selected samples. The data was then scaled to the $[-1,+1]$ range in order to have all the features in the same order of magnitude. Grid-based cross-validation was used to select the optimal penalty C the RBF kernel parameter $\gamma$ for the training set. The training set was trained to build the model using the RBF kernel and the test set was classified using the obtained model.

*2.3.1  Case Study: Barnase*

Figure 4 shows the prediction of critical residues using the SVM classifier, evolutionary traces and rigidity, respectively, with respect to the experimental data from the Protherm database for barnase (PDB:1bni). The Protherm database contains experimental data for 47 residues. 38 of them (80.1 %) are critical and 9 are not critical according to our criteria outlined above. The SVM approach correctly predicted 38 out of 47 residues (80.1 %) to be critical or non-critical. 30 residues out of the 38 were true positives and 8 true negatives. Out of the rest, eight were false positives and one false negative.

The ET-based score correctly predicted 27 residues (57.5 %) and the rigidity analysis correctly predicted 30 residues (63.8 %). There is only partial overlap between the residues identified by the three methods, and the SVM classifier had much better prediction ability than any of the methods separately. Both the conservation and the rigidity based approach showed weaker positive correlation with the experimental data (correlation coefficients of 0.31

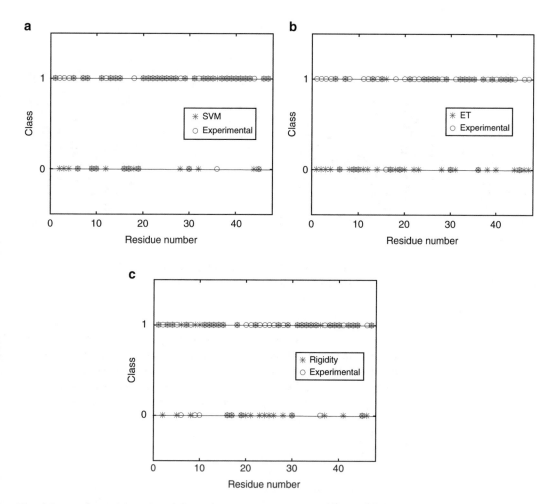

**Fig. 4** Comparison of experimentally available criticality data with our SVM based approach (**a**) conservation (**b**) and rigidity analysis (**c**) for Barnase (PDB:1bni). The *bottom line* (0) indicates non-critical residues and the *top line* (1) indicates critical residues. An × and a *circle* at the same position show an agreement between computational and experimental data. The *x*-axis is a serial residue number and is not necessarily the residue number in the protein

and 0.18, respectively), but the SVM classifier showed much higher correlation with experiment (correlation coefficient of 0.57). It should be noted that the majority of residues for which experimental information exists are critical, so the test set as well as the SVM-based model are biased towards critical, rather than non-critical residues. See [39] for more details. Figure 5 shows the protein structure with the critical residues highlighted, both for the experimentally detected residues and the true positive critical residues detected by the SVM classifier. It can be seen that the classifier missed several residues but was able to detect most of them, especially on the surface.

a

b

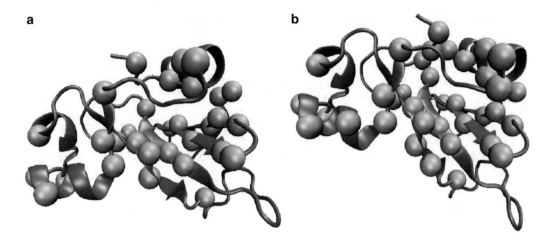

**Fig. 5** Illustration of Barnase (PDB:1bni) with critical residues *highlighted* in *spheres*. (**a**) Experimentally determined critical residues. (**b**) Residues determined to be critical by our classifier

*2.3.2 Case Study: Critical Residues on Binding Sites*

Analysis of experimental data shows that known critical residues may have different percentages of solvent accessibility. This is not surprising since buried critical residues play an important role in maintaining the protein structure, while critical residues on the surface are related to binding sites. To further validate this assumption, we searched the PiSite Database [47] for binding sites and interaction partners. We found that Bovine Pancreatic Trypsin Inhibitor (PDB:1bpi) has six different binding partners and ten binding states. The number of binding partners for each known critical residue is shown in the last column of Table 2. Out of 13 solvent accessible critical residues that have $\Delta\Delta G$ less than $-1.0$, 11 residues had at least one binding partner, which means they are on the binding interface. The SVM classifier correctly predicted most of these residues as critical or not, and as seen in the table, most of the incorrect predictions are associated with borderline $\Delta\Delta G$ values (as mentioned above, we defined a residue as critical if its $\Delta\Delta G$ was $-0.5$ or lower).

These results are very promising since detecting critical residues on the interface would be very helpful for scientists working on the docking problem. Halperin et al. [17] mentioned that binding sites are typically part rigid and part flexible, with far greater extent of movements in the interface than in any other exposed parts of the structure. Hence, information about critical residues on the surface would not just help in reducing the search space but also in detecting residues that are critical for flexibility on the surface. Protein binding can then be modeled more realistically with the flexible residues on the binding site for a more compact docking.

**Table 2**
**Rigidity analysis and conservation score analysis for protein bovine pancreatic trypsin inhibitor (PDB:1bpi) with residue mutations to alanine**

| Mutation | WT residue SASA (Å$^2$) | $\Delta\Delta G$ | Number of binding partners | SVM label |
|---|---|---|---|---|
| K46A | 177.11 | 0.1 | 2 | −1 (TN) |
| R53A | 174.71 | −0.1 | 2 | −1 (TN) |
| T54A | 68.66 | −0.1 | 2 | 1 (FP) |
| T32A | 114.38 | −0.1 | 2 | −1 (TN) |
| E49A | 116.65 | −0.2 | 1 | −1 (TN) |
| G56A | 20.42 | −0.2 | 2 | −1 (TN) |
| G57A | 39.32 | −0.2 | 0 | −1 (TN) |
| R17A | 211.65 | −0.3 | 5 | −1 (TN) |
| K15A | 196.87 | −0.4 | 5 | −1 (TN) |
| K41A | 105.59 | −0.4 | 2 | −1 (TN) |
| D50A | 51.92 | −0.4 | 1 | 1 (FP) |
| R42A | 167.75 | −0.5 | 2 | 1 (TP) |
| Q31A | 79.04 | −1.0 | 1 | −1 (FN) |
| G28A | 41.29 | −1.0 | 1 | 1 (TP) |
| Y35A | 14.74 | −1.1 | 2 | 1 (TP) |
| P13A | 70.66 | −1.2 | 4 | 1 (TP) |
| Y10A | 73.8 | −1.2 | 1 | −1 (FN) |
| V34A | 117.65 | −1.2 | 3 | 1 (TP) |
| I18A | 98.24 | −1.5 | 4 | 1 (TP) |
| S47A | 35.24 | −1.6 | 1 | 1 (TP) |
| M52A | 122.96 | −1.7 | 2 | 1 (TP) |
| G12A | 16.54 | −1.8 | 4 | 1 (TP) |
| R20A | 36.99 | −1.8 | 2 | 1 (TP) |
| F22A | 21.02 | −2.0 | 0 | 1 (TP) |
| G36A | 0.25 | −2.1 | 4 | 1 (TP) |
| I19A | 158 | −2.1 | 3 | 1 (TP) |
| N24A | 35.71 | −2.2 | 0 | 1 (TP) |
| G37A | 36.14 | −2.3 | 4 | 1 (TP) |
| N44A | 19.98 | −3.3 | 2 | 1 (TP) |

WT = wild type, TP = true positive, TN = true negative, FP = false positive, FN = false negative
The table rows are ordered by $\Delta\Delta G$; the mutations that are least destabilizing are at the top of the table, while the mutations that are most destabilizing are towards the bottom of the table

## 3  Notes and Conclusions

Specific amino acids in proteins play a critical role in its structural stability and dynamics. Being able to detect these amino acids is very useful, as it can help in structural analysis, the simulation of protein motions and the discovery of protein-protein and protein-drug interactions and binding modes. There is increasing evidence that binding interfaces in proteins are highly conserved and there are many experimental and computational methods that detect clusters of conserved residues or "hotspots" on protein surfaces. In this chapter we introduced our work in discovering amino acids that may be critical for protein structure and binding. First, we showed a method for protein-protein docking and refinement using a combination of geometric complementarity, physicochemical interactions and evolutionary conservation. Our goal was to bias the docking search and ranking stages towards clusters of conserved residues on the protein surface. We show that this approach indeed helps reducing the computational cost and improve the prediction of binding interfaces. In a subsequent work we devised a machine learning classifier to predict the importance of amino acids in proteins. The features we used were based on a graph-based method to detect rigid and flexible regions in proteins, evolutionary conservation, amino acid type and SASA. We were able to achieve high levels of prediction, higher than each one of the features separately. More recently, we devised an artificial intelligence (AI)-based method to predict and refine docked complexes [53, 54]. The AI-based method uses more features and seems to give very good results in predicting protein-protein interactions. While the work described here focuses primarily on protein-protein interactions, predicting binding interface and incorporating binding site knowledge into docking methods has many useful applications in drug design, virtual screening, and analyzing protein dynamics.

## Acknowledgements

The work described here was partially funded by NSF grant CCF-1116060. The author thanks Dr. Bahar Akbal-Delibas, Dr. Filip Jagodzinski, Dr. Amarda Shehu, and Irina Hashmi for their collaboration. The computations were carried out in part using the UMB research cluster.

## Glossary

| | |
|---|---|
| AI | Artificial intelligence |
| lRMSD | Least root mean square deviation |
| PDB | Protein Data Bank |
| SVM | Support vector machine |
| VdW | van der Waals |

## References

1. Goodsell DS, Olson AJ (2000) Structural symmetry and protein function. Annu Rev Biophys Biomol Struct 29(1):105–153

2. Braun P, Gingras A-C (2012) History of protein-protein interactions: from egg-white to complex networks. Proteomics 12 (10):1478–1498

3. Jones S, Thornton JM (1995) Protein-protein interactions: a review of protein dimer structures. Prog Biophys Mol Biol 63(1):31–65

4. Young L, Jernigan RL, Covell DG (1994) A role for surface hydrophobicity in protein-protein recognition. Protein Sci 3(5):717–729

5. Moreira IS, Fernandes PA, Ramos MJ (2007) Hot spots – a review of the protein-protein interface determinant amino-acid residues. Protein Struct Funct Bioinform 68 (4):803–812

6. Andrew A (1998) Bogan and Kurt S Thorn. Anatomy of hot spots in protein interfaces. J Mol Biol 280(1):1–9

7. Hu Z, Ma B, Wolfson H, Nussinov R (2000) Conservation of polar residues as hot spots at protein interfaces. Protein Struct Funct Bioinform 39(4):331–342

8. Brückner A, Polge C, Lentze N, Auerbach D, Schlattner U (2009) Yeast two-hybrid, a powerful tool for systems biology. Int J Mol Sci 10 (6):2763–2788

9. Srinivasa Rao V, Srinivas K, Sujini GN, Sunand Kumar GN (2014) Protein-protein interaction detection: methods and analysis. Int J Proteom 12:2014

10. Engin Cukuroglu H, Engin HB, Gursoy A, Gursoy O (2014) Hot spots in protein-protein interfaces: towards drug discovery. Prog Biophys Mol Biol 116:165–173

11. Ofran Y, Rost B (2003) Predicted protein-protein interaction sites from local sequence information. FEBS Lett 544(1-3):236–239

12. Assi SA, Tanaka T, Rabbitts TH, Fernandez-Fuentes N (2010) Pcrpi: presaging critical residues in protein interfaces, a new computational tool to chart hot spots in protein interfaces. Nucleic Acids Res 38(6):e86

13. Lichtarge O, Bourne HR, Cohen FE (1996) An evolutionary trace method defines binding surfaces common to protein families. J Mol Biol 257(2):342–358

14. Wilkins AD, Bachman BJ, Erdin S, Lichtarge O (2012) The use of evolutionary patterns in protein annotation. Curr Opin Struct Biol 22 (3):316–325

15. Halperin I, Wolfson H, Nussinov R (2003) Sitelight: binding-site prediction using phage display libraries. Protein Sci 12(7):1344–1359

16. Engelen S, Ladislas AT, Sacquin-More S, Lavery R, Carbone A (2009) Joint evolutionary trees: a large-scale method to predict protein interfaces based on sequence sampling. PLoS Comp Bio 5(1):e1000267

17. Halperin I, Ma B, Wolfson H, Nussinov R (2002) Principles of docking: an overview of search algorithms and a guide to scoring functions. Protein Struct Funct Bioinform 47 (4):409–443

18. Huang S-Y (2014) Search strategies and evaluation in protein–protein docking: principles, advances and challenges. Drug Discov Today 19(8):1081–1096

19. Camacho CJ, Vajda S (2005) Protein-protein association kinetics and protein docking. Curr Opin Struct Biol 12(1):36–40

20. Kozakov D, Beglov D, Bohnuud T, Mottarella SE, Xia B, Hall DR, Vajda S (2013) How good is automated protein docking? Protein Struct Funct Bioinform 81(12):2159–2166

21. Morris GM, Huey R, Lindstrom W, Sanner MF, Belew RK, Goodsell DS, Olson AJ (2009) Autodock4 and autodocktools4: automated docking with selective receptor flexibility. J Comput Chem 30(16):2785–2791

22. Fernandez-Recio J (2011) Prediction of protein binding sites and hot spots. Wiley Interdiscip Rev Comput Mol Sci 1(5):680–698

23. Tress M, de Juan D, Graña O, Gomez MJ, Gomez-Puertas P, Gonzalez JM, Lopez G, Valencia A (2005) Scoring docking models with evolutionary information. Protein Struct Funct Bioinform 60(2):275–280

24. Kanamori E, Murakami Y, Tsuchiya Y, Standley D, Nakamura H, Kinoshita K (2007) Docking of protein molecular surfaces with evolutionary trace analysis. Protein Struct Funct Bioinform 69(4):832–838

25. Hashmi I, Akbal-Delibas B, Haspel N, Shehu A (2012) Guiding protein docking with geometric and evolutionary information. J Bioinform Comput Biol 10(3):1242008

26. Akbal-Delibas B, Hashmi I, Shehu A, Haspel N (2012) An evolutionary conservation based method for refining and re-ranking protein complex structures. J Bioinform Comput Biol 10(3):1242002

27. Connolly ML (1983) Analytical molecular surface calculation. J Appl Cryst 16(5):548–558

28. Norel R, Lin SL, Wolfson HJ, Nussinov R (1999) Examination of shape complementarity in docking of unbound proteins. Protein Struct Funct Genet 36(3):307–317

29. Dominguez C, Boelens R, Bonvin A (2003) Haddock: a protein-protein docking approach based on biochemical orbiophysical information. J Am Chem Soc 125(1):1731–1737

30. Fischer D, Lin SL, Wolfson HL, Nussinov R (2005) A geometry-based suite of molecular docking processes. J Mol Biol 248(2):459–477

31. Wolfson H, Rigoutsos I (1997) Geometric hashing: an overview. IEEE Comp Sci and Eng 4(4):10–21

32. Akbal-Delibas B, Haspel N (2013) A conservation and biophysics guided stochastic approach to refining docked multimeric proteins. BMC Struct Biol 13(Suppl 1):S7

33. Phillips JC, Braun R, Wang W, Gumbart J, Tajkhorshid E, Villa E, Chipot C, Skeel RD, Kale L, Schulten K (2005) Scalable molecular dynamics with NAMD. J Comput Chem 26:1781–1802

34. Craig JJ (1989) Introduction to robotics. Mechanics and control, Electrical and computer engineering: control engineering. Addison Wesley, Reading, MA

35. Akbal-Delibas B, Hashmi I, Shehu A, Haspel N (2011) Refinement of docked protein complex structures using evolutionary traces. In: 2011 I.E. international conference on bioinformatics and biomedicine workshops (BIBMW). IEEE, Washington, DC, pp 400–404

36. Duan Y, Wu C, Chowdhury S, Lee MC, Xiong G, Zhang W, Yang R, Cieplak P, Luo R, Lee T, Caldwell J, Wang J, Kollman P (2003) A point-charge force field for molecular mechanics simulations of proteins based on condensed-phase quantum mechanical calculations. J Comput Chem 24(16):1999–2012

37. Wilkins A, Erdin S, Lua R, Lichtarge O (2012) Evolutionary trace for prediction and redesign of protein functional sites. Methods Mol Biol 819:29–42

38. Akbal-Delibas B, Jagodzinski F, Haspel N (2013) A conservation and rigidity based method for detecting critical protein residues. BMC Struct Biol 13(Suppl 1):S6

39. Jagodzinski F, Akbal-Delibas B, Haspel N (2013) An evolutionary conservation & rigidity analysis machine learning approach for detecting critical protein residues. In: CSBW (Computational Structural Bioinformatics Workshop), in proc of ACM-BCB (ACM International conference on Bioinformatics and Computational Biology). ACM, New York, NY, pp 780–786

40. Jagodzinski F, Hardy J, Streinu I (2012) Using rigidity analysis to probe mutation-induced structural changes in proteins. J Bioinform Comput Biol 10(3):1242010

41. Jacobs DJ, Rader AJ, Thorpe MF, Kuhn LA (2001) Protein flexibility predictions using graph theory. Proteins 44:150–165

42. Jacobs DJ, Thorpe MF (1995) Generic rigidity percolation: the pebble game. Phys Rev Lett 75:4051–4054

43. Lee A, Streinu I (2008) Pebble game algorithms and sparse graphs. Discret Math 308 (8):1425–1437

44. Jacobs DJ, Hendrickson B (1997) An algorithm for two-dimensional rigidity percolation: the pebble game. J Comput Phys 137:346–365

45. Fox N, Jagodzinski F, Li Y, Streinu I (2011) KINARI-Web: a server for protein rigidity analysis. Nucleic Acids Res 39(Web Server Issue):W177–W183

46. Kumar MD, Bava KA, Gromiha MM, Prabakaran P, Kitajima K, Uedaira H, Sarai A (2005) Protherm and pronit: thermodynamic databases for proteins and protein–nucleic acid interactions. Nucleic Acids Res 34(suppl 1): D204–D206

47. Higurashi M, Ishida T, Kinoshita K (2009) PiSite: a database of protein interaction sites using multiple binding states in the PDB. Nucleic Acids Res 37(suppl 1):D360–D364

48. Chih C. Chang, Chih J. Lin. 2011. LIBSVM: a library for support vector machines. ACM Trans Intell Syst Technol 2(3):1–27

49. Cheng J, Randall A, Baldi P (2006) Prediction of protein stability changes for single-site mutations using support vector machines. Protein Struct Funct Bioinform 62:1125–1132

50. Lise S, Buchan D, Pontil M, Jones DT (2011) Predictions of hot spot residues at protein-protein interfaces using support vector machines. PLoS One 6(2):e16774

51. Worth CL, Preissner R, Blundell L (2011) SDM-a server for predicting effects of

mutations on protein stability and malfunction. Nucleic Acids Res 39(Web Server Issue): W215–W222

52. Xavier Suresh M, Michael Gromiha M, Suwa M (2015) Development of a machine learning method to predict membrane protein-ligand binding residues using basic sequence information. Adv Bioinform 2015:7

53. Akbal-Delibas B, Pomplun M, Haspel N (2014) AccuRMSD: a machine learning approach to predicting structure similarity of docked protein complexes. In: Proceedings of ACM-BCB (5th ACM International conference on Bioinformatics and Computational Biology). ACM, New York, NY, pp 289–296

54. Akbal-Delibas B, Pomplun M, Haspel N. AccuRefiner: a machine learning guided refinement method for protein-protein docking. In: Proc of BICoB (7th international conference on Bioinformatics and Computational Biology), Honolulu, Hawaii, March 2015

Methods in Pharmacology and Toxicology (2016): 153–166
DOI 10.1007/7653_2015_62
© Springer Science+Business Media New York 2015
Published online: 23 April 2016

# MDock: An Ensemble Docking Suite for Molecular Docking, Scoring and In Silico Screening

## Chengfei Yan and Xiaoqin Zou

## Abstract

Molecular docking refers to computational methods for the prediction of the binding mode and binding affinity between two molecules. Over decades of development, protein–ligand docking methods have been widely used for in silico screening of molecular libraries for drug candidates, serving as a valuable tool in structure-based drug design. MDock is a protein–ligand docking suite originally released from our laboratory in 2007, which incorporates the iteratively derived knowledge-based scoring function and the ensemble docking method. In this chapter, we describe the methodology and usage of MDock for molecular docking and in silico screening. The MDock suite is freely available to academic users through applications at http://zoulab.dalton.missouri.edu/mdock.htm.

Keywords: Molecular docking, Scoring function, In silico screening, Binding affinity

## 1   Introduction

Molecular docking refers to an approach that predicts the binding mode and affinity between two interacting molecules. This approach has been widely applied to protein–ligand binding, protein–protein binding, and protein–nucleic acid binding. Molecular docking is also an important tool for structure-based drug design [1–6]. Given a potential drug target with a known three-dimensional atomic structure, a key step for drug design is to find small molecules that can bind tightly to a specific site on the target and enhance (or inhibit) the function of the target. Due to its high efficiency and low cost, molecular docking is often used for the screening of large chemical libraries for drug candidates. The top-ranked compounds from in silico screen are normally evaluated in biological assays; the confirmed active compounds are advanced for further lead optimization.

One of the examples of molecular docking tools is MDock, a protein–ligand docking suite released by our laboratory in 2007 [7]. MDock docks a rigid ligand to the protein by matching a subgroup of the ligand atomic centers to the sphere points that represent the negative image of the binding pocket, a strategy that was proposed by Kuntz and co-workers [8, 9]. Each docked pose is scored in combination with local optimization by using ITScore, an iteratively derived knowledge-based scoring function [10–12]. The pose with the lowest score is considered as the predicted binding mode, and the corresponding score is considered as the predicted binding energy score. Specifically, to account for ligand flexibility, multiple low-energy ligand conformers are pre-generated, and each conformer is docked to the protein independently. The docked conformer with the lowest score among all the conformers being docked is set as the predicted binding mode for the ligand, and the corresponding score is the predicted binding energy score.

To account for protein structural variations during ligand binding, MDock also allows users to dock a ligand simultaneously to multiple protein structures (up to 99 structures), a procedure referred to as ensemble docking. The ensemble docking algorithm in MDock is computationally efficient, with a computational time comparable to single protein docking [7, 13].

In this chapter, we will describe the methodology and the usage of MDock for molecular docking and in silico screening in detail. To further illustrate the usage of MDock for in silico screening, we will use the designed ligands for spleen tyrosine kinase (SYK), which were donated by GlaxoSmithKline (GSK) to the Community Structure-Activity Resource (CSAR) 2014 benchmark (http://www.csardock.org/) [14–16], for a case study.

## 2 Materials

### 2.1 The MDock Package

The MDock suite is freely available to academic users through application at http://zoulab.dalton.missouri.edu/mdock.htm. MDock is an open source software written in Fortran. For users who prefer to modify MDock's source code, the Intel Fortran compiler is required for compiling the executables. For users who apply MDock directly to docking studies, the pre-compiled executable files (*MDock, clu_sph,* and *get_sph*) are provided in the *bin* directory of the MDock package and are ready for use. Here, *MDock* is the command for docking, *get_sph* is for selecting the sphere points that cover the binding region, and *clu_sph* is for clustering the sphere points from multiple protein structures for ensemble docking. The source codes are placed under the *Source_codes* directory. The documentation and the demo parameter files are under the *Manual* directory. The tutorial files are under the *Tutorial* directory. Linux users can run the programs directly after *MDock* is installed and the *bin* directory is added (e.g., by typing *source Install_MDock* or by adding the path manually). For windows users, a Windows Linux emulator Cygwin (https://www.cygwin.com/) is recommended.

**2.2   The Overview of the MDock Methodology**

MDock implements a similar method to UCSF DOCK [17] to orient the rigid ligand to the binding pocket by exhaustively matching [7] the ligand atomic centers to the sphere points that represent the negative image of the binding pocket. The uniqueness of MDock lies in its iteratively derived scoring function (referred to as ITScore) and its ensemble docking method. MDock is convenient for in silico screening.

*2.2.1   The Iterative Scoring Function*

ITScore is a knowledge-based scoring function that was originally developed in our laboratory in 2006 [10, 11]. The main idea for the extraction of ITScore is to iteratively adjust the pairwise potentials by comparing the experimentally observed pair distribution functions ($g_{ij}^{obs}(r)$) derived from the native structures and the predicted pair distribution functions ($g_{ij}^k(r)$) derived from the sampled decoys (including the native structures), with each decoy carrying a Boltzmann weight calculated from the interaction potentials of the current step. Finally, ($g_{ij}^k(r)$) converge to ($g_{ij}^{obs}(r)$) with all the native structures having the lowest energies in comparison with their decoys. The idea is described by the following equations:

$$u_{ij}^{k+1}(r) = u_{ij}^k(r) + \Delta u_{ij}^k(r), \quad \Delta u_{ij}^k(r) = \frac{1}{2} K_B T[g_{ij}^k(r) - g_{ij}^{obs}(r)], \quad (1)$$

where $i$ and $j$ represent the atom types of an atom pair, respectively, and $r$ is the distance between the atom pair. $K_B$ is the Boltzmann constant, and $T$ is the temperature. $\{u_{ij}^k(r)\}$ are the pairwise potentials in the $k$th step, and $\{u_{ij}^{k+1}(r)\}$ are the updated potentials for the next step. Given a set of initial potentials $\{u_{ij}^0(r)\}$, the potentials are updated using the above iterative equation, until $\{g_{ij}^k(r)\}$ converge to $\{g_{ij}^{obs}(r)\}$ and all the native structures are associated with the lowest energies compared to their corresponding decoys. The detailed description of the iterative method is provided in [10].

It should be noted that we recently improved the scoring function by using the refined set of PDBbind 2012 [18, 19] as the new training set, which is much larger than the original training set [20]. To reproduce the results of the case study in this chapter, one should use the latest version of MDock (Ver. 2.0).

*2.2.2   The Ensemble Docking*

MDock implements the ensemble docking method to account for protein structural variations during ligand binding. Specifically, multiple protein structures are superimposed with the protein conformational state treated as an additional dimension for parameter optimization. The energy function for parameter optimization is defined as

$$E = E(x, y, z, \phi, \theta, \psi, n), \quad (2)$$

where $x$, $y$, and $z$ stand for the coordinates of the center of mass of the ligand, and $\phi$, $\theta$, and $\psi$ stand for the three Euler angles, respectively. $n$ represents the $n$th protein structure in the protein ensemble. MDock simultaneously optimizes the ligand coordinates and the protein conformational variable $n$ to automatically select the optimal protein structure that best fits the ligand.

*2.2.3 The In Silico Screening*

MDock can be easily applied to in silico screening. For a given chemical database, the user is required to prepare a mol2 format file that provides the coordinates and Sybyl atom types of the chemical compounds. The charge and hydrogen information is not needed for MDock. The effect of charges is implicitly considered in the pairwise interaction potentials of MDock through atom types. MDock will then serially dock all the compounds onto the given target protein, predict the binding modes, and rank these compounds according to the predicted binding affinities. The top candidates can be assayed for experimental verification.

**2.3 Software Dependencies**

Several additional tools are also needed for file preparation for MDock. All these tools are free for academic users.

1. UCSF Chimera [21]:
   Chimera is used for preparing the protein and ligand files and for analyzing the docking results. The software can be downloaded directly from the website http://www.cgl.ucsf.edu/chimera

2. DMS (optional):
   DMS is used for building the molecular surface. DMS can be obtained from the website http://www.cgl.ucsf.edu/Overview/software.html#dms. An alternative option is to use the *Write DMS* tool in Chimera.

3. Sphgen_cpp:
   Sphgen_cpp is an accessory tool of the UCSF Dock program suite [17]. Sphgen_cpp is used for generating sphere points based on the molecular surface files. Sphgen_cpp can be downloaded from the website http://dock.compbio.ucsf.edu/Contributed_Code/sphgen_cpp.htm.

4. OMEGA (optional) [22, 23]
   The OMEGA is a program suite released by OpenEye Scientific Software (Santa Fe, NM, USA, http://www.eyesopen.com/). The software is free for academic users. OMEGA is used for generating multiple conformations for a given ligand. The input for OMEGA can be either three-dimensional (3D) structures in pdb format or SMILES strings in smi format. One may also use other programs to sample different ligand conformers.

# 3    Methods

MDock requires the 3D structure of the protein target (or an ensemble of protein structures), the 3D structure of the ligand, and the file that contains the sphere points which represent the negative image of the binding pocket. The preparation of these files is described as follows:

## 3.1    Preparation of the Protein and Ligand Files

The structures of the protein and the ligand can be either the experimentally determined or theoretically modeled structures. MDock uses the SYBYL mol2 format files for docking. However, for the preparation of the aforementioned sphere points, the pdb file of the protein structure is also required. The pdb file and mol2 file can be easily converted from one to the other using Chimera. Multiple structures of the ligand or multiple ligands can be stored in a single mol2 file. MDock docks the multiple structures in the ligand mol2 file one by one. For ensemble docking, the multiple structures of the protein need to be superimposed together, which can be done by the *MatchMaker* tool in Chimera. The protein structures for ensemble docking can be NMR models, protein structures bound with different ligands, or conformations sampled by computational techniques such as Molecular Dynamics (MD) or Monte Carlo (MC) simulations.

It is noted that solvent molecules, ions, and other co-bound small molecules should be deleted when preparing the protein structures for docking. MDock does not require the addition of hydrogens and charges for the protein and the ligand. The hydrogen and the charge information in the input files is automatically ignored.

## 3.2    Generation and Selection of Sphere Points for Docking

It takes the following steps to generate and select sphere points for docking purpose:

1. Generating the molecular surface of the protein structure. The molecular surface of the protein structure can be generated using the following command:

    *dms protein.pdb −a −n −o protein.ms*

    where *dms* is taken from the molecular surface generation software DMS, *protein.pdb* is the pdb file of the protein structure, and *protein.ms* is the output file which contains the coordinates of the dots representing the molecular surface of the protein. Alternatively, Chimera's Write DMS tool can also be used for sphere point generation.

2. Generating sphere points based on the molecular surface of the protein structure.

The file contains the sphere points for the protein structure can be generated by

$$sphgen\_cpp \ -i \ protein.ms \ -o \ protein.sph$$

where *sphgen_cpp* is the executable of the Sphgen_cpp program in the UCSF Dock software. The output *protein.sph* file contains the coordinates of the sphere points of the protein structure.

3. Defining the putative binding site.

A pdb-format file (denoted as "*site.pdb*") that locates the putative binding site is required to prepare for the selection of the sphere points that cover the binding region. For a protein structure with known binding pocket, this pdb file can be either the coordinates of the residues close to the center of the binding pocket or the coordinates of the co-crystallized ligand(s). For a protein structure with no prior knowledge of its binding pocket, users can use any binding site prediction tools or servers, such as Q-SiteFinder [24], 3DligandSite [25], and GalaxySite [26], to predict the binding pocket.

4. Selecting the sphere points that adequately cover the binding region.

The sphere points which cover all the binding region can be selected using the following command:

$$get\_sph \ site.pdb \ protein.sph$$

where *get_sph* is an accessory command in the *bin* directory, which selects all the sphere points within a specified distance (default: 3.0 Å) from the atoms in "*site.pdb*." The default output files are *recn.sph*, *recn.pdb*, and *sph.par*. *recn.sph* contains the selected sphere points that will be used by MDock in the docking calculations. *recn.pdb* is for the display of the sphere points in *recn.sph* using Chimera. *sph.par* saves the record of the parameters used by *get_sph*.

Users should display *recn.pdb* in Chimera to examine whether the binding region was adequately covered. If not, users should use a larger cutoff for sphere points selection. The cutoff distance for sphere points selection and other parameters for *get_sph* can be specified in two ways:

1. Run *get_sph* interactively:

$$get\_sph \ site.pdb \ protein.sph \ -param$$

Users will be asked to provide a value for each parameter. If users decide to use the default value for a parameter, simply hit "Enter." The parameters will be output in the sph.par file.

2. Run *get_sph* with parameters defined in a parameter file, say, sph.par:

*get_sph site.pdb protein.sph −param sph.par*

All the parameters will then be read from this parameter file.

A detailed explanation of the parameters in *get_sph* is provided in the manual of *MDock*.

For molecular docking against a single protein structure, the sphere points in *recn.sph* will be directly used for molecular docking. The preparation is more complicated for molecular docking against multiple protein structures. Specifically, the sphere points should be prepared for each protein structure independently. Then, these sphere points generated from individual protein structures are combined and clustered as follows:

*cat */recn.sph > all.sph*
*clu_sph all.sph recn.sph*

The output file, "*recn.sph*", comprises the coordinates of the sphere points to be used for ensemble docking.

### 3.3 Molecular Docking

#### 3.3.1 Single (Protein) Docking

The docking command, *MDock*, can be executed in three ways:

1. Run *MDock* using default parameters:

*MDock protein.mol2 ligand(s).mol2*

The *ligand(s).mol2* file contains a single ligand conformer or multiple conformers of a ligand or multiple ligands. MDock automatically docks all the conformers to the protein. This method requires the sphere point file *recn.sph* as a standard input. The default parameters will be used for the docking calculation, the values of the parameters will be output in a parameter file named *MDock.par*.

2. Run *MDock* interactively:

*MDock protein.mol2 ligand(s).mol2 −param*

*MDock* will interactively ask users to provide a value for each parameter. If users prefer the default value, hit "Enter" key. The input values of the parameters will be saved in a parameter file named *MDock.par*.

3. Run *MDock* by using the parameters pre-defined in a parameter file, say, *MDock.par*:

*MDockprotein.mol2 ligand(s).mol2 −param MDock.par*

*MDock* will search in *MDock.par* for the required docking parameters. If any required parameter is missing, MDock will interactively ask the user to specify the value for the parameter.

Besides its application to molecular docking, *MDock* can also be applied to binding mode optimization, scoring, and even target selectivity. For detailed descriptions of the parameters for *MDock*, the user can refer to the MDock manual.

*3.3.2  Ensemble Docking*

For ensemble docking, the *mol2* files for the multiple protein structures should be under the same directory, with their file names sharing a user-defined prefix followed by a double-digit number (from 01 to 99) to label the protein structures. For example, if we have eight protein structures for ensemble docking, we define the prefix as *PKA*, then the eight *mol2* files will be named *PKA01.mol2*, *PKA02.mol2*, ..., and *PKA08.mol2*. The command to run *MDock* against multiple protein structures is

*MDock PKA ligand(s).mol2*

Similar to single docking, ensemble docking also requires the sphere point file, "recn.sph", and can be run interactively with user-defined parameters or with the parameters defined in a parameter file.

*3.3.3  The Output Files of MDock*

*MDock* creates three files: a mol2 file that lists the docked modes including their coordinates and energy scores (default: MDock. mol2), an output file that lists the energy scores of the docked modes (for ensemble docking, the corresponding protein structure number for each docked mode is also included) (default: MDock. out), and a file that records the information about the consumed CPU time and the number of processed ligand conformers (default: MDock.log).

# 4    The Case Study

The target SYK with its 276 ligands in the CSAR 2014 benchmark is used for the case study. The CSAR benchmark provides the SMILES strings of the ligands in an *smi*-format file (*SYK_set.smi*). The $pIC_{50}$ values of all the ligands for SYK and the complex structures (in pdb format) for eight ligands (GTC000222 to GTC000226, GTC000233, GTC000249 and GTC000250) are also released in the benchmark.

In our docking study, up to 500 conformers for each ligand were generated from its SMILES string using Omega 2.4.6 using the following command:

*omega2 -in SYK_set.smi -out ligs.mol2 -warts true -fromCT true -strictfrags true -maxconfs 500 -flipper true*

A total of 108,981 3D conformers for 276 ligands were generated and stored in *mol2* files (*ligs.mol2*). Both single docking and ensemble docking were performed. Specifically, the protein

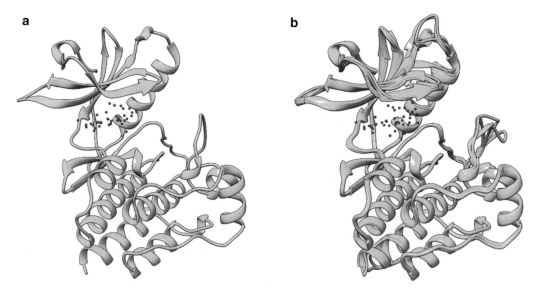

**Fig. 1** (**a**) The protein structure with the sphere points for single (protein) docking. (**b**) The protein structures with the sphere points for ensemble docking

structure from the SYK-GTC000222 complex was used for single docking. As for ensemble docking, the protein structures from the eight released complexes were superimposed with Chimera, using the protein from the SYK-GTC000222 complex as the reference structure; these eight structures formed the protein conformational ensemble.

The files containing the sphere points for single docking and ensemble docking were prepared as described in Sect. 3.2. For sphere point selection, we used the ligand coordinates (*site.pdb*) from the PDB entry 1XBC [27], which contains SYK bound with a small molecule that binds to the same binding pocket as those 276 ligands. 1XBC was also superimposed to the SYK-GTC000222 complex using Chimera.

Figure 1a, b show typical views of the protein structures and the sphere points being selected for single docking and ensemble docking, respectively. The parameter files used for single docking and ensemble docking are identical and are shown in Fig. 2. For each ligand conformer, up to 1000 poses were rigidly sampled followed by local optimization and scoring. Only the best scored pose for each conformer was saved. The computations were performed using a single 3.40 GHz Intel Core i7 CPU. Single docking took 56,265 s, whereas ensemble docking took 27,103 s. Ensemble docking is more efficient in this case study because by using multiple protein structures, the local optimization was more easily to converge, and because with more protein conformers, ensemble docking requires fewer than 1000 ligand poses to exhaustively sample the possible binding poses.

```
clash_potential_penalty        |  3.0
orient_ligand (yes/no)         |  yes
minimize_ligand (yes/no)       |  yes
maximum_orientations           |  1000
gridded_score (yes/no)         |  yes
grid_spacing (0.3~0.5)         |  0.3
sort_orientations (yes/no)     |  yes
write_score_total              |  1
write_orientations (yes/no)    |  yes
minimization_cycles (1~3)      |  1
ligand_selectivity (yes/no)    |  no
output_filename_prefix         |  mdock_dock
box_filename (optional)        |
grid_box_size                  |  8.0
sphere_point_filename          |  recn.sph
```

**Fig. 2** The parameter file used for single (protein) docking and ensemble docking

For each ligand, the best-scored binding mode (i.e., the mode with the lowest score) among all the docked conformers was considered as the predicted binding mode, and the corresponding score was considered as the predicted binding energy score. The root-mean-square-deviation (RMSD) of the heavy atoms between the predicted binding mode and the native binding mode was used as the metric for evaluating the performance of binding mode prediction, whereas the Pearson correlation coefficient ($r$) between the predicted binding energy scores and the $-pIC50$ values was used to evaluate the performance of the binding affinity prediction. Table 1 lists the RMSDs of the best predicted binding mode (with the lowest RMSD) for the top 1 prediction and for the top 3 predictions, respectively, for the eight ligands with released complex structures. The results of single docking and ensemble docking are also shown, respectively.

It can be seen from Table 1 that single docking and ensemble docking show comparable performances. An example of successful ensemble docking for binding mode prediction is shown in Fig. 3: The top prediction for the ligand GTC000222 achieved an RMSD of 0. 866 Å compared with the native binding mode. For binding affinity prediction, ensemble docking shows a better performance than single docking: In the score versus $-pIC50$ plot shown in Fig. 4, the predicted binding affinities for the 276 ligands with ensemble docking achieved a higher correlation with the $-pIC50$ values (0. 72) than the correlation achieved from single docking (0. 51).

Other applications of MDock can be found in our publications [13, 20, 28, 29].

**Table 1**
**Results of binding mode prediction on SYK with single (protein) docking and ensemble docking**

| Ligand | Single docking (Å) | | Ensemble docking (Å) | |
|---|---|---|---|---|
| | Top 1[a] | Top 3[b] | Top 1 | Top 3 |
| GTC000222 | 0.864 | 0.864 | 0.866 | 0.866 |
| GTC000223 | 0.942 | 0.942 | 2.124 | 0.965 |
| GTC000224 | 3.198 | 2.555 | 2.705 | 2.705 |
| GTC000225 | 1.318 | 1.008 | 1.685 | 1.032 |
| GTC000226 | 2.268 | 2.049 | 2.172 | 2.023 |
| GTC000233 | 1.967 | 1.310 | 1.877 | 0.894 |
| GTC000249 | 0.656 | 0.656 | 1.698 | 1.698 |
| GTC000250 | 0.799 | 0.799 | 3.422 | 0.748 |

[a] This column presents the *RMSD* between the native binding mode and the predicted binding mode of the ligand when only the top prediction is considered
[b] This column shows the *RMSD* between the native binding mode and best predicted binding mode within the top three predictions

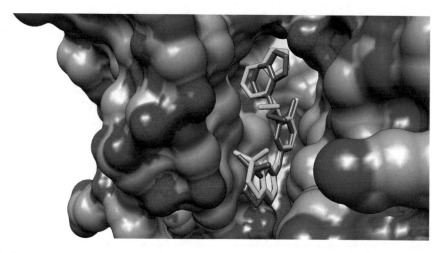

**Fig. 3** The binding mode of the ligand GTC000222 was successfully predicted by ensemble docking, with an RMSD of 0.866 Å from the native binding mode. The protein is represented by its molecular surface. The native ligand is in *cyan*, and the predicted binding mode is in *magenta*

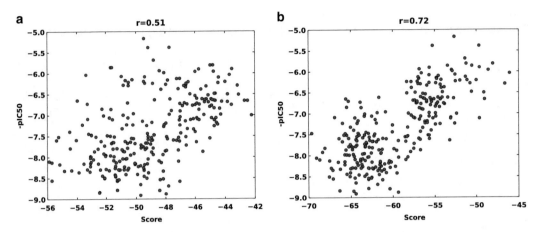

**Fig. 4** (**a**) The score versus − *pIC*50 plot for single (protein) docking. (**b**) The score versus − *pIC*50 plot for ensemble docking

## 5 Notes

1. For the preparation of the protein structures for docking, solvent molecules, ions and co-bound small molecules should be removed.

2. MDock does not need to add hydrogens and charges for the protein and the ligand. The information about hydrogens and charges in the input protein and ligand files is automatically ignored.

3. For ensemble docking, the multiple protein structures should be superimposed for preparing the sphere points and docking calculation.

4. For sphere point selection, users should manually examine the sphere points to make sure that the whole binding region is adequately covered by the sphere points. Otherwise, the value of the cutoff distance should be increased to include more sphere points.

## Acknowledgements

Xiaoqin Zou is supported by NIH grant R01GM088517, NSF CAREER Award DBI0953839, and American Heart Association (Midwest Affiliate) 13GRNT16990076. The computations were performed on the HPC resources at the University of Missouri Bioinformatics Consortium (UMBC).

# References

1. Brooijmans N, Kuntz ID (2003) Molecular recognition and docking algorithms. Annu Rev Biophys Biomol Struct 32(1):335–373

2. Kitchen DB, Decornez H, Furr JR, Bajorath J (2004) Docking and scoring in virtual screening for drug discovery: methods and applications. Nat Rev Drug Discov 3(11):935–949

3. Huang S-Y, Zou X (2010) Advances and challenges in protein-ligand docking. Int J Mol Sci 11(8):3016–3034

4. Huang S-Y, Grinter SZ, Zou X (2010) Scoring functions and their evaluation methods for protein–ligand docking: recent advances and future directions. Phys Chem Chem Phys 12 (40):12899–12908

5. Sousa SF, Ribeiro AJM, Coimbra JTS, Neves RPP, Martins SA, Moorthy NSHN, Fernandes PA, Ramos MJ (2013) Protein-ligand docking in the new millennium – a retrospective of 10 years in the field. Curr Med Chem 20 (18):2296–2314

6. Grinter SZ, Zou X (2014) Challenges, applications, and recent advances of protein-ligand docking in structure-based drug design. Molecules 19(7):10150–10176

7. Huang S-Y, Zou X (2007) Ensemble docking of multiple protein structures: considering protein structural variations in molecular docking. Proteins Struct Funct Bioinf 66(2):399–421

8. Kuntz ID, Blaney JM, Oatley SJ, Langridge R, Ferrin TE (1982) A geometric approach to macromolecule-ligand interactions. J Mol Biol 161(2):269–288

9. Ewing TJA, Kuntz ID (1997) Critical evaluation of search algorithms for automated molecular docking and database screening. J Comput Chem 18(9):1175–1189

10. Huang S-Y, Zou X (2006) An iterative knowledge-based scoring function to predict protein–ligand interactions: I. Derivation of interaction potentials. J Comput Chem 27 (15):1866–1875

11. Huang S-Y, Zou X (2006) An iterative knowledge-based scoring function to predict protein–ligand interactions: II. Validation of the scoring function. J Comput Chem 27 (15):1876–1882

12. Huang S-Y, Zou X (2011) Scoring and lessons learned with the CSAR benchmark using an improved iterative knowledge-based scoring function. J Chem Inf Model 51(9):2097–2106

13. Huang S-Y, Zou X (2007) Efficient molecular docking of NMR structures: application to HIV-1 protease. Protein Sci 16(1):43–51

14. Dunbar JB Jr, Smith RD, Yang C-Y, Ung PM-U, Lexa KW, Khazanov NA, Stuckey JA, Wang S, Carlson HA (2011) CSAR benchmark exercise of 2010: selection of the protein–ligand complexes. J Chem Inf Model 51 (9):2036–2046

15. Damm-Ganamet KL, Smith RD, Dunbar JB Jr, Stuckey JA, Carlson HA (2013) CSAR benchmark exercise 2011–2012: evaluation of results from docking and relative ranking of blinded congeneric series. J Chem Inf Model 53 (8):1853–1870

16. Dunbar JB Jr, Smith RD, Damm-Ganamet KL, Ahmed A, Esposito EX, Delproposto J, Chinnaswamy K, Kang Y-N, Kubish G, Gestwicki JE, Stuckey JA, Carlson HA (2013) CSAR data set release 2012: ligands, affinities, complexes, and docking decoys. J Chem Inf Model 53 (8):1842–1852

17. Moustakas DT, Lang PT, Pegg S, Pettersen E, Kuntz ID, Brooijmans N, Rizzo RC (2006) Development and validation of a modular, extensible docking program: Dock 5. J Comput Aided Mol Des 20(10–11):601–619

18. Wang R, Fang X, Lu Y, Yang C-Y, Wang S (2005) The PDBbind database: methodologies and updates. J Med Chem 48(12):4111–4119

19. Cheng T, Li X, Li Y, Liu Z, Wang R (2009) Comparative assessment of scoring functions on a diverse test set. J Chem Inf Model 49 (4):1079–1093

20. Yan C, Grinter SZ, Merideth BR, Ma Z, Zou X (2015) Iterative knowledge-based scoring functions derived from rigid and flexible decoy structures: evaluation with the 2013 and 2014 CSAR benchmarks. J Chem Inf Model. doi:10.1021/acs.jcim.5b00504

21. Pettersen EF, Goddard TD, Huang CC, Couch GS, Greenblatt DM, Meng EC, Ferrin TE (2004) UCSF chimera—a visualization system for exploratory research and analysis. J Comput Chem 25(13):1605–1612

22. Hawkins PCD, Skillman AG, Warren GL, Ellingson BA, Stahl MT (2010) Conformer generation with omega: algorithm and validation using high quality structures from the protein databank and Cambridge structural database. J Chem Inf Model 50(4):572–584

23. Hawkins PCD, Nicholls A (2012) Conformer generation with omega: learning from the data set and the analysis of failures. J Chem Inf Model 52(11):2919–2936

24. Laurie ATR, Jackson RM (2005) Q-sitefinder: an energy-based method for the prediction of

protein–ligand binding sites. Bioinformatics 21 (9):1908–1916

25. Wass MN, Kelley LA, Sternberg MJE (2010) 3DLigandSite: predicting ligand-binding sites using similar structures. Nucleic Acids Res. doi:10.1093/nar/gkq406

26. Heo L, Shin W-H, Lee MS, Seok C (2014) Galaxysite: ligand-binding-site prediction by using molecular docking. Nucleic Acids Res 42(W1):W210–W214

27. Atwell S, Adams JM, Badger J, Buchanan MD, Feil IK, Froning KJ, Gao X, Hendle J, Keegan K, Leon BC et al (2004) A novel mode of gleevec binding is revealed by the structure of spleen tyrosine kinase. J Biol Chem 279 (53):55827–55832

28. Grinter SZ, Liang Y, Huang S-Y, Hyder SM, Zou X (2011) An inverse docking approach for identifying new potential anti-cancer targets. J Mol Graph Model 29(6):795–799

29. Grinter SZ, Yan C, Huang S-Y, Jiang L, Zou X (2013) Automated large-scale file preparation, docking, and scoring: evaluation of ITScore and STScore using the 2012 community structure-activity resource benchmark. J Chem Inf Model 53(8):1905–1914

Methods in Pharmacology and Toxicology (2016): 167–188
DOI 10.1007/7653_2015_46
© Springer Science+Business Media New York 2015
Published online: 22 September 2015

# Pharmacophore Modeling: Methods and Applications

## David Ryan Koes

## Abstract

A pharmacophore represents the essential features of a molecular interaction and are an integral part of modern computational drug discovery. This review provides an introduction into the basic concepts and approaches of pharmacophore-based drug design using a practical example. Recently developed approaches and tools for utilizing pharmacophores are also reviewed.

**Keywords** Pharmacophore, Virtual screening, Computer-aided drug design, Structure-based drug design, Rational design, Protein–ligand interactions, Drug discovery

## 1   Introduction

Pharmacophores play an essential role in modern computational drug discovery. Hundreds of reports of pharmacophore-based virtual screens are reported every year [1], and pharmacophore modeling is integrated in a number of commercial virtual screening software packages such as Discovery Studio [2], MOE [3], SYBYL-X [1], Phase [4], and LigandScout [2]. As the topic has been expertly and comprehensively reviewed previously [5–12], here we focus on reviewing basic concepts and recent developments within the context of a practical example. For our running example we use the ligand binding domain of estrogen receptor alpha (ERα) as this system remains of clinical interest [13] and has a large amount of structural and binding data available. The details of the datasets used and how they are assessed are provided in Box 1. Using this system and freely available tools, we describe how pharmacophores are typically formulated, demonstrate some methods for elucidating pharmacophores from structural and chemical data, explain how pharmacophore matching is performed, and discuss additional considerations when integrating pharmacophore matching into a broader virtual screening workflow.

**Box 1**:
ERα Example

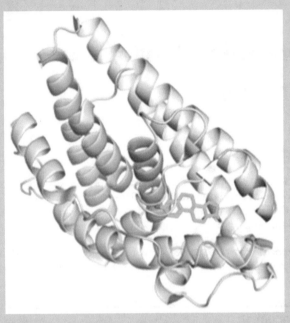

The structure of the ERα ligand binding domain with the agonist estradiol (PDB 1QKU)

For developing our pharmacophore models for ERα we use a training set of compounds with known activity and test our models using a distinct test set of compounds. For a training set, we use compounds from PubChem assay 629. This assay measures the binding of the SRC-1 nuclear receptor interaction domain to the ligand binding domain of ERα. Compounds identified as active are either direct antagonists of ERα or inhibitors of the ERα/SRC-1 interaction. For our training set we consider only those compounds that demonstrated activity in a confirmatory assay (PubChem assay 713) as active compounds and only compounds that did not exhibit activity in the primary assay (629) as inactive. Compounds with activity in the primary assay that was not reproduced in the confirmatory assay are ignored. The resulting set consists of 84,875 unique compounds of which 221 (0.26 %) are active.

For our test set we use the esr1 target of the DUD-E [14] database. This set is assembled from multiple sources and is designed to support retrospective virtual screening. There are 21,068 compounds of which 383 (1.82 %) are active. Importantly, the active compounds include both antagonists and agonists. This allows us to test predictions of protein–ligand binding

(continued)

**Box 1 (continued)**

without concern for the phenotype of the compound, which is particularly relevant for ERα since agonists and antagonists bind in the same active site.

For each compound in both sets we generated a maximum of 20 conformations, three-dimensional structures that realistically sample the internal torsions of the molecule. We used RDKit [15], which is one of the best performing open-source conformer generators [16], and the Universal Force Field (UFF) [17]. From these conformers we created searchable pharmacophore indices using Pharmer [18]. In reporting the performance of our models we report the number of true positives (TP), false positives (FP), precision, recall, F1 score, enrichment factor (EF), and p-value of enrichment (pEF). The F1 score is the harmonic mean of the precision and the recall and provides a balanced assessment of screening performance, the enrichment factor is the precision divided by the percentage of positives in the input set, and the p-value of enrichment is the probability of obtaining an enrichment at least as good as the observed enrichment by chance (calculated using a hypergeometric test). A compound is considered to match a pharmacophore model if any of its conformers is a match.

## 2  What Is a Pharmacophore?

The concepts behind pharmacophores date back more than 100 years to the ideas of Paul Ehrlich, although these nascent concepts substantially evolved over time to yield the current modern definition [19]. The official modern definition of a pharmacophore is provided by the International Union of Pure and Applied Chemistry [20]:

A pharmacophore is the ensemble of steric and electronic features that is necessary to ensure the optimal supramolecular interactions with a specific biological target structure and to trigger (or to block) its biological response.

A pharmacophore does not represent a real molecule or a real association of functional groups, but a purely abstract concept that accounts for the common molecular interaction capacities of a group of compounds towards their target structure. The pharmacophore can be considered as the largest common denominator shared by a set of active molecules.

Put more simply, a pharmacophore is a spatial arrangement of generic molecular interactions that concisely explains the biological activity of a ligand molecule. Typically the biological activity in question is protein–ligand binding.

Intrinsic to the pharmacophore concept is the three dimensional arrangement of features. It is not only *what* features are included in the pharmacophore, but also *how* these features are presented to the receptor that matters. An ideal pharmacophore describes a minimal arrangement of features that is necessary to induce activity; however, it is not, by itself, a sufficient condition for activity as molecules that match a pharmacophore may have additional properties that prevent activity. Realistically, for any given system there will be an assortment of reasonable pharmacophores as there may be a variety of possible binding modes and mechanisms of action (e.g., competitive vs allosteric) that can induce the same biological activity.

## 3   Feature Definition and Annotation

The most common features used to define pharmacophores are hydrogen bond donors/acceptors, negative/positive charges, hydrophobic regions, and aromatic rings. Excluded volumes, which specify regions of space the molecule does not overlap, or inclusion volumes, which specify regions of space a molecule must overlap, may also be used to provide purely steric constraints. More specific interaction features, such as metal interactions [21], may also be specified. Highly specific features that map directly to specific functional groups (e.g., mimics of protein side chains [22]) violate the strict definition of a pharmacophore, but may still be useful for virtual screening purposes.

Equally important as what features are specified is their arrangement in space. For both pharmacophore elucidation and matching, molecules must be annotated with pharmacophore feature points that specify a precise location that represents the feature. A pharmacophore model or query specifies a range of possible geometries for a set of pharmacophore feature points. This is typically represented using tolerance spheres. A pharmacophore model for ERα is shown in Fig. 1. We consider this pharmacophore the 'canonical' pharmacophore for ERα binding [23]. A molecule can be said to match a pharmacophore model if there exists a reasonable pose and conformation of the molecule that places the necessary features of the molecule within the specified tolerance spheres (e.g., a ring center should lie within an aromatic tolerance sphere).

Although feature definition and annotation may seem straightforward, in practice comparative studies of different pharmacophore modeling packages [24–26] found substantial differences in how molecules are annotated with pharmacophore features. Different software packages may identify different protonation states of a molecule, resulting in different hydrogen bond features. Weak hydrogen bond acceptors/donors (e.g., ester oxygens or thiols) may or may not be annotated. The direction of hydrogen bond

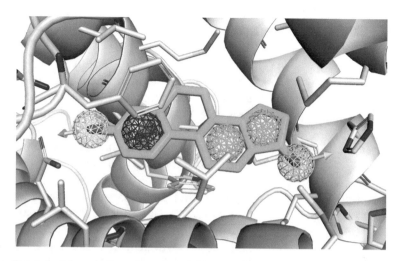

**Fig. 1** A pharmacophore for estradiol binding to the ligand binding domain of ERα. This pharmacophore model was constructed from a crystal structure (PDB 1QKU) and literature reports [23]. The hydroxyl groups at either end of estradiol make hydrogen bonds to the receptor. A hydrogen acceptor interaction is represented with an *orange mesh sphere* and a hydrogen donor interaction is represented by a *white mesh sphere*. Additionally, these interactions have a direction, indicated by the *arrows*. The core of estradiol is hydrophobic and buried in a hydrophobic cavity. These interactions are represented with *green mesh spheres*. The aromatic ring also contributes to binding, and this interaction is indicated with a *purple mesh sphere*. All spheres have a radius of 1 Å. Image generated with PyMOL [39] using the `load_query` plugin from Pharmer [18]

features is necessarily approximate when annotating a single molecule as the true orientation of the bond depends on the geometry of the full complex. Charged features are likewise dependent on protonation states and different choices can be made as to the center of a multi-atom charged group. Hydrophobic feature annotation displays the most variance across packages [25, 26] as there is no clear canonical way to reduce hydrophobic regions to a minimal set of informative points. As a consequence of the different annotation schemes, care should be taken when attempting to transition pharmacophore models between different modeling environments.

For our ERα running example, we will use the open-source Pharmer [18] pharmacophore software to identify pharmacophore features in molecules. Pharmer uses OpenBabel [27] to assign protonation states and formal charges to molecules and identifies pharmacophore features using a set of SMARTS [28] expressions, which can be customized by the user if desired. If a feature consists of multiple atoms, the feature point is placed at the geometric center of the matched atoms. Groups of hydrophobic features that are all within 2 Å of each other (i.e., they form a clique) are merged into a single feature.

## 4  Elucidating Pharmacophores

Assigning pharmacophore features is the first step in elucidating a pharmacophore model. The challenge of pharmacophore elucidation is to determine the subset of possible features of a molecule (or molecules) that best explains the observed biological activity. Pharmacophore elucidation methods are broadly categorized as ligand-based, receptor-based, and ligand-receptor based depending on the type of data they use as input.

### 4.1  Ligand-Based Pharmacophore Elucidation

Ligand-based pharmacophore elucidation takes as input a set of known actives: molecules that demonstrate the desired biological activity such as enzyme inhibition. The structure of the receptor and the three-dimensional binding mode of the ligands are not presumed to be known. These methods typically work by enumerating and overlaying conformations of the input molecules in an attempt to find those pharmacophores that are shared by the largest set of molecules. As the molecular alignment problem is computationally challenging and the objective for ranking alignments is unclear, several approaches have been proposed [5, 10]. We summarize the most recently proposed approaches here.

GAPE [29] improves upon the genetic algorithm based GASP [30] program by updating the scoring function and supporting partial matching of pharmacophore features, which allows the elucidated pharmacophore to contain features that aren't present across all input ligands. Similarly, multiobjective genetic algorithm (MOGA) [31] was enhanced by adding partial feature matching, including a clique detection based alignment initialization procedure, and biasing the conformational search to prefer torsions that are common in known structures. A novel fingerprint based approach [32] decomposes generated conformers into triangles that are then discretized into fingerprints to support efficient overlay generation. An alternative combinatorial optimization strategy for pharmacophore elucidation is growing neural gas optimization (GNG). GNG is the basis of PENG [33], which generally achieves better alignments than the default MOE [3] algorithm and was successfully used in a prospective pharmacophore screen for leukotriene A4 hydrolase. Ant colony optimization has also been proposed a viable optimization method [34] while distance geometry provides an alternative to rigid alignment methods [35].

Instead of reducing molecules to pharmacophore interaction *points*, a potentially more sophisticated and informative approach (but more computationally demanding) is to compute molecular interaction *fields* (MIFs) [36]. FLAPpharm [37] is a recent example of an MIF based approach to pharmacophore elucidation.

As an example of ligand-based pharmacophore elucidation, we applied the freely available PharmaGist [38] webserver to our training set. PharmaGist performs multiple flexible alignments of the input ligands to produce a series of ranked pharmacophores. As PharmaGist is limited to a maximum of 32 input ligands, we provided the 32 highest affinity ligands from our training set. The highest ranked five feature model is shown in Fig. 1a and the results of screening our test set with different sized models is shown in Fig. 1b. With this input set, PharmaGist failed to identify the canonical pharmacophore model, and the models that were identified did not result in a significant enrichment. This should not be seen as an indictment of PharmaGist, as it performs well in other contexts [40], but it does illustrate the challenges inherent in deriving a pharmacophore model from only ligand data.

The success of ligand-based methods is highly dependent on the nature of the provided input set, and comparing such methods requires a standardized benchmark. Such benchmarks for evaluating pharmacophore elucidation and molecular alignment algorithms were recently published [41, 42], however the methods discussed here have yet to be comprehensively and comparatively evaluated. Previous evaluations of older methods [43, 44] found that automatic pharmacophore elucidation can be successful, but benefits from expert intervention, particularly in the choice of the set of molecules used as input.

**4.2  Receptor-Based Pharmacophore Elucidation**

If ligand-binding information is not available (or is limited), but the structure of the protein target is known, receptor-based pharmacophore elucidation can be used. Even in the absence of a known structure, homology models may be productively used, as has been done for serotonin transporters [45] and G-protein-coupled receptors [46, 47]. Receptor-based elucidation was recently comprehensively reviewed [48]. The primary tasks are identifying pharmacophore features in the ligand-space from the receptor and selecting the most important features.

Geometric rules can be used to project receptor features (e.g., a hydrogen acceptor) into ligand space (e.g., a complementary hydrogen donor). As these projections are necessarily imprecise, they can be complemented (or replaced) by more sophisticated methods that compute grid energies [49], dock molecular fragments [50], or perform simulations. Simulation methods, such as Site-Identification by Ligand Competitive Saturation (SILCS) [51, 52], use molecular dynamics to simulate the target protein in solution. As the dynamics of the receptor are simulated, even an unbound, *apo*, structure may sample bound-like states. The simulated environment includes probe molecules, which may be as simple as the water molecules themselves [53], or may be a selection of organic fragments with different chemical properties, as with SILCS. Regions where a probe appears frequently are likely interaction points. For example, a hydrophobic probe, such as benzene, will disproportionately favor a hydrophobic pocket on the protein.

**a**

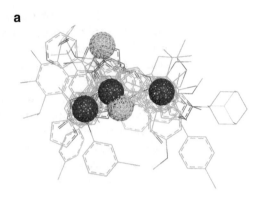

**b**

| Features | Ligands | TP | FP | Precision | Recall | F1 | EF | pEF |
|---|---|---|---|---|---|---|---|---|
| 5 | 9 | 1 | 178 | 0.56% | 0.26% | 0.004 | 0.309 | 0.961 |
| 4 | 18 | 41 | 2166 | 1.86% | 10.70% | 0.032 | 1.041 | 0.418 |
| 3 | 27 | 131 | 8083 | 1.59% | 34.20% | 0.031 | 0.892 | 0.958 |

**Fig. 2** (**a**) The alignment found by PharmaGist from the 32 highest affinity members of our training set. The five feature pharmacophore ranked highest by PharmaGist is shown. This identifies a generally linear and planar set of aromatic features (*purple*), that might correspond to the hydrophobic core of the canonical pharmacophore, but the hydrogen acceptor features (*orange*) are not clear matches to the canonical pharmacophores. (**b**) The results of using the top ranked five, four, and three feature pharmacophores to screen our test set. The resulting enrichments are not significant

Docking methods are less computationally demanding than simulation methods as they usually do not account for protein flexibility (or, if they do, limit themselves to side-chain flexibility [54]). These methods dock chemical probes and cluster and score the results to identify binding 'hot spots' that can be converted to pharmacophore features based on the chemical properties of the probe. A probe can be as simple as water [55] for identifying hydrogen bond interactions or a panel of chemically diverse probe molecules can be used. For example, the FTMap webserver [56] uses 16 different probe molecules. The application of FTMap to both bound and unbound ERα structures is shown in Fig. 2. We generate consensus pharmacophores by merging like features that are within 3 Å of each other and only retaining those features that match a majority of probes (i.e., more than 8). For both structures, the top FTMap clusters correctly identify the estradiol binding site from the full protein analysis. However, the canonical interactions are best captured in the analysis of the bound structure. On the other hand, the unbound structure analysis reveals a third interaction site that, while not relevant to the agonist estradiol, is frequently the target of antagonists. As shown in Fig. 2c, both consensus pharmacophores generate significant enrichments, although the unbound-based pharmacophore lacks generality as it matches a total of 18 compounds. These results indicate how dependent receptor-only methods are on the receptor structure and illustrate the appeal of simulation methods that consider the dynamics of the protein rather than rely on a single structure. They also show the amount of implicit information present in a bound receptor structure, even in the absence of the cognate ligand.

**4.3 Ligand-Receptor Pharmacophore Elucidation**

A protein–ligand complex provides the most direct method for elucidating a pharmacophore. Given a complex, straightforward rules can be applied to identify all the interacting features of a ligand [4, 57–59]. For example, a hydrogen donor on the ligand must be an appropriate distance and angle removed from a hydrogen acceptor on the receptor, or a hydrophobic group on the ligand must be buried in a hydrophobic pocket. However, identifying all the interacting features is not sufficient to identify a usable pharmacophore as the pharmacophore should consist of only the most essential features, and pharmacophore models with too many features will be overly selective and possibly not match any compounds.

Interacting features can be prioritized for inclusion in a pharmacophore model by computing the energetic contributions of the corresponding functional group [60], or cross-referencing with the results of a receptor-based analysis. For instance, interactions that are present in the protein–ligand complex, but are not picked up by docking or simulation methods, are likely less relevant. Simulation can also be used to refine the positions of the interacting features to partially account for receptor flexibility [61].

If ligand activity data is available, then an excellent way to elucidate an informative pharmacophore from a set of interacting features is to simply enumerate all possible pharmacophore models and evaluate them on a well constructed training set. We demonstrate this approach applied to ERα in Fig. 3. We generated all possible combinations of three, four, and five features from the nine interacting pharmacophore features identified by Pharmer from the bound ERα (PDB 1QKU) structure. All features were represented by directionless 1 Å tolerance spheres. The best performing models of each size, as determined by the F1 score on the training set, are shown in Fig. 3. All three models capture components of the canonical pharmacophore. The three feature model consists of the major polar contacts, the four feature model adds in a hydrophobic center, and the five feature model adds an aromatic interaction and exchanges a hydrogen donor for an additional hydrophobic feature. All three models have excellent performance on our test set, as shown in Fig. 3d. Enrichments are highly significant and range from 22X to 78X while even the most selective five feature pharmacophore retrieves 18.5 % of the actives in the test set.

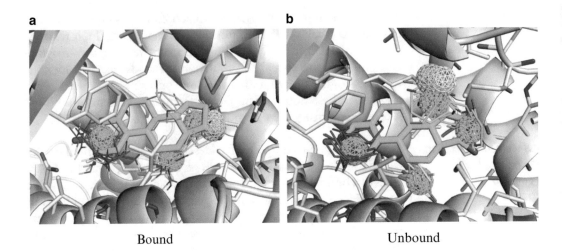

Bound                                    Unbound

**c**

|  | Features | TP | FP | Precision | Recall | F1 | EF | pEF |
|---|---|---|---|---|---|---|---|---|
| Bound | 5 | 54 | 265 | 16.93% | 14.10% | 0.154 | 11.209 | $<10^{-10}$ |
| Unbound | 6 | 5 | 13 | 27.78% | 1.31% | 0.025 | 21.157 | $10^{-5}$ |

**Fig. 3** (**a** and **b**) The results of running FTMap on a bound (PDB 1QKU) and unbound (PDB 2B23) ERα receptor structure. The top ranked clusters of chemical probes identified by FTMap are shown overlaid estradiol (*green*). Consensus pharmacophore features derived from these clusters are shown as mesh spheres. Hydrophobic features are *green*, hydrogen donors *white*, and hydrogen acceptors *orange*. The top two clusters are shown as *magenta* (*left*) and *cyan* (*right*) sticks and overlap the polar contacts from the canonical pharmacophore (Fig. 1). In the unbound structure, HIS-524 (*right*) is flipped away from the binding site resulting in a less compact cluster that, unlike the bound structure cluster, does not clearly identify the canonical polar contact. In the unbound structure a third cluster (*yellow*) identifies a hydrophobic pocket that is often filled by antagonists. These clusters serve to both identify the binding site and characterize the most likely interactions and pharmacophore features in the absence of ligand binding data or protein–ligand structures. (**c**) The results of using these pharmacophore models to screen our test set. Both result in significant enrichments, but the pharmacophore derived from the bound structure retrieved substantially more active compounds

## 5    Identifying Pharmacophore Matches

Pharmacophore search identifies those library compounds that match a pharmacophore. Pharmacophore search technologies can be categorized as fingerprint-based or alignment-based. Fingerprint-based approaches [62–64] use a variety of methods to reduce the spatial relationship between pharmacophore features in a database conformer to a Boolean or numeric fingerprint. For example, all distances between pharmacophore features can be assigned into discrete bins (e.g., distances of 1–2 Å between a hydrophobic and hydrogen donor feature) where each bin corresponds to a unique position in a Boolean fingerprint. Alternatively, distance information can be directly stored within a numeric fingerprint, as is done with FLAP [64], to eliminate the error introduced by discretizing distances at a cost of decreased computational efficiency. Numeric fingerprints may also consist of histograms of distances, as is the case with Triplets of Interaction fingerprints [65] and Atom Pair 2D-fingerprints (APfps) [66]. APfps is also noteworthy since it computes topological distances in the 2D molecule (i.e., the number of bonds between atoms) and so does not depend on the generation of molecular conformations. This simpler approach still produces reasonable correlations with three-dimensional shape similarities. Another example of a 2D pharmacophore search tool is PhAST [67] which uses a novel string alignment approach.

Fingerprint-based approaches are typically used as similarity measures. For example, the fingerprint of a molecule is compared to the fingerprint of a model using a Tanimoto (Jaccard) similarity coefficient. These approaches generally are not capable of generating an alignment of a matching molecule to the model, nor is there necessarily any guarantee that such an alignment is feasible. Nonetheless, pharmacophore similarity measures naturally integrate with other fingerprint-based methods [68] and, in addition to their utility in virtual screening, are useful for other purposes such as assessing binding site similarity [69, 70] and "target fishing" for novel targets of known ligands [58].

Alignment-based approaches perform a three-dimensional alignment between the pharmacophore model and a molecule, often by solving maximum common subgraph problems [71]. This is typically done using rigid conformations of database compounds (as with our example workflow), but flexible alignment methods, where the conformation of the compound is fit 'on-the-fly' to the target pharmacophore model, are also used. However, flexible alignment methods are computationally more expensive and it is not clear that they provide superior results [72]. Alignment methods can be used as similarity metrics by computing the volumetric overlap of pharmacophore features [73], but their primary advantage is that they produce poses of the matching molecules aligned to the pharmacophore model.

Both fingerprint and alignment approaches typically evaluate every possible molecule (conformer) in the search database and search times scale with the size of the database. More recently, index-based methods of searching, which scale with the breadth and complexity of the query, not the database size, were developed for searching and aligning libraries of rigid conformers. AnchorQuery [22] is limited to chemical spaces containing a predefined 'anchor' fragment that is used to define the coordinate system of the molecule. Pharmacophore features of rigid conformations are then stored in a spatial index at these anchor-oriented coordinates. Pharmer [18], used in our workflow, is a general purpose pharmacophore search tool that stores geometric triplets of pharmacophore features in a specialized KD-tree data structure. Searches are performed by looking up the component triangles of a pharmacophore model in this index, which is a sublinear time operation with respect to the size of the database.

A number of pharmacophore tools are freely available online as web applications. The iDrug website [74, 75] supports binding site analysis, pharmacophore elucidation, and pharmacophore search of more than 800,000 compounds using a semi-flexible alignment approach. It can also be used to search small, user-provided databases. PharmMapper [76] searches over 7000 receptor-based pharmacophores for matches to a provided query ligand. That is, the query is a ligand and the results are pharmacophore models that correspond to targets the ligand might bind. AnchorQuery [22, 77] integrates with PocketQuery [78] to support the analysis of protein–protein interaction structures and structure-based pharmacophore elucidation. It has a search database of more than two billion conformations of over 31 million synthetically accessible molecules, all designed to contain an amino acid analog. ZINC-Pharmer [59, 79] uses Pharmer [18] to search the purchasable subset of the ZINC database [80], which currently consists of more than 22 million molecules. Its interface is shown in Fig. 4 during a search for the pharmacophore of Fig. 3c. This search

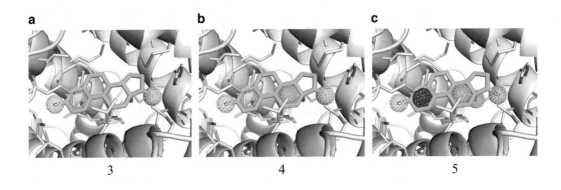

| Features | Train F1 | TP | FP | Precision | Recall | F1 | EF | pEF |
|---|---|---|---|---|---|---|---|---|
| 3 | 0.189 | 214 | 537 | 28.50% | 55.87% | 0.377 | 21.921 | $<10^{-10}$ |
| 4 | 0.301 | 140 | 139 | 50.18% | 36.55% | 0.423 | 55.404 | $<10^{-10}$ |
| 5 | 0.326 | 71 | 50 | 58.68% | 18.54% | 0.282 | 78.111 | $<10^{-10}$ |

**Fig. 4 (a–c)** The best performing pharmacophore models of three different sizes on our ERα training set, as determined by their F1 score on the training set. All possible subsets of three, four, and five interacting features from the ERα bound structure, PDB 1QKU, were generated and evaluated. (**d**) Applying these models to our test set results in highly significant enrichments. As a total of 336 models were evaluated, these enrichments remain statistically significant after applying the Bonferroni multiple test correction

took less than 8 s to identify 80,000 matches out of more than 215 million conformations.

## 6   Using the Results of Pharmacophore Search

Pharmacophore search is often successful at creating enriched subsets, as in Fig. 3. However, this is rarely the final result as often there are more hits than it is feasible to screen. Furthermore, the nature of a pharmacophore is that it identifies the existence of beneficial features, not the presence of disadvantageous features. For example, a compound may match a pharmacophore, but still exhibit severe steric or electrostatic clashes with the receptor. Additional processing of the pharmacophore hits can eliminate clearly undesirable compounds while prioritizing compounds for screening.

Metrics derived directly from the pharmacophore match, such as the root mean squared deviation (RMSD) between matched features, have a limited ability to adequately prioritize compounds, particularly when the initial pharmacophore model is already specified using small tolerances. Figure 5 shows this for the results of

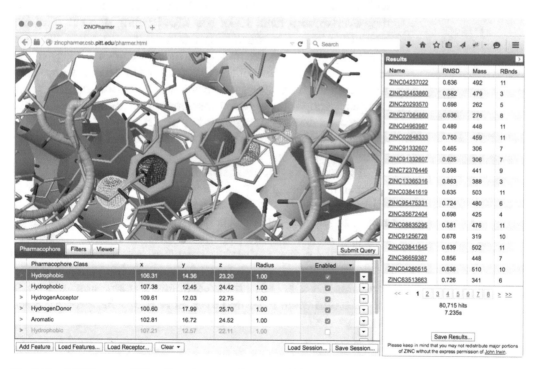

**Fig. 5** The ZINCPharmer [79] online pharmacophore search interface with the pharmacophore from Fig. 3c shown. The search of the 22 million compounds of the ZINC purchasable subset identified more than 80,000 matches and took less than 8 s

the three point pharmacophore of Fig. 3. When ranked by RMSD, the distribution of actives in the result set has no clear bias toward lower ranked, lower RMSD, compounds.

A more effective method of ranking hits is to fully use the structure of the receptor to optimize the pharmacophore aligned pose in the binding site. This can be done by docking the compounds to the binding site [81]. Alternatively, if an alignment-based method of search is used, the resulting aligned pose can be energy minimized using the same scoring functions used in docking to find a pose near the pharmacophore that is at a local minimum. We applied this approach to the 751 compounds of the test set that matched the three feature pharmacophore shown in Fig. 3. We used the minimization software smina [82], a fork of AutoDock Vina [83] that is customized to better support energy minimization and scoring function development. When minimized against the estradiol bound structure (PDB 1QKU), there is a substantial improvement in the ranking of the true actives, as shown in Fig. 5b. Of the top 100 compounds, 66 are active. However, there is also a noticeable anti-enrichment where many active compounds are ranked poorly. Inspection of the pharmacophore aligned poses of these compounds shows that many antagonists have unresolvable clashes with the agonist-bound receptor. Specifically, as shown in Fig. 6, they overlap with helix 12 of the ERα binding domain. This is a common binding mode of ERα antagonists. In these cases, as shown by the antagonist-bound structure shown in Fig. 6, the receptor adopts a substantially different conformation where helix 12 is shifted which allows larger ligands in the binding site. When our pharmacophore aligned compounds are minimized and ranked with respect to this antagonist-bound receptor, the result is an impressive prioritization of active compounds as shown in Fig. 5c. Of the top 100 compounds, 99 are active.

Although using docking scoring functions to minimize and rank pharmacophore aligned poses is an effective and computationally efficient approach, the inverse approach, where pharmacophores are used to filter or guide docking algorithms have also been successfully applied. For example, pharmacophores have been applied as a post-processing step to docking when targeting VEGFR-2 [84] and hLTC4S [85]. The integration of pharmacophore similarity measures into DOCK [86] produced dramatic improvements in pose reproduction when measured over more than 1000 protein–ligand complexes [87].

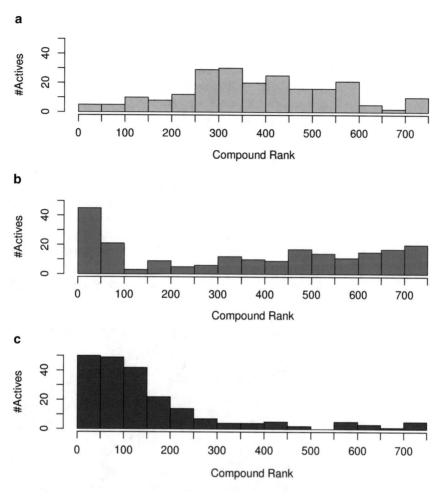

**Fig. 6** The distribution of active compounds among the 751 compounds matched by the three feature pharmacophore of Fig. 3 in our test set when ranked by different methods. (**a**) Ranked By pharmacophore RMSD. (**b**) Minimized and ranked against agonist bound receptor (PDB 1QKU). (**c**) Minimized and ranked against antagonist bound receptor (PDB 3ERT)

## 7  Discussion

We have demonstrated, through our ERα running example, that a pharmacophore-oriented screening process can be remarkably effective. However, we cannot claim the success we demonstrated with ERα generalizes to other targets. First and foremost, this is a retrospective evaluation: it is easier to arrive at the right answer when the right answer is already known. In particular, we purposely selected a target that is extensively studied and has a well-established pharmacophore [23]. It was no coincidence that the structures we developed our models from contained this known pharmacophore. There may also be a historical bias present in our compound sets as the discovery of some of the active compounds may have been guided by knowledge of this pharmacophore. Furthermore, our test set was constructed as a benchmark set and contained both agonists and antagonists. This allowed us to predict binding without concern for the ultimate phenotype.

An additional concern is the possibility of overlap between our training and test sets. Although they contained distinct sets of compounds, a high degree of chemical similarity between training and test sets can result in overly optimistic assessments of predictive performance [88]. When projected onto a two-dimensional surface, as shown in Fig. 7, the active compounds in our training and test sets do have some degree of overlap. Importantly, however, the active compounds found to match our three feature pharmacophore of Fig. 3 are not limited to this overlapping region. In fact,

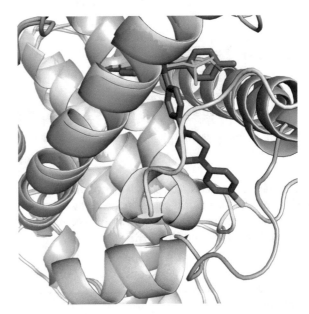

**Fig. 7** Agonist-bound (PDB 1QKU) and antagonist-bound (PDB 3ERT) structures of ERα shown with estradiol (*green*) and an inhibitor (*magenta*) that ranked nearly last when its pharmacophore aligned pose was minimized against the agonist-bound receptor but in the top ten when minimized against the antagonist-bound receptor. The main difference in the bound receptors is the movement of helix 12, shown in *yellow* in the agonist-bound conformation and *orange* in the antagonist-bound conformation. This helix is displaced in the antagonist-bound form and, consequently, inhibitors that bind to this conformation clash severely with the agonist-bound receptor

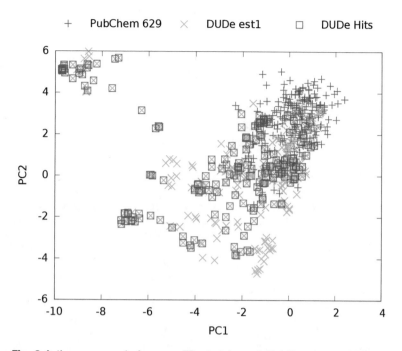

**Fig. 8** Active compounds from our ERα training set (PubChem assay 629) and test set (the est1 benchmark of DUD-E [14]) mapped onto a two dimension space. Principal components analysis (PCA) was used to reduce the OpenBabel [27] FP2 fingerprints of the full set of active compounds to the two main principal components (PC1 and PC2). Although the training set does overlap the test set, most compounds in the test set are not in this overlapping region. More importantly, the compounds identified as hits in Fig. 5 span the space, indicating that pharmacophores are not limited to the chemical space they are trained on (e.g., they are suitable for scaffold hopping)

they span the full space of active compounds in our DUD-E test set. This demonstrates that pharmacophores can generalize across a diversity of chemotypes and underlines their applicability to scaffold hopping.

We have reviewed the fundamental concepts, most recent advances, and common approaches to using pharmacophores in computational drug discovery and shown that a pharmacophore-centered workflow can achieve impressive virtual screening hit rates on an example ERα target. With the recent advances of index-based pharmacophore search methods and the availability of online tools for searching millions of commercially available compounds within seconds, there is no better time to integrate pharmacophore approaches into drug discovery projects.

## Acknowledgements

We would like to thank Lee McDermott, Dan Zuckerman, and Jocelyn Sunseri for their insightful feedback during the preparation of the manuscript. This work was supported by the National Institute of Health [R01GM108340]. The content is solely the responsibility of the author and does not necessarily represent the official views of the National Institutes of Health.

## References

1. Braga RC, Andrade CH (2013) Assessing the performance of 3d pharmacophore models in virtual screening: how good are they? Curr Top Med Chem 13(9):1127–1138

2. Guner O, Clement O, Kurogi Y (2004) Pharmacophore modeling and three dimensional database searching for drug design using catalyst: recent advances. Curr Med Chem 11 (22):2991–3005

3. Chemical Computing Group (2015) Molecular Operating Environment (MOE) version 2013.08. Chemical Computing Group, Inc.

4. Dixon S, Smondyrev A, Knoll E, Rao S, Shaw D, Friesner R (2006) PHASE: a new engine for pharmacophore perception, 3D QSAR model development, and 3D database screening: 1. Methodology and preliminary results. J Comput Aided Mol Des 20(10):647–671. doi:10.1007/s10822-006-9087-6, PubMed:17124629

5. Leach AR, Gillet VJ, Lewis RA, Taylor R (2009) Three-dimensional pharmacophore methods in drug discovery. J Med Chem 53 (2):539–558. doi:10.1021/jm900817u, PubMed:19831387

6. Yang S-Y (2010) Pharmacophore modeling and applications in drug discovery: challenges and recent advances. Drug Discov Today 15 (11–12):444–450

7. Dragos H (2011) Pharmacophore-based virtual screening. In: Bajorath J (ed) Chemoinformatics and computational chemical biology, vol 672, Methods in molecular biology. Humana Press, New York, pp 261–298

8. Mason JS, Good AC, Martin EJ (2001) 3-D pharmacophores in drug discovery. Curr Pharm Des 7(7):567–597

9. Langer T, Krovat EM (2003) Chemical feature-based pharmacophores and virtual library screening for discovery of new leads. Curr Opin Drug Discov Devel 6(3):370–376, PubMed:12833670

10. Seidel T, Ibis G, Bendix F, Wolber G (2010) Strategies for 3D pharmacophore-based virtual screening: 3D pharmacophore elucidation and virtual screening. Drug Discov Today Technol 7(4):e221–e228

11. Van Drie JH (2013) Generation of three-dimensional pharmacophore models. WIREs Comput Mol Sci 3(5):449–464

12. Martin YC (2007) 4.06 - Pharmacophore modeling: 1 methods. In: Comprehensive medicinal chemistry {II}. Elsevier, Oxford, pp 119–147

13. Chen GG, Zeng Q, Tse GMK (2008) Estrogen and its receptors in cancer. Med Res Rev 28 (6):954–974

14. Mysinger MM, Carchia M, Irwin JJ, Shoichet BK (2012) Directory of useful decoys, enhanced (DUD-E): better ligands and decoys for better benchmarking. J Med Chem 55 (14):6582–6594. doi:10.1021/jm300687e, PubMed:22716043. PubMed Central: PMC3405771

15. RDKit: open-source cheminformatics. http://www.rdkit.org. Accessed 4 Sep 2012

16. Ebejer J-P, Morris GM, Deane C (2012) Freely available conformer generation methods: how good are they? J Chem Inf Model. doi:10.1021/ci2004658, PubMed:22482737

17. Rappe AK, Casewit CJ, Colwell KS, Goddard WA, Skiff WM (1992) Uff, a full periodic table force field for molecular mechanics and molecular dynamics simulations. J Am Chem Soc 114 (25):10024–10035

18. Koes DR, Camacho CJ (2011) Pharmer: efficient and exact pharmacophore search. J Chem Inf Model 51(6):1307–1314. doi:10.1021/ci200097m, PubMed:21604800. PubMed Central:PMC3124593

19. Güner OF, Phillip Bowen J (2014) Setting the record straight: the origin of the pharmacophore concept. J Chem Inf Model 54 (5):1269–1283

20. Wermuth CG, Ganellin CR, Lindberg P, Mitscher LA (1998) Glossary of terms used in medicinal chemistry (IUPAC Recommendations 1998). Pure Appl Chem 70(5):1129

21. Hou X, Du J, Liu R, Zhou Y, Li M, Xu W, Fang H (2015) Enhancing the sensitivity of pharmacophore-based virtual screening by incorporating customized zbg features: a case study using histone deacetylase 8. J Chem Inf Model 55 (4):861–871

22. Koes D, Khoury K, Huang Y, Wang W, Bista M, Popowicz GM, Wolf S, Holak TA, Dömling A, Camacho CJ (2012) Enabling large-scale design, synthesis and validation of small molecule protein-protein antagonists. PLoS One 7 (3):e32839 EP. doi:10.1371/journal.pone. 0032839, PubMed:22427896. PubMed Central:PMC3299697

23. Anstead GM, Carlson KE, Katzenellenbogen JA (1997) The estradiol pharmacophore: ligand structure-estrogen receptor binding affinity relationships and a model for the receptor binding site. Steroids 62(3):268–303, PubMed:9071738

24. Sanders MPA, Barbosa AJM, Zarzycka B, Nicolaes GAF, Klomp JPG, de Vlieg J, Del Rio A (2012) Comparative analysis of pharmacophore screening tools. J Chem Inf Model 52 (6):1607–1620

25. Spitzer GM, Heiss M, Mangold M, Markt P, Kirchmair J, Wolber G, Liedl KR (2010) One concept, three implementations of 3D pharmacophore-based virtual screening: distinct coverage of chemical search space. J Chem Inf Model 50(7):1241–1247. doi:10.1021/ci100136b, PubMed:20583761

26. Wolber G, Seidel T, Bendix F, Langer T (2008) Molecule-pharmacophore superpositioning and pattern matching in computational drug design. Drug Discov Today 13(1–2):23–29. doi:10.1016/j.drudis.2007.09.007, Epub 2007 Nov 5

27. O'Boyle NM, Banck M, James CA, Morley C, Vandermeersch T, Hutchison GR (2011) Open Babel: an open chemical toolbox. J Cheminform 3:33. doi:10.1186/1758-2946-3-33, PubMed:21982300. PubMed Central: PMC3198950

28. Daylight theory manual, daylight version 4.9 ed. Feb 2008. Daylight Chemical Information Systems, Inc., Aliso Viejo, CA

29. Jones G (2010) Gape: an improved genetic algorithm for pharmacophore elucidation. J Chem Inf Model 50(11):2001–2018

30. Jones G, Willet P, Glen R (2000) GASP: genetic algorithm superimposition program. In: Güner OF (ed) Pharmacophore perception, development, and use in drug design, vol 2.

International University Line, La Jolla, CA, pp 85–106

31. Gardiner EJ, Cosgrove DA, Taylor R, Gillet VJ (2009) Multiobjective optimization of pharmacophore hypotheses: bias toward low-energy conformations. J Chem Inf Model 49 (12):2761–2773

32. Taylor R, Cole JC, Cosgrove DA, Gardiner EJ, Gillet VJ, Korb O (2012) Development and validation of an improved algorithm for overlaying flexible molecules. J Comput Aided Mol Des 26(4):451–472

33. Moser D, Wittmann SK, Kramer J, Blöcher R, Achenbach J, Pogoryelov D, Proschak E (2015) Peng: a neural gas-based approach for pharmacophore elucidation. method design, validation, and virtual screening for novel ligands of lta4h. J Chem Inf Model 55 (2):284–293

34. Korb O, Monecke P, Hessler G, Stützle T, Exner TE (2010) Pharmacophore: multiple flexible ligand alignment based on ant colony optimization. J Chem Inf Model 50 (9):1669–1681

35. Binns M, de Visser SP, Theodoropoulos C (2012) Modeling flexible pharmacophores with distance geometry, scoring, and bound stretching. J Chem Inf Model 52(2):577–588

36. Artese A, Cross S, Costa G, Distinto S, Parrotta L, Alcaro S, Ortuso F, Cruciani G (2013) Molecular interaction fields in drug discovery: recent advances and future perspectives. WIREs Comput Mol Sci 3(6):594–613

37. Cross S, Baroni M, Goracci L, Cruciani G (2012) Grid-based three-dimensional pharmacophores i: Flappharm, a novel approach for pharmacophore elucidation. J Chem Inf Model 52(10):2587–2598

38. Schneidman-Duhovny D, Dror O, Inbar Y, Nussinov R, Wolfson HJ (2008) PharmaGist: a webserver for ligand-based pharmacophore detection. Nucleic Acids Res 36: W223–W228. doi:10.1093/nar/gkn187, PubMed:18424800. PubMed Central: PMC2447755

39. The PyMOL Molecular Graphics System, Version 1.6. Schrödinger, LLC, August. http://www.pymol.org/

40. Schneidman-Duhovny D, Dror O, Inbar Y, Nussinov R, Wolfson HJ (2008) Deterministic pharmacophore detection via multiple flexible alignment of drug-like molecules. J Comput Biol 15(7):737–754. doi:10.1089/cmb.2007. 0130, PubMed:18662104. PubMed Central: PMC2699263

41. Giangreco I, Cosgrove DA, Packer MJ (2013) An extensive and diverse set of molecular

overlays for the validation of pharmacophore programs. J Chem Inf Model 53(4):852–866

42. Cross S, Ortuso F, Baroni M, Costa G, Distinto S, Moraca F, Alcaro S, Cruciani G (2012) Grid-based three-dimensional pharmacophores ii: Pharmbench, a benchmark data set for evaluating pharmacophore elucidation methods. J Chem Inf Model 52 (10):2599–2608

43. Patel Y, Gillet VJ, Bravi G, Leach AR (2002) A comparison of the pharmacophore identification programs: catalyst, DISCO and GASP. J Comput Aided Mol Des 16(8):653–681, PubMed:12602956

44. Tiikkainen P, Markt P, Wolber G, Kirchmair J, Distinto S, Poso A, Kallioniemi O (2009) Critical comparison of virtual screening methods against the MUV data set. J Chem Inf Model 49(10):2168–2178. doi:10.1021/ci900249b, PubMed:19799417

45. Manepalli S, Geffert LM, Surratt CK, Madura JD (2011) Discovery of novel selective serotonin reuptake inhibitors through development of a protein-based pharmacophore. J Chem Inf Model 51(9):2417–2426

46. Sanders MPA, Verhoeven S, de Graaf C, Roumen L, Vroling B, Nabuurs SB, de Vlieg J, Klomp JPG (2011) Snooker: a structure-based pharmacophore generation tool applied to class A GPCRs. J Chem Inf Model 51 (9):2277–2292

47. Klabunde T, Giegerich C, Evers A (2009) Sequence-derived three-dimensional pharmacophore models for g-protein-coupled receptors and their application in virtual screening. J Med Chem 52(9):2923–2932

48. Sanders MPA, McGuire R, Roumen L, de Esch IJP, de Vlieg J, Klomp JPG, de Graaf C (2012) From the protein's perspective: the benefits and challenges of protein structure-based pharmacophore modeling. Med Chem Commun 3:28–38

49. Bingjie H, Lill MA (2013) Exploring the potential of protein-based pharmacophore models in ligand pose prediction and ranking. J Chem Inf Model 53(5):1179–1190

50. Rafał K, Bojarski AJ (2013) New strategy for receptor-based pharmacophore query construction: a case study for 5-ht7 receptor ligands. J Chem Inf Model 53(12):3233–3243

51. Wenbo Y, Lakkaraju SK, Raman EP, MacKerell AD Jr (2014) Site-identification by ligand competitive saturation (silcs) assisted pharmacophore modeling. J Comput Aided Mol Des 28(5):491–507

52. Wenbo Y, Lakkaraju SK, Raman EP, Fang L, MacKerell AD (2015) Pharmacophore

modeling using site-identification by ligand competitive saturation (silcs) with multiple probe molecules. J Chem Inf Model 55 (2):407–420

53. Bingjie H, Lill MA (2012) Protein pharmacophore selection using hydration-site analysis. J Chem Inf Model. doi:10.1021/ci200620h, PubMed:22397751. PubMed Central: PMC3422394

54. Grove LE, Hall DR, Beglov D, Vajda S, Kozakov D (2013) Ftflex: accounting for binding site flexibility to improve fragment-based identification of druggable hot spots. Bioinformatics 29(9):1218–1219

55. Ross GA, Morris GM, Biggin PC (2012) Rapid and accurate prediction and scoring of water molecules in protein binding sites. PLoS One 7 (3):e32036. doi:10.1371/journal.pone. 0032036, PubMed:22396746. PubMed Central:PMC3291545

56. Kozakov D, Grove LE, Hall DR, Bohnuud T, Mottarella SE, Luo L, Xia B, Beglov D, Vajda S (2015) The FTMap family of web servers for determining and characterizing ligand-binding hot spots of proteins. Nat Protoc 10 (5):733–755

57. Wolber G, Langer T (2004) LigandScout: 3-D pharmacophores derived from protein-bound ligands and their use as virtual screening filters. J Chem Inf Model 45(1):160–169. doi:10. 1021/ci049885e, PubMed:15667141

58. Meslamani J, Li J, Sutter J, Stevens A, Bertrand HO, Rognan D (2012) Protein-ligand-based pharmacophores: generation and utility assessment in computational ligand profiling. J Chem Inf Model 52(4):943–955

59. Koes DR, Camacho CJ (2012) ZINCPharmer: pharmacophore search of the ZINC database. Nucleic Acids Res 40:W409–W414. doi:10. 1093/nar/gks378, PubMed:22553363. PubMed Central:PMC3394271

60. Salam NK, Nuti R, Sherman W (2009) Novel method for generating structure-based pharmacophores using energetic analysis. J Chem Inf Model 49(10):2356–2368

61. Bowman AL, Makriyannis A (2011) Approximating protein flexibility through dynamic pharmacophore models: application to fatty acid amide hydrolase (faah). J Chem Inf Model 51(12):3247–3253

62. Mason JS, Morize I, Menard PR, Cheney DL, Hulme C, Labaudinieres RF (1999) New 4-point pharmacophore method for molecular similarity and diversity applications: overview of the method and applications, including a novel approach to the design of combinatorial libraries containing privileged substructures.

J Med Chem 42(17):3251–3264. doi:10. 1021/jm9806998, PubMed:10464012

63. Mason JS, Cheney DL (2000) Library design and virtual screening using multiple 4 point pharmacophore fingerprints. Pac Symp Biocomput 5:576–587, PubMed:10902205

64. Baroni M, Cruciani G, Sciabola S, Perruccio F, Mason JS (2007) A common reference framework for analyzing/comparing proteins and ligands. Fingerprints for Ligands and Proteins (FLAP): theory and application. J Chem Inf Model 47(2):279–294. doi:10.1021/ci600253e, PubMed:17381166

65. Desaphy J, Raimbaud E, Ducrot P, Rognan D (2013) Encoding protein-ligand interaction patterns in fingerprints and graphs. J Chem Inf Model 53(3):623–637

66. Awale M, Reymond J-L (2014) Atom pair 2d-fingerprints perceive 3d-molecular shape and pharmacophores for very fast virtual screening of zinc and gdb-17. J Chem Inf Model 54 (7):1892–1907

67. Hähnke V, Schneider G (2011) Pharmacophore alignment search tool: influence of scoring systems on text-based similarity searching. J Comput Chem 32(8):1635–1647

68. Cereto-Massagué A, Ojeda MJ, Valls C, Mulero M, Garcia-Vallvé S, Pujadas G (2015) Molecular fingerprint similarity search in virtual screening. Methods 71:58–63

69. Wood DJ, de Vlieg J, Wagener M, Ritschel T (2012) Pharmacophore fingerprint-based approach to binding site subpocket similarity and its application to bioisostere replacement. J Chem Inf Model 52(8):2031–2043

70. Desaphy J, Azdimousa K, Kellenberger E, Rognan D (2012) Comparison and druggability prediction of protein-ligand binding sites from pharmacophore-annotated cavity shapes. J Chem Inf Model 52(8):2287–2299

71. Raymond JW, Willett P (2002) Maximum common subgraph isomorphism algorithms for the matching of chemical structures. J Comput Aided Mol Des 16(7):521–533, PubMed:12510884

72. Dror O, Schneidman-Duhovny D, Inbar Y, Nussinov R, Wolfson HJ (2009) Novel approach for efficient pharmacophore-based virtual screening: method and applications. J Chem Inf Model 49(10):2333–2343

73. Vilar S, Tatonetti NP, Hripcsak G (2015) 3D pharmacophoric similarity improves multi adverse drug event identification in pharmacovigilance. Sci Rep 5

74. Wang X, Chen H, Yang F, Gong J, Li S, Pei J, Liu X, Jiang H, Lai L, Li H (2014) idrug: a web-accessible and interactive drug discovery and design platform. J Cheminform 6(1):28

75. iDrug - an online interactive drug discovery and design platform. http://lilab.ecust.edu. cn/idrug. Accessed 4 May 2015

76. Liu X, Ouyang S, Yu B, Liu Y, Huang K, Gong J, Zheng S, Li Z, Li H, Jiang H (2010) PharmMapper server: a web server for potential drug target identification using pharmacophore mapping approach. Nucleic Acids Res 38: W609–W614. doi:10.1093/nar/gkq300, PubMed:20430828. PubMed Central: PMC2896160

77. AnchorQuery. http://anchorquery.csb.pitt. edu. Accessed 4 May 2015

78. Ryan Koes D, Camacho CJ (2012) PocketQuery: protein-protein interaction inhibitor starting points from protein-protein interaction structure. Nucleic Acids Res. doi:10.1093/nar/gks336, PubMed:22523085. PubMed Central:PMC3394328

79. ZINCPharmer. http://zincpharmer.csb.pitt. edu. Accessed 4 May 2015

80. Irwin JJ, Sterling T, Mysinger MM, Bolstad ES, Coleman RG (2012) ZINC: a free tool to discover chemistry for biology. J Chem Inf Model 52(7):1757–1768. doi:10.1021/ci3001277, Epub 2012 Jun 15

81. Drwal MN, Griffith R (2013) Combination of ligand- and structure-based methods in virtual screening. Drug Discov Today Technol 10(3): e395–e401

82. Koes DR, Baumgartner MP, Camacho CJ (2013) Lessons learned in empirical scoring with smina from the CSAR 2011 benchmarking exercise. J Chem Inf Model 53 (8):1893–1904

83. Trott O, Olson AJ (2010) AutoDock Vina: improving the speed and accuracy of docking with a new scoring function, efficient optimization, and multithreading. J Comput Chem 31 (2):455–461, http://www.ncbi.nlm.nih.gov/pubmed/19499576

84. Planesas JM, Claramunt RM, Teixidó J, Borrell JI, Pérez-Nueno VI (2011) Improving vegfr-2 docking-based screening by pharmacophore postfiltering and similarity search postprocessing. J Chem Inf Model 51 (4):777–787

85. Thangapandian S, John S, Sakkiah S, Lee KW (2011) Molecular docking and pharmacophore filtering in the discovery of dual-inhibitors for human leukotriene a4 hydrolase and leukotriene c4 synthase. J Chem Inf Model 51 (1):33–44

86. Moustakas DT, Lang PT, Pegg S, Pettersen E, Kuntz ID, Brooijmans N, Rizzo RC (2006) Development and validation of a modular, extensible docking program: Dock 5. J Comput Aided Mol Des 20(10-11):601–619

87. Jiang L, Rizzo RC (2015) Pharmacophore-based similarity scoring for dock. J Phys Chem B 119(3):1083–1102

88. Kramer C, Gedeck P (2010) Leave-cluster-out cross-validation is appropriate for scoring functions derived from diverse protein data sets. J Chem Inf Model 50(11):1961–1969, 10.1021/ci100264e

89. Certara. SYBYL-X. http://www.certara.com/products/molmod/sybyl-x/

Methods in Pharmacology and Toxicology (2016): 189–215
DOI 10.1007/7653_2015_51
© Springer Science+Business Media New York 2015
Published online: 10 February 2016

# Computational Fragment-Based Drug Design

## Chunquan Sheng, Guoqiang Dong, and Chen Wang

### Abstract

Fragment-based drug design (FBDD) is a promising approach for drug discovery. Experimental FBDD faces some intrinsic limitations and challenges such as the high requirements for the quality of target proteins and biophysical techniques. Computational FDBB can be used independently or in parallel with experimental FBDD to significantly improve the efficiency and success rate of lead discovery and optimization. In this chapter, we describe the protocols of computational FBDD, the recent advances in new algorithms and some successful examples. Both the advantages and the limitations of various computational methods are also discussed.

Keywords: Computational fragment-based drug design, Fragment informatics, Fragment docking, Fragment-based de novo design

## 1 Experimental Fragment-Based Drug Design

The key step in drug discovery is to discover small molecules that bind to a biological target with high affinity and selectivity. Conventionally, high-throughput screening (HTS) is a routine method to identify initial hit or lead compounds in the pharmaceutical industry [1]. However, HTS has several limitations such as small coverage of drug-like chemical space [2] ($10^6$–$10^7$ screening compounds versus $10^{60}$ drug-like molecules), low hit rates and unfavorable physico-chemical properties (e.g., large molecular weight and high hydrophobicity) [3]. Thus, the optimization of HTS-derived hits into drug-like candidates could be a difficult task with low efficiency.

As an alternative approach, fragment-based drug design (FBDD) is becoming an efficient method for drug discovery [4]. FBDD constructs novel drug-like lead compounds from small fragments by taking advantages of both random screening and structure-based drug design (SBDD). Compared to HTS, FBDD has several advantages, including sampling a larger chemical space (higher chemical diversity), higher hit rates, and higher ligand efficiency (LE = $-\log$ IC$_{50}$/number of heavy atoms) [5, 6]. The workflow of FBDD is depicted in Fig. 1. The first step of FBDD is to detect weak to moderate binders (5 mM to 1 μM) of the desired target by screening a library containing hundreds to thousands of

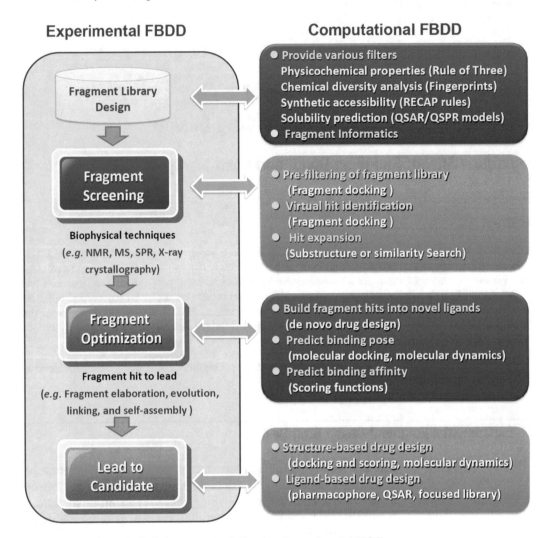

**Fig. 1** The complementarity between computational and experimental FBDD

fragments at a high concentration [7, 8]. The detection methods for fragment screening include nuclear magnetic resonance (NMR) [9, 10], mass spectroscopy (MS) [11, 12], X-ray crystallography [13], and surface plasmon resonance (SPR) spectroscopy [14, 15]. These biophysical techniques are highly sensitive to the relatively weak fragment binders. Then, on the basis of the structural information of the target-fragment complex, various optimization strategies, such as fragment linking, fragment evolution, fragment optimization, and fragment self-assembly, can be used separately or in combination to increase the affinity and drug-likeness of fragment hits [16]. Finally, the lead-to-candidate optimization is technically similar to that of conventional drug design methods [4].

Although FBDD has made a great success in drug discovery [17–19], it still faces some intrinsic limitations and challenges.

Firstly, the sampling of a larger region of drug-like space is still required. Despite its better performance than HTS, a FBDD study using a typical library of $10^3$ fragments can only sample approximately the chemical diversity space of $10^9$ molecules. Secondly, current fragment screening methods depend largely on high quality target proteins, expensive equipment, and specific expertise [20], which limits their application to a broader range of targets. For example, the application of FBDD to membrane proteins (e.g., G-protein coupled receptors, GPCRs) remains a significant challenge because of the high demand on the amount, purity and solubility of target proteins for labeling or crystallization [21]. Thirdly, it is difficult for current FBDD methods to treat flexibility and selectivity during fragment detection and optimization [22, 23] because the conformation and key interactions of the original fragment hits may be changed once they are constructed into a new molecule. Therefore, most of the FBDD methods need to be improved to take ligand specificity or selectivity into account.

## 2   Computational Fragment-Based Drug Design

To overcome the limitations of experimental FBDD, computational approaches provide an alternative to improve the efficiency and success rate of drug discovery. The protocol for computational FBDD includes (Fig. 1): (1) construction of a virtual fragment library; (2) fragment-based active site mapping and characterization; (3) fragment docking to identify initial hits; (4) hit-to-lead-to-candidate optimization [24–31]. The computational FBDD process can be used as a integrated workflow. Any single step in this process can also be used as a complementary method to assist experimental FBDD in an efficient and cost-effective manner (Fig. 1).

As compared with experimental FBDD, computational approaches have several advantages. First, high quality fragment libraries can be constructed by computational approaches. Various computational filters can be designed to improve the chemical diversity, physicochemical properties, solubility and synthetic accessibility of the fragment library [7, 8, 32]. Computational methods are also useful to exclude fragments with unwanted chemical groups and incorporate drug-like fragments, such as the most frequently occurring fragments from known drugs. Secondly, larger fragment databases can be explored by computational tools. Unlike the low-throughput nature of experimental FBDD, virtual fragment screening can identify potent hits without using complicated detection techniques. Molecular docking can be used as a prescreen tool to reduce experimental efforts of FBDD. Thirdly, computational approaches provide efficient and flexible optimization strategies to improve the activity and drug-likeness of the fragment hits. Substructure search and similarity-based search can be used to accelerate hit expansion and obtain structure–activity relationship (SAR) information for a secondary design [33, 34]. Moreover, totally new compounds can be designed using fragment hits as "seeds." The selection of most promising fragment hits for the subsequent optimization is facilitated by computational analysis of the structural information of the protein-hit complex. In silico SBDD methods are also able to build up or assemble the fragment hits into a new molecule with improved potency and drug-likeness. For example, an appropriate linker to join fragment hits can be virtually screened by de novo drug design algorithms [35, 36]. For the designed molecules, their binding affinities and binding poses are predicted by molecular docking and molecular dynamics simulations, and the best compounds can be subjected for chemical synthesis and biological assaying [37, 38]. Computational SBDD tools now play an important role in fragment-to-lead and lead-to-candidate optimization studies and have led to several clinical candidates [28, 29].

## 3 Construction of a Fragment Library

### 3.1 The Definition of a Fragment

It is difficult to give a precise definition for the term 'fragment'. Generally, a fragment is a substructure of a more complex molecule, which has low molecular weight, high solubility and weak binding affinity with the target protein. In FBDD, fragments are often used as building blocks to design lead compounds with improved biological activity. The most well-accepted definition of fragments is the "rule of three" (RO3) [39]. The physicochemical properties of a fragment should meet the criteria: (1) MW $\leq$ 300 Da; (2) hydrogen bond donors (HBA) and acceptors (HBD) $\leq$ 3; (3) LogP $\leq$ 3. Additional physicochemical properties for a fragment include: (1) rotatable bonds $\leq$ 3, (2) polar surface area (PSA) $\leq$ 60 Å$^2$. According to the literatures, a typical fragment hit in FBDD has the MW in the range of 120–250 and the binding affinity in the range 30 μM to 1 mM [16]. More recently, modifications or extensions of the RO3 have been suggested [40–42].

### 3.2 How to Construct a Virtual Fragment Library

Library design for experimental FBBD can be referred to several recent papers [7, 43, 44]. Herein, the construction of a virtual fragment library was focused on. The first step is to break molecules into fragments by in silico fragmentation methods. The publicly or commercially available databases, such as PubChem [45], eMolecules [46], WOMBAT [47], ZINC [48], WDI [49], Medchem [50], MDDR [51], and CMC [52], provide rich sources for fragmentation and fragment library design. Computational fragmentation approaches can be classified as substructure methods and building block methods. The substructure approaches treat fragment as a substructure of the molecule and completely analyze all possible fragments [53]. They are not specific fragmentation methods and are often used in similarity searches. The building block methods use predefined breaking rules to dissect molecules into chemically meaningful fragments (e.g., rings, functional groups, side-chains, and linkers) and have broad applications in computational FBDD. For example, our group built drug-like fragment libraries by decomposition of the molecules in MDDR database [51] into rings, linkers, and side chains [54]. Virtual retro-synthesis is another efficient way for fragmentation. RECAP is the most widely used method that employs several common chemical reactions as the rules to break structures and the bonds formed by one of these reactions are cleaved [55]. RECAP has been successfully used to explore drug-like fragments in marketed drugs [56, 57] and construct synthetically feasible fragment libraries [58]. However, RECAP only covers a very limited number of generally applicable reactions. Lessel et al. used the Ftrees-FS (Feature Trees Fragment Space Search) method [59, 60] to generate a huge fragment library encoding about $5 \times 10^{11}$ compounds based on more synthetic protocols [61] Unlike RECAP, several methods constructed fragment libraries that avoid using retro-synthetic rules. For example, Cramer's group developed Topomer search methodologies, such as ChemSpace [62] and AllChem [63], to navigate fragment space through known chemistry [64]. The maximum number of permitted bond deletions per iteration and the total number of iterations determine the average size of fragments and the composition of the fragment population. According to Schulz's evaluation of six computational tools for the construction of a fragment library, the best method to design a diverse fragment library is the iteratively removal protocol [44].

### 3.3 Major Fragment Libraries for FBDD

The major fragment libraries and their key features are listed in Table 1. These libraries can be freely downloaded in different file formats (e.g., SDF, MDL, SMILE). Most of them meet the criteria of the RO3 and can be used for both experimental and computational FBDD. However, the HBA and HBD criteria have not been widely adopted [65]. Therefore, the ChemDiv fragment library used softened filters for HBD ($\leq 7$) and HBA ($\leq 7$). Notably, the majority of commercially available libraries are predominantly populated with flat (hetero)aromatic fragments. However, the protein–ligand interaction is three-dimensional (3D). Thus, the design of fragment library with enhanced 3D characteristics would help to increase the fragment chemical space and discover ligand-efficient, medicinally attractive, and chemically tractable fragment hits [66]. $Fsp^3$ parameter, the number of $sp^3$-hybridized carbons in total carbon count, is an important criterion to evaluate the 3D properties of a compound library. ChemDiv (http://www.chemdiv.com/) constructed a 3D fragment library ($Fsp^3 \geq 0.4$ and/or at least one chiral centers in structure) featured with bridged-fragments and

**Table 1**
**Major fragment libraries and their key features**

| Name | Number of fragments | Key features |
|------|---------------------|--------------|
| ZINC Fragment Library | 847,909 | RO3 compliance and virtual library |
| Maybridge Fragment Libraries | 2500 | RO3 compliance, computationally engineered diversity, and commercial availability |
| ChemBridge's Fragment Library | >7000 | RO3 compliance and commercial availability |
| Enamine Golden Fragment Library | 1300 | RO3 compliance, chemical diversity (coefficient = 0.885), and commercial availability |
| ChemDiv Fragment Library | >15,700 | Softened filters of RO3 (HBA and HBD $\leq$ 7), chemical diversity (coefficient = 0.87), and commercial available |
| ChemDiv 3D Fragment Library | >4400 | Softened filters of RO3 (HBA $\leq$ 5 and HBD $\leq$ 8), at least one chiral center, spiro and bridged fragments |

spiro-fragments. Recently, several UK not-for-profit drug discovery groups formed the 3D Fragment Consortium (http://www.3DFrag.org) to build a shared library of between 500 and 3000 fragments with a complementary set of 3D fragments. Young's group constructed a unique set of 3D fragments containing highly sp$^3$-rich skeletons by diversity-oriented synthesis (DOS) [67]. Waldmann's group built a natural-product-derived fragment library containing 2000 structurally diverse molecules that are rich in sp3-configured centers by the computational analysis of more than 180,000 natural products [68]. This 3D fragment library successfully yielded novel phosphatases inhibitors and stabilizers of inactive conformations of p38a MAP kinase. Despite the advantages of 3D fragment library, Jhoti et al. cautioned that there was a tendency to increase fragment size in 3D fragment libraries, and fragments should be simple enough to probe the basic architecture of all proteins [65].

### 3.4 Fragment Space

Fragment space means combinations of molecular fragments and their connection rules. Due to the "combinatorial explosion," a rather small number of fragments can span a large chemical space [59]. The generation of drug-like and chemically tractable fragment space provides basis to discover active compounds against a large variety of targets [69]. Fragmentation and chemoinformatic analysis of the large chemical database is the most commonly used method to generate fragment space. For example, on the basis of RECAP-based fragmentation of the WDI 2004 [49] and the Medchem03 [50] databases, Mauser et al. generated 1000-size fragment space containing a subset with the most frequently occurring fragments (2039 fragments) and a substructure-based diverse subset (1923 fragments) [70]. The two subsets are complementary to each other and their combination covers a larger part of the drug-like chemical space. Tanaka et al. extracted fragments from the ZINC database, performed network analysis of fragment libraries and proposed an efficient compound-prioritization method for fragment linking [48].

### 3.5 Fragment Frequency Analysis and Fragment Mining

Molecular fragments can be used as descriptors for chemoinformatics analysis (e.g., similarity searches, diversity analysis) and are associated with specific biological activities, and ADME/T (absorption, distribution, metabolism, excretion, and toxicity) profiles [71–73]. Thus, analysis of distribution of fragments types, their frequency of occurrence and co-occurrence in existing or virtual compound databases provides important information for understanding the nature of fragment–activity and fragment–drug-likeness relationships. Chemoinformatics analysis of the most frequently occurred fragments in drugs is helpful to fragment library design and fragment optimization. Fragment frequency analysis has also been used to build predictive models for biological activity and ADME/T prediction [74–76].

Fragment frequency analysis includes occurrence and co-occurrence analysis. Occurrence analysis characterizes fragment distributions in large databases, while co-occurrence analysis compares fragment sets in a pairwise manner. Bemis and Murcko performed pioneering work on the analysis of drug-like fragments [56, 57], in which frequently occurred molecular frameworks and side chains were identified in the CMC drug sets. Similar strategies have been used to analyze other databases (e.g., MDDR, NCI) to find drug-like fragments [76–81]. The resulted drug-like fragment libraries and their correlations can inspire medicinal chemists with innovative ideas for drug design and assist the investigation of unexplored parts of chemical space. Moreover, fragment frequency analysis has been extended to identify the privileged fragments in oral drugs (with good bioavailability) [82], multi-targeting fragments [83, 84], and the most popular fragment replacements in drug-like molecules [85–87].

Bajorath's group introduced a new concept named "fragment profile" that was used to evaluate molecular similarity relationships [88]. Fragment profiles are generated by MolBlaster which randomly deletes chemical bonds of molecules in connectivity tables and makes quantitative comparisons using entropy-based metrics. Unlike molecular fingerprint, fragment profile is randomly generated and does not depend on predefined chemical descriptors, and thus it can encode sufficient information for similarity evaluation. On the basis of fragment profile, a new tool for ligand-based virtual screening was developed [89]. Furthermore, a new methodology to identify unique fragment signatures for molecular sets with similar activities and then map the fragment pathways of biologically active molecules was developed by the same group [90]. More recently, Lounkine et al. developed FragFCA which uses chemically intuitive queries of varying complexity to identify molecular fragments and their combinations that are either specific for compounds with different activity profiles or are unique to highly potent molecules [91].

## 4    Fragment-Based Active Site Mapping

The second step in computational FBDD is to identify and characterize important regions (hot spots) that can bind drug-like fragments and contribute substantially to the binding free energy in the binding pocket of the drug target. Such hot regions can be identified and characterized by fragment-based approaches. Multiple solvent crystal structures (MSCS) is an experimental tool to predict ligand-binding sites of target proteins [92, 93]. MSCS determines consensus sites on the protein's surface by exposing a crystalline protein to various organic solvents (smaller fragments) in the case that potential ligand binding regions can be co-localized with multiple solvent molecules. However, MSCS and other experimental methods require an expensive investment in equipment and resources. Thus, various fragment-based computational approaches were developed to provide alternatives to predict the ligand-binding sites of a protein (Table 2) [94].

Geometric algorithms and probe mapping/docking algorithms are two major classes of methods for active site mapping [95]. For the latter, fragments are used as molecular probes to detect hot spots. GRID (a module in Molecular Discovery software package) [96, 97] and multiple copy simultaneous search (MCSS, a module in InsightII software package) [98] are two well-accepted methods. GRID identifies favorable sites for small functional groups in protein binding sites by calculating 3D energy maps. MCSS determines the most energetically favorable position of thousands of copies of small functional groups, which are randomly placed into the binding site and subject to energy minimization [99]. The copies with the lowest energies can be regarded as "hot spots" of ligand binding.

Beside GRID and MCSS, a number of computational methods have been reported [100, 101]. Several recent methods will be highlighted in the following sections. CS-Map is a fragment-based computational mapping program using a three-step algorithm [84, 91]. First, regions with favorable electrostatics and solvation are determined by rigid body search. Then, the regions are refined by free energy calculation and docking. Finally, potential regions are clustered, scored and ranked. CS-Map has the advantages of better sampling of regions with favorable desolvation and electrostatics by taking into account desolvation effect in its scoring

**Table 2**
**Summary fragment-based computational tools for active site mapping**

| Method | Key features | Refs |
|---|---|---|
| GRID | Global search of the entire protein surface, requires empirical parametrization, and lack of water molecules in the model. | [106, 107] |
| MCSS | The most established method with broad applications, incorporation of physicochemical potential functions and molecular simulation, and no consideration for the cooperative effects of water and locating minimum enthalpy poses. | [98, 99] |
| CS-Map | The ability of better sampling, finding small buried pockets and desolvation term in the free energy calculation, different dielectric constants for different targets. | [91] |
| FTMap | A fast approach but lack of water molecules in the model. | [83] |
| 3D-RISM-based method | A realistic model including the coexistence of water and the influence of ligand concentrations on binding modes, no consideration of protein structural change induced by ligand binding. | [71] |
| Grand canonical Monte Carlo simulation | Fast and simple parameters without prior knowledge and calibration, lack of complete validation, and case sensitive. | [103] |
| Barril's method | The ability of detecting hot spots for both small molecules and macromolecules, nonparametric, applicable to any target class, computationally expensive, and limited sampling. | [72] |

function and using average free energies to cluster and rank the positions of the docked ligands. Another new algorithm FTMAP was developed by the same group as to CS-Map, which uses the fourier transform correlation method for sampling protein–probe complexes in combination with a highly accurate energy function [83]. FTMAP is more efficient than CS-Map and free to academic users (http://ftmap.bu.edu/login.php). As compared to the experimental method MSCS, FTMap not only could duplicate the MSCS data for two targets of Parkinson's disease, but can also discover hot spots that are not found in the MSCS experiments [102].

Imai et al. developed 3D-RISM (three-dimensional reference interaction site model) to identify the most favorable orientations and positions of fragments on a protein surface [71]. A unique feature of this method is its ability to achieve "entire ligand mapping" on a protein surface in a real solution system by considering ligands and water at the same level in terms of the site distribution. In addition, the influence of ligand concentration on the binding mode can be investigated in the 3D-RISM-based method. Molecular dynamics simulation, Monte Carlo simulation and other computationally expensive methods have also been used for fragment mapping, clustering and ranking. For example, Clark et al. used grand canonical Monte Carlo simulation to compute binding free energies of a large number of fragment poses on the entire protein surface and predict the affinities and preferred binding poses of small molecular fragments [103]. Barril's group used first-principles molecular simulations to detect binding sites by quantifying the maximal binding affinity of a ligand [72]. This method can efficiently evaluate the druggability of the target and be applicable to any target class because it is not trained on a specific data set. Although these methods are computationally expensive, they can provide very detailed information for the interaction preferences of the binding sites.

## 5   Fragment Docking and Virtual Fragment Screening

Experimental FBDD only screens hundreds to thousands of fragments. However, there are at least 250,000 commercially available fragments [104], most of which remain untested. As a complementary approach, virtual fragment screening by molecular docking can test a large portion of commercially available fragments. Carlsson's group performed parallel NMR-based biophysical screening and docking-based screening of fragment libraries against the A2A adenosine receptor ($A_{2A}AR$) [105]. The results highlighted the complementarily between biophysical and computational-based fragment screens because there was no overlap between the hits identified from the NMR- and docking-based screens. Siegal's results also supported that experimental and computational fragment screening approaches could be pragmatically combined to increasing chemical space coverage and discovering novel and potent fragment hits [106]. In fact, fragment docking has already been applied in combination with experimental fragment screening for drug discovery purposes. For example, Brough et al. discovered Hsp90 molecular chaperone inhibitors of by merging structural features of various hits derived from both parallel fragment screening and fragment docking [107].

The main challenge for virtual fragment screening is the accuracy for fragment docking and scoring. First, it is difficult to determine the accurate binding pose and binding mode of fragments. Since fragments are small in size and have low internal degrees of freedom, a fragment might be accommodated by a number of pockets on protein surfaces during docking calculations, which can lead to falsely docked positions. It is also difficult to predict the binding poses of a fragment even if it is placed into the correct pocket, because alternative binding might yield similar docking scores or calculated binding energies [108]. Secondly, most of the scoring functions were developed and optimized for larger drug-like molecules, which are not accurate enough to differentiate an weakly active fragments among many non-active fragments [109].

**5.1 Docking Software Used for Fragment Docking**

Several commercially available docking software, such as DOCK, Glide and AutoDock, have been successfully used in fragment docking and screening (Table 3). For example, Shoichet's group identified fragment-like AmpC β-lactamase inhibitors by docking and ranking a library of 137,639 fragments using DOCK [110]. The hit rate is 48 % and the accuracy of the binding poses was further validated by solving the crystal structures of fragment–enzyme complexes. Glide [111, 112] is also efficient in fragment docking [113, 114]. A study from AstraZeneca indicated that GlideSP with its default settings provided a good enrichment in virtual screening of fragment inhibitors of DNA ligase and prostaglandin D2 synthase [113]. Another evaluation study suggested that Glide had good performance in sampling efficacy of fragment docking, but its scoring functions remained to be further improved [114]. AutoDock Vina was successfully used to discover dengue virus (DENV) protease inhibitors by in silico fragment screening of a library of 149,151 fragments [115, 116]. Fragment docking was also implemented into several de novo drug design software (e.g., LUDI [97] and SEED [117]), which dock fragments into the correct pocket of the active site and evolve them into new molecules. For example, the program DAIM [92] developed by Caflisch's group can automatically decompose molecules into fragments and then use the docking algorithms from SEED to select the anchor fragments for docking [93, 96, 117]. Recently, this fragment-based docking protocol was implemented into the CHARMMing Web user interface [118].

**5.2 Strategies to Improve the Accuracy of Fragment Docking**

Although several docking software has achieved good hit rate and docking accuracy, the fragment docking algorithm and scoring function remain to be further improved. Currently, strategies to improve the accuracy of fragment docking and scoring mainly include: (1) using computationally intensive tools to the post-docking process; (2) development of fragment-specific scoring functions; (3) making the fragments larger during docking; (4) docking multiple fragments simultaneously.

**Table 3**
**Common programs used in fragment docking**

| Program | Provider | URL |
| --- | --- | --- |
| Dock | Brian K. Schoichet | www.dock.compbio.ucsf.edu/DOCK3.7/ |
| Glide | Schrodinger | www.schrodinger.com |
| AutoDock | Arthur J. Olson | www.autodock.scripps.edu |
| LUDI | Accelrys/Discovery Studio 4.0 | www.accelrys.com |
| DAIM/SEED | Amedeo Caflish | www.biochem-caflisch.uzh.ch/download/ |
| RosettaLigand | Rosetta Commons | www.rosettacommons.org/software |

It was reported that the incorporation of intensive computational tools (e.g., MM/PBSA, MM/GBSA, and QM/MM) to reoptimize and rescore binding poses of fragments could improve the docking accuracy of fragment-like kinase inhibitors [119]. In contrast, Kawatkar's work indicated that such computationally intensive procedures could not improve the enrichment [113]. Thus, the success of these computationally expensive rescoring strategies might depend on specific targets.

In fragment docking, current scoring functions often fail to distinguish the correct binding mode from the incorrect ones [120]. One possible solution is to develop fragment-specific scoring functions [114]. The binding nature of fragments, such as less functional groups and fewer specific interactions, should be taken into account during the parameterization of currently available scoring functions. Moreover, force field-based scoring algorithm as well as other more advanced methods for the evaluation of protein–ligand interaction energies might be helpful to improve the fragment-specific scoring functions [120]. Marcou's study revealed that the application of interaction fingerprints (IFP) for posing and prioritizing fragments was statistically superior to conventional scoring functions [121].

In some cases, docking enlarged fragments can improve the accuracy of fragment docking. Fukunishi et al. developed the replica generation (FSRG) method that uses a set of larger molecules (replica molecules) generated by adding side chains to the fragment to optimize fragment docking. During docking, only complementarily between the surface of ligand and protein was evaluated [122]. The efficiency of FSRG in finding active fragments from the decoys was validated in six target proteins. However, successful examples are still very limited. On the other hand, docking multiple fragments simultaneously can simulate the real cases of fragment binding because multiple fragments are always involved in the process of molecular recognition. For example, Li's group developed the MLSD strategy for multiple ligand simultaneous docking, which can improve the sampling of docking poses and scoring of binding energy by mimicking the real molecular binding processes [123]. Moreover, fragments docked at different pockets of the target protein can be linked to generate a new ligand. This multiple fragments docking and linked strategy was successfully used to the discovery of novel STAT3 (signal transducer and activator of transcription 3) inhibitors [124].

Considering receptor flexibility as well as ligand flexibility is also important to predict the binding mode and affinity of fragments and increase the success rate of FBDD [23]. The use of protein side chain rotamer libraries [125] and multiple receptor conformations [126] is the most commonly used approaches to address flexibility. RosettaLigand is a docking algorithm that can handle full ligand and receptor flexibility simultaneously by using

Monte-Carlo sampling and Rosetta full-atom energy function [127]. Its advantage in fragment virtual screening was validated in retrospective tests [128].

Moreover, preparing the protein structure carefully and choosing appropriate parameters are also important for accurate fragment docking [98]. Kumar's work indicated that the availability of information about active inhibitors, protein–ligand interaction, program parameters, and screening protocols for drug-like ligands is helpful to improve fragment screening performance [128]. Molecular dynamics simulation is an efficient tool to investigate the conformational space of the target proteins and provide reasonable conformation or conformational ensembles for subsequent fragment docking. Ekonomiuk's study indicated that using molecular dynamics snapshots of NS3 protease for fragment-based docking could identify small-molecule inhibitors that could not be identified by simply using the X-ray structure [129].

**5.3 Case Study: Discovery of Novel Coagulation Factor VIIa Inhibitors by Fragment-Based Virtual Screening**

Coagulation factor VIIa is a new antithrombotic target. Most of the factor VIIa inhibitors bound with the S1 pockets contains both hydrophobic and cationic groups, leading to poor membrane permeability and oral absorption. In order to discover neutral S1-targeting inhibitors and improve pharmacokinetic profiles, Cheney et al. performed a fragment-based virtual screening study (Fig. 2a) [130]. The first step was to construct a fragment library. The Available Chemicals Directory (ACD) database was filtered on the basis of drug-likeness, number of heavy atoms and rotatable bonds, yielding about 18,000 fragments. This library was then screened by the molecular docking program Glide and the protein flexibility was considered by using protein ensemble docking. As a result, 250 compounds were finally selected and assayed. NMR binding assays identified 28 initial hits and their binding mode was determined by X-ray crystallography. As shown in Fig. 2c, the representative hit **2** ($K_i = 8.9$ mM) bound to factor VIIa S1 pocket and formed a hydrogen bond with Gly218. Based on the binding mode of lactam **2**, a number of analogues with good inhibitory potency and improved permeability were discovered. For example, compound **5** was cellular permeable and had a $K_i$ value of 130 nM. Other successful examples of fragment-based virtual screening are listed in Table 4.

# 6    From Fragment Hits to Drug Leads

**6.1 Computational Approaches to Evolve Fragments to Leads**

A key step in FBDD is to evolve fragment hits into drug leads or candidates by various structure-based design strategies [16]. Computational approaches have been extensively used in fragment optimization, fragment linking and fragment assembly. Moreover, fragment-based de novo drug design can be seen as the virtual

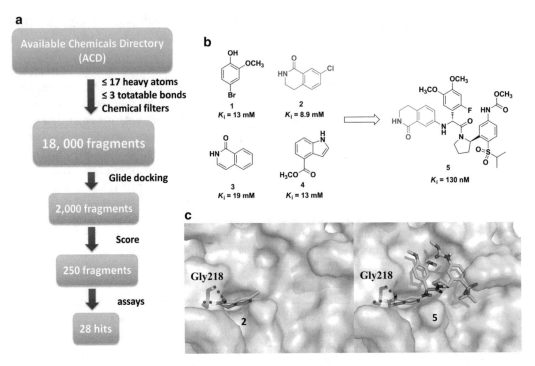

**Fig. 2** Discovery of novel coagulation factor VIIa inhibitors by fragment docking. (**a**) The protocol for fragment-based virtual screening; (**b**) Fragment hits of virtual screening and fragment optimization; (**c**) Binding mode of fragment hit 2 and optimized inhibitor 5

process of FBDD. Both approaches use small fragments (building blocks) as starting points to design drug-like compounds. De novo drug design [137] is complementary to HTS and FBDD because it is time and cost effective and capable of exploring larger chemical space. As compared to experimental FBDD methods, de novo design can provide potential solutions and reduce experimental costs. Moreover, de novo design tools are helpful to overcome the limitations of experimental FBDD. For example, at the stage of fragment linking, it is difficult to predict the effects of the linkers on the whole binding conformation. De novo design methods are able to suggest reasonable linkers and predict the binding conformation of the resulting molecules by docking and scoring. De novo design contributes to computational FBDD by a procedure involving compound buildup, docking/scoring, and optimization. Up to now, more than 30 de novo design tools have been developed [36, 58]. New methods focus on improving the efficiency in the sampling of the chemical space, the accuracy of scoring functions, synthetic feasibility and drug likeness [36].

**6.2 Strategies to Assemble and Optimize Fragments**

Fragment-based growing/linking and fragment hybridization are two major strategies to assemble fragments into novel molecules. It is difficult to evaluate all the solutions in a reasonable

**Table 4**
**Recent examples of fragment docking and virtual screening**

| Target | Fragment library | Docking method | Hit rate | Fragment hit | Activity | Ref |
|--------|------------------|----------------|----------|--------------|----------|-----|
| Dopamine D3 receptor | In-house library (12,905 fragments) | Glide | 27 % | **6** | $K_i = 0.17\ \mu M$ | [131] |
| Histamine H4 receptor | In-house library (12,905 fragments) | Glide | 18 % | **7** | $K_i = 8.4\ \mu M$ | [131] |
| A2A adenosine receptor | In-house library (328,000 fragments) | DOCK | 64 % | **8** | $K_i = 2.2\ \mu M$ | [105] |
| Bromodomain 4 | ZINC-based library (238,408 fragments) | In-house tool | 10 % | **9** | $IC_{50} = 7.0\ \mu M$ | [132] |
| Aurora kinase A | In-house library (125 fragments) | Libdock and Glide | 17 % | **10** | $IC_{50} = 852\ nM$ | [133] |
| β-lactamase | ZINC (67,489 fragments) | DOCK | 14 % | **11** | $K_i = 3.1\ \mu M$ | [134] |

(continued)

**Table 4**
**(continued)**

| Target | Fragment library | Docking method | Hit rate | Fragment hit | Activity | Ref |
|---|---|---|---|---|---|---|
| Pneumococcal Surface Antigen A | In-house library (1519 fragments) | FlexX | 3 % | **12** | 39.5% inhibition at 500 μM | [135] |
| Group X secreted phospholipase A2 | In-house library (300,000 fragments) | Glide | 10 % | **13** | $IC_{50} = 20$ μM | [136] |

computational time because the drug-like search space is about $10^{60}$ molecules. De novo drug design aims to efficiently find "good" solutions rather than the best solutions. Advanced optimization algorithms, such as particle swarm optimization (PSO), evolutionary algorithms [138], and ant colony optimization (ACO) [139], can improve the sampling efficiency of the huge chemical space [140].

For fragment growth, predefined conformation of a seed (fixed scaffold) in the binding pocket of the receptor should be obtained from structural biology or molecular docking. Then, the seed grows fragment-by-fragment to fit the active site geometrically and energetically. At each step, docking software was used for binding pose prediction and the acceptance or rejection of the fragment growth is guided by scoring functions. Early methods of this type include: SmoG [141, 142], SPROUT [143], GrowMol [144], GroupBuild [145], and GROW [146]. FlexNovo [147] was developed by the incremental construction algorithm of docking software FlexX [148] and was implemented into a comprehensive software package named NovoBench [149]. FlexNovo can explore thousands of fragments and incorporate various filters including physicochemical properties and diversity. Moreover, NovoBench also integrates a number of tools to meet the various demands of computational FBDD including generation of fragment space (Colibri [150] and FragView), property-based (FragEnum [151]), and ligand-based (Ftrees-FS [59]) search algorithms.

During fragment growth, most of the methods treat the "seed" as a fixed fragment. However, the conformation of the new molecule may be changed. AutoGrow can tackle the problem by re-docking each generated new compound during fragment addition and generating new poses for each molecule [152]. An evolutionary algorithm is used to evaluate the docking results of every population and select the best one for subsequent generation. Fragment optimized growth (FOG) algorithm improves the efficiency of fragment growth by using the frequency of specific fragment-fragment connections [153]. In addition, FOG can be trained to grow new molecules with chemical and topological features similar to a specific class of compounds (e.g., natural products and drugs) by the Topology Classifier (TopClass) algorithm [153].

For fragment linking, fragments bound with different binding pockets are linked to build new molecules. A number of de novo design methods, such as CONCERTS [154], LUDI [155, 156], CAVEAT [157], NEWLEAD [158], DLD [159], BUILDER [160], and SKELGEN [161], can link fragments into a new molecule, which is expected to have higher binding affinity than the individual fragments. However, overall conformation of the generated molecules may be changed and key interactions between the initial fragment and target might be lost. Thus, re-docking the new ligands is necessary in the post-processing step. GANDI is a new de novo design tool for automatically linking fragments and uses multi-objective evolutionary optimization strategy to simultaneously optimize the force field energy [162]. Lai's group developed LigBuilder [163, 164], which uses a genetic algorithm to construct ligands iteratively by fragment linking or growing. Moreover, synthetic accessibility and drug-likeness are taken into account in LigBuilder [165]. Notably, GANDI (http://www.biochem-caflisch.uzh.ch/download/) and LigBuilder (http://ligbuilder.org/) are freely available to academic users.

### 6.3 Scoring Functions and Multi-objective Optimization

In the fragment optimization process, scoring functions are crucial to evaluate the binding affinity. Due to the huge number of iterations, scoring functions are required to have the balance of speed and accuracy. Scoring functions from molecular docking are widely used, which can discriminate between inactive and active compounds rather than rank the ligands with similar chemotypes [166]. In this case, physics-based approaches, such as MM-GBSA/PBSA [167, 168], free-energy perturbation (FEP) [169, 170], grand canonical Monte Carlo (GCMC) simulations [103], single-step perturbation [171], and thermodynamic integration (TI) [172], can accurately predict binding free energies but require high computational sources. Even though, they are very helpful to improve the success rate by reevaluating in the post-processing stage. With the dramatic increase of the computational ability (e.g., cloud computing), physics-based scoring functions will have broader application in computational FBDD.

Single objective optimization only focuses on the interaction scores. In contrast, the multi-objective optimization strategies is more efficient to improve the quality of the designed molecules. For example, MEGA combines graph-theory with evolutionary techniques to achieve an efficient global search for good solutions [173]. Its optimization process includes binding affinity scorers, molecular similarity scorers, and chemical structure scorers. Thus, the molecules designed by MEGA may possess structural diversity, good binding affinity and drug-like properties.

**6.4 Synthetic Accessibility and Drug-Likeness**

Synthetic accessibility is one of the important issues that remain to be addressed in computational FBDD. The synthetic accessibility of computer-designed structures can be improved by two approaches. The first approach uses synthesizable building blocks and connection rules to design new molecules. Synthesizable building blocks can be obtained from commercially available resources. Moreover, virtual retro-synthesis rules can be used to decompose compound databases to generate synthesizable building blocks. Such rules (e.g., RECAP [55]) are based on commonly used organic synthesis reactions [174, 175]. SYNOPSIS [175] was developed to cover more types connection rules (70 selected organic reactions) and the building blocks are selected from the ACD database [176]. The second approach uses scoring functions to evaluate the synthesizability of the generated molecules (e.g., SYLVIA [165]) in the post-processing step. Other computer-aided organic synthesis design methods, such as Route Designer [177] and DOGS [58, 178] can suggest synthetic routes for the designed molecules.

Drug-likeness is another important constraint in every stage of computational FBDD. The fragment libraries are often constructed by decomposition of the drug or drug-like database. In the post-processing stage, Lipinski's "rule of five" [179] is broadly used as the filter before synthesis and biological evaluation. Moreover, recent progress in computational ADMET prediction [180] is helpful to reevaluate the candidate molecules in a cost-effective manner.

**6.5 Case Study: Novel Activated Factor XI Inhibitors Through Fragment Docking and Structure-Based Fragment Linking and Expansion**

Activated factor XI (FXIa) inhibitors are anticipated to possess both anticoagulant and profibrinolytic effects with a low risk of bleeding [181]. A research group from AstraZeneca applied a computational FBDD approach including virtual fragment screening, X-ray crystallography, structure-based fragment optimization, and biological assays to discover highly potent FXIa inhibitors [182]. The binding pockets of FXIa can be divided into S1–S4 and S1′–S2′ and the S1 pocket is the most prominent and probable site for fragment binding.

An in-house library of AstraZeneca containing about 65,000 fragments were docked into the FXIa X-ray structure (PDB code: 1ZSJ) using the Glide software. After Glide scoring and visual inspection, a total of 1800 structures were selected for experimental screening. In the screening cascade, 1D NMR spectroscopy was first used to identify primary fragment hits, followed by SPR and enzymatic assays to determine $K_D$ and $IC_{50}$ values, respectively. Initially, 13 neutral or weakly basic fragment hits were discovered by NMR. Subsequent similarity search yielded another 37 hits.

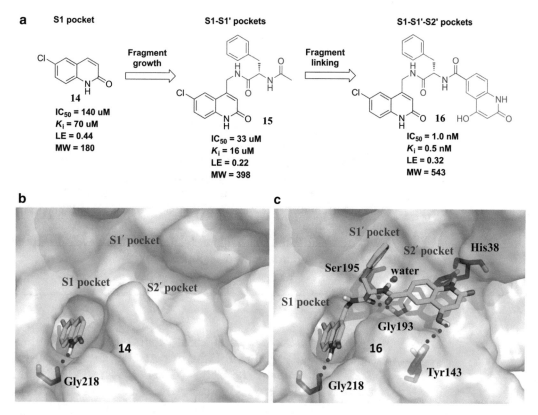

**Fig. 3** Discovery of novel FXIa inhibitors through fragment docking and structure-based fragment linking and expansion. (**a**) The process of fragment growth and fragment linking; (**b** and **c**) Binding mode of fragment hit **14** and optimized inhibitor **16** with the active site of FXIa

Among them, the crystal structure of the representative hit 14 (6-chloro-3,4-dihydro-1H-quinolin-2-one, Fig. 3a) in complex with FXIa were solved.

Fragment **14** was located into the S1 pocket and displayed a $IC_{50}$ value of 140 μM. Its quinolinone NH group forms a hydrogen bond with the backbone carbonyl of Gly218 (Fig. 3b). Guided by the binding mode, fragment **14** was further optimized to improve the inhibitory activity. The first step is to extend fragment **14** to interact with the S1′ site (Fig. 3a). The linkers and extension groups were designed by Glide docking and visual inspection. As a result, compound **15** was synthesized, which showed minor improvement in potency ($IC_{50} = 33$ μM) and decrease in LE to 0.22. Further addition of an S2′ binding group led to substantial increase of the activity. Compound **16** has an $IC_{50}$ of 1 nM and a LE of 0.32, which interacts with S1–S1′–S2′ binding pockets (Fig. 3c).

# 7    Conclusion

Computational approaches play a synergistic role to experimental FDBB by improving its performance. Computational FBDD can also be used independently in lead discovery and optimization. Fragment-based virtual screening and de novo design have been widely used in drug discovery and have led to promising results. Developing new docking and scoring methods that can accurately predict the binding poses and the binding free energy of fragments is of key importance to computational FBDD. Moreover, taking the advantages of both computational and experimental FBDD and merging them into an integrated drug design process will maximize the efficiency of drug discovery. Therefore, future research on computational FBDD should be focused on the development of new docking and integration methods.

# Acknowledgements

We gratefully acknowledge financial support from the National Basic Research Program of China (grant 2014CB541800), the 863 Hi-Tech Program of China (Grant 2014AA020525), the National Natural Science Foundation of China (Grant 81222044).

# References

1. Mayr LM, Bojanic D (2009) Novel trends in high-throughput screening. Curr Opin Pharmacol 9:580–588

2. Bohacek RS, McMartin C, Guida WC (1996) The art and practice of structure-based drug design: a molecular modeling perspective. Med Res Rev 16:3–50

3. Gribbon P, Sewing A (2005) High-throughput drug discovery: what can we expect from HTS? Drug Discov Today 10:17–22

4. Hajduk PJ, Greer J (2007) A decade of fragment-based drug design: strategic advances and lessons learned. Nat Rev Drug Discov 6:211–219

5. Chessari G, Woodhead AJ (2009) From fragment to clinical candidate–a historical perspective. Drug Discov Today 14:668–675

6. Bembenek SD, Tounge BA, Reynolds CH (2009) Ligand efficiency and fragment-based drug discovery. Drug Discov Today 14:278–283

7. Schuffenhauer A, Ruedisser S, Marzinzik AL, Jahnke W, Blommers M, Selzer P, Jacoby E (2005) Library design for fragment based screening. Curr Top Med Chem 5:751–762

8. Siegal G, Ab E, Schultz J (2007) Integration of fragment screening and library design. Drug Discov Today 12:1032–1039

9. Lepre CA, Moore JM, Peng JW (2004) Theory and applications of NMR-based screening in pharmaceutical research. Chem Rev 104:3641–3676

10. Shuker SB, Hajduk PJ, Meadows RP, Fesik SW (1996) Discovering high-affinity ligands for proteins: SAR by NMR. Science 274:1531–1534

11. Swayze EE, Jefferson EA, Sannes-Lowery KA, Blyn LB, Risen LM, Arakawa S, Osgood SA, Hofstadler SA, Griffey RH (2002) SAR by MS: a ligand based technique for drug lead discovery against structured RNA targets. J Med Chem 45:3816–3819

12. Erlanson DA, Wells JA, Braisted AC (2004) Tethering: fragment-based drug discovery. Annu Rev Biophys Biomol Struct 33:199–223

13. Hartshorn MJ, Murray CW, Cleasby A, Frederickson M, Tickle IJ, Jhoti H (2005)

Fragment-based lead discovery using X-ray crystallography. J Med Chem 48:403–413

14. Danielson UH (2009) Fragment library screening and lead characterization using SPR biosensors. Curr Top Med Chem 9:1725–1735

15. Neumann T, Junker HD, Schmidt K, Sekul R (2007) SPR-based fragment screening: advantages and applications. Curr Top Med Chem 7:1630–1642

16. Rees DC, Congreve M, Murray CW, Carr R (2004) Fragment-based lead discovery. Nat Rev Drug Discov 3:660–672

17. Murray CW, Rees DC (2009) The rise of fragment-based drug discovery. Nat Chem 1:187–192

18. Congreve M, Chessari G, Tisi D, Woodhead AJ (2008) Recent developments in fragment-based drug discovery. J Med Chem 51:3661–3680

19. Zartler ER, Shapiro MJ (2005) Fragonomics: fragment-based drug discovery. Curr Opin Chem Biol 9:366–370

20. Warr W (2011) A. Fragment-based drug discovery: what really works. An interview with Sandy Farmer of Boehringer Ingelheim. J Comput Aided Mol Des 25:599–605

21. Fruh V, Zhou Y, Chen D, Loch C, Ab E, Grinkova YN, Verheij H, Sligar SG, Bushweller JH, Siegal G (2010) Application of fragment-based drug discovery to membrane proteins: identification of ligands of the integral membrane enzyme DsbB. Chem Biol 17:881–891

22. Bamborough P, Brown MJ, Christopher JA, Chung CW, Mellor GW (2011) Selectivity of kinase inhibitor fragments. J Med Chem 54:5131–5143

23. Babaoglu K, Shoichet BK (2006) Deconstructing fragment-based inhibitor discovery. Nat Chem Biol 2:720–723

24. Desjarlais RL (2011) Using computational techniques in fragment-based drug discovery. Methods Enzymol 493:137–155

25. Gozalbes R, Carbajo RJ, Pineda-Lucena A (2010) Contributions of computational chemistry and biophysical techniques to fragment-based drug discovery. Curr Med Chem 17:1769–1794

26. Hoffer L, Renaud JP, Horvath D (2011) Fragment-based drug design: computational & experimental state of the art. Comb Chem High Throughput Screen 14:500–520

27. Hubbard RE, Chen I, Davis B (2007) Informatics and modeling challenges in fragment-based drug discovery. Curr Opin Drug Discov Dev 10:289–297

28. Law R, Barker O, Barker JJ, Hesterkamp T, Godemann R, Andersen O, Fryatt T, Courtney S, Hallett D, Whittaker M (2009) The multiple roles of computational chemistry in fragment-based drug design. J Comput Aided Mol Des

29. Vangrevelinghe E, Rudisser S (2007) Computational approaches for fragment optimization. Curr Comput Aided Drug Des 3:69–83

30. Villar HO, Hansen MR (2007) Computational techniques in fragment based drug discovery. Curr Top Med Chem 7:1509–1513

31. Zoete V, Grosdidier A, Michielin O (2009) Docking, virtual high throughput screening and in silico fragment-based drug design. J Cell Mol Med 13:238–248

32. Makara GM (2007) On sampling of fragment space. J Med Chem 50:3214–3221

33. Fejzo J, Lepre C (1999) A.; Peng, J. W.; Bemis, G. W.; Ajay; Murcko, M. A.; Moore, J. M. The SHAPES strategy: an NMR-based approach for lead generation in drug discovery. Chem Biol 6:755–769

34. Lepre C (2007) Fragment-based drug discovery using the SHAPES method. Expert Opin Drug Discov 2:1555–1566

35. Chung S, Parker JB, Bianchet M, Amzel LM, Stivers JT (2009) Impact of linker strain and flexibility in the design of a fragment-based inhibitor. Nat Chem Biol 5:407–413

36. Schneider G, Fechner U (2005) Computer-based de novo design of drug-like molecules. Nat Rev Drug Discov 4:649–663

37. Zhu Z, Sun ZY, Ye Y, Voigt J, Strickland C, Smith EM, Cumming J, Wang L, Wong J, Wang YS, Wyss DF, Chen X, Kuvelkar R, Kennedy ME, Favreau L, Parker E, McKittrick BA, Stamford A, Czarniecki M, Greenlee W, Hunter JC (2010) Discovery of cyclic acyl-guanidines as highly potent and selective beta-site amyloid cleaving enzyme (BACE) inhibitors: Part I–inhibitor design and validation. J Med Chem 53:951–965

38. Johnson MC, Hu Q, Lingardo L, Ferre RA, Greasley S, Yan J, Kath J, Chen P, Ermolieff J, Alton G (2011) Novel isoquinolone PDK1 inhibitors discovered through fragment-based lead discovery. J Comput Aided Mol Des 25:689–698

39. Congreve M, Carr R, Murray C, Jhoti H (2003) A 'rule of three' for fragment-based lead discovery? Drug Discov Today 8:876–877

40. Card GL, Blasdel L, England BP, Zhang C, Suzuki Y, Gillette S, Fong D, Ibrahim PN, Artis DR, Bollag G, Milburn MV, Kim SH, Schlessinger J, Zhang KY (2005) A family of

phosphodiesterase inhibitors discovered by cocrystallography and scaffold-based drug design. Nat Biotechnol 23:201–207

41. Davies DR, Mamat B, Magnusson OT, Christensen J, Haraldsson MH, Mishra R, Pease B, Hansen E, Singh J, Zembower D, Kim H, Kiselyov AS, Burgin AB, Gurney ME, Stewart LJ (2009) Discovery of leukotriene A4 hydrolase inhibitors using metabolomics biased fragment crystallography. J Med Chem 52:4694–4715

42. Law RJ (2009) Tetrabromobisphenol A: investigating the worst-case scenario. Mar Pollut Bull 58:459–460

43. Boyd SM, de Kloe GE (2010) Fragment library design: efficiently hunting drugs in chemical space. Drug Discov Today Technol 7:e147–e202

44. Schulz MN, Landstrom J, Bright K, Hubbard RE (2011) Design of a Fragment Library that maximally represents available chemical space. J Comput Aided Mol Des 25:611–620

45. PubChem database, pubchem.ncbi.nlm.nih.gov.

46. eMolecules, www.emolecules.com.

47. Oprea TI, Blaney JM (2006) Cheminformatics approaches to fragment-based lead discovery. In: Jahnke W, Erlanson DA (eds) Fragment-based approaches in drug discovery, vol 34. Wiley, Weinheim, pp 91–111

48. Tanaka N, Ohno K, Niimi T, Moritomo A, Mori K, Orita M (2009) Small-world phenomena in chemical library networks: application to fragment-based drug discovery. J Chem Inf Model 49:2677–2686

49. World Drug Index (2002) V. T. P., PA

50. MedChem03 database. BioByte, Claremont, C., and Daylight Chemical Information Systems, Inc., Aliso Viejo, CA

51. MDL Drug Data Report. Symyx Technologies, Inc., Sunnyvale, CA

52. Chen H, Gao J, Lu Y, Kou G, Zhang H, Fan L, Sun Z, Guo Y, Zhong Y (2008) Preparation and characterization of PE38KDEL-loaded anti-HER2 nanoparticles for targeted cancer therapy. J Control Release 128:209–216

53. Horst EVD, IJzerman AP (2008) Computational approaches to fragment and substructure discovery and evaluation. In: Zartler ER, Shapiro MJ (eds) Fragment-based drug discovery: a practical approach. Wiley, New York, pp 199–222

54. Zhang M, Sheng C, Xu H, Song Y, Zhang W (2007) Constructing virtual combinatorial fragment libraries based upon MDL Drug

Data Report database. Sci China Ser B 50:364–371

55. Lewell XQ, Judd DB, Watson SP, Hann MM (1998) RECAP–retrosynthetic combinatorial analysis procedure: a powerful new technique for identifying privileged molecular fragments with useful applications in combinatorial chemistry. J Chem Inf Comput Sci 38:511–522

56. Bemis G, Murcko MA (1999) Properties of known drugs. 2. Side chains. J Med Chem 42:5095–5099

57. Bemis G, Murcko MA (1996) The properties of known drugs. 1. Molecular frameworks. J Med Chem 39:2887–2893

58. Hartenfeller M, Schneider G (2011) De novo drug design. Methods Mol Biol 672:299–323

59. Rarey M, Stahl M (2001) Similarity searching in large combinatorial chemistry spaces. J Comput Aided Mol Des 15:497–520

60. Rarey M, Dixon JS (1998) Feature trees: a new molecular similarity measure based on tree matching. J Comput Aided Mol Des 12:471–490

61. Lessel U, Wellenzohn B, Lilienthal M, Claussen H (2009) Searching fragment spaces with feature trees. J Chem Inf Model 49:270–279

62. Andrews KM, Cramer RD (2000) Toward general methods of targeted library design: topomer shape similarity searching with diverse structures as queries. J Med Chem 43:1723–1740

63. Cramer RD, Soltanshahi F, Jilek R, Campbell B (2007) AllChem: generating and searching 10(20) synthetically accessible structures. J Comput Aided Mol Des 21:341–350

64. Jilik RJ, Cramer RD (2004) Topomers: a validated protocol for their self-consistent generation. J Chem Inf Comput Sci 44:1121–1127

65. Jhoti H, Williams G, Rees DC, Murray CW (2013) The 'rule of three' for fragment-based drug discovery: where are we now? Nat Rev Drug Discov 12:644–645

66. Morley AD, Pugliese A, Birchall K, Bower J, Brennan P, Brown N, Chapman T, Drysdale M, Gilbert IH, Hoelder S, Jordan A, Ley SV, Merritt A, Miller D, Swarbrick ME, Wyatt PG (2013) Fragment-based hit identification: thinking in 3D. Drug Discov Today 18:1221–1227

67. Hung AW, Ramek A, Wang Y, Kaya T, Wilson JA, Clemons PA, Young DW (2011) Route to three-dimensional fragments using diversity-oriented synthesis. Proc Natl Acad Sci U S A 108:6799–6804

68. Over B, Wetzel S, Grutter C, Nakai Y, Renner S, Rauh D, Waldmann H (2013) Natural-

product-derived fragments for fragment-based ligand discovery. Nat Chem 5:21–28

69. Carr RA, Congreve M, Murray CW, Rees DC (2005) Fragment-based lead discovery: leads by design. Drug Discov Today 10:987–992

70. Mauser H, Stahl M (2007) Chemical fragment spaces for de novo design. J Chem Inf Model 47:318–324

71. Bondensgaard K, Ankersen M, Thogersen H, Hansen BS, Wulff BS, Bywater RP (2004) Recognition of privileged structures by G-protein coupled receptors. J Med Chem 47:888–899

72. Schnur DM, Hermsmeier MA, Tebben AJ (2006) Are target-family-privileged substructures truly privileged? J Med Chem 49:2000–2009

73. Clark M, Wiseman JS (2009) Fragment-based prediction of the clinical occurrence of long QT syndrome and torsade de pointes. J Chem Inf Model 49:2617–2626

74. Kho R, Hodges JA, Hansen MR, Villar HO (2005) Ring systems in mutagenicity databases. J Med Chem 48:6671–6678

75. Kazius J, Nijssen S, Kok J, Back T, Ijzerman AP (2006) Substructure mining using elaborate chemical representation. J Chem Inf Model 46:597–605

76. Sutherland JJ, Higgs RE, Watson I, Vieth M (2008) Chemical fragments as foundations for understanding target space and activity prediction. J Med Chem 51:2689–2700

77. Lee ML, Schneider G (2001) Scaffold architecture and pharmacophoric properties of natural products and trade drugs: application in the design of natural product-based combinatorial libraries. J Comb Chem 3:284–289

78. Siegel MG, Vieth M (2007) Drugs in other drugs: a new look at drugs as fragments. Drug Discov Today 12:71–79

79. Grabowski K, Schneider G (2007) Properties and architecture of drugs and natural products revisited. Curr Chem Biol 1:115–127

80. Wang J, Hou T (2010) Drug and drug candidate building block analysis. J Chem Inf Model 50:55–67

81. Lameijer EW, Kok JN, Back T, Ijzerman AP (2006) Mining a chemical database for fragment co-occurrence: discovery of "chemical cliches". J Chem Inf Model 46:553–562

82. Vieth M, Siegel M (2006) Structural fragments in marketed oral drugs. In: Erlanson DA, Jahnke W (eds) Fragment-based approaches in drug discovery. Wiley, Weinheim, pp 113–124

83. Morphy R, Rankovic Z (2005) Designed multiple ligands. An emerging drug discovery paradigm. J Med Chem 48:6523–6543

84. Sheridan RP (2003) Finding multiactivity substructures by mining databases of drug-like compounds. J Chem Inf Comput Sci 43:1037–1050

85. Sheridan RP (2002) The most common chemical replacements in drug-like compounds. J Chem Inf Comput Sci 42:103–108

86. Ertl P (2003) Cheminformatics analysis of organic substituents: identification of the most common substituents, calculation of substituent properties, and automatic identification of drug-like bioisosteric groups. J Chem Inf Comput Sci 43:374–380

87. Haubertin DY, Bruneau P (2007) A database of historically-observed chemical replacements. J Chem Inf Model 47:1294–1302

88. Batista J, Godden JW, Bajorath J (2006) Assessment of molecular similarity from the analysis of randomly generated structural fragment populations. J Chem Inf Model 46:1937–1944

89. Batista J, Bajorath J (2007) Chemical database mining through entropy-based molecular similarity assessment of randomly generated structural fragment populations. J Chem Inf Model 47:59–68

90. Batista J, Bajorath J (2007) Mining of randomly generated molecular fragment populations uncovers activity-specific fragment hierarchies. J Chem Inf Model 47:1405–1413

91. Lounkine E, Auer J, Bajorath J (2008) Formal concept analysis for the identification of molecular fragment combinations specific for active and highly potent compounds. J Med Chem 51:5342–5348

92. Mattos C, Bellamacina CR, Peisach E, Pereira A, Vitkup D, Petsko GA, Ringe D (2006) Multiple solvent crystal structures: probing binding sites, plasticity and hydration. J Mol Biol 357:1471–1482

93. Mattos C, Ringe D (1996) Locating and characterizing binding sites on proteins. Nat Biotechnol 14:595–599

94. Leis S, Schneider S, Zacharias M (2010) In silico prediction of binding sites on proteins. Curr Med Chem 17:1550–1562

95. Laurie AT, Jackson RM (2006) Methods for the prediction of protein-ligand binding sites for structure-based drug design and virtual ligand screening. Curr Protein Pept Sci 7:395–406

96. Goodford PJ (1985) A computational procedure for determining energetically favorable

binding sites on biologically important macromolecules. J Med Chem 28:849–857

97. von Itzstein M, Wu WY, Kok GB, Pegg MS, Dyason JC, Jin B, Van Phan T, Smythe ML, White HF, Oliver SW et al (1993) Rational design of potent sialidase-based inhibitors of influenza virus replication. Nature 363:418–423

98. Miranker A, Karplus M (1991) Functionality maps of binding sites: a multiple copy simultaneous search method. Proteins 11:29–34

99. Schubert C, Stultz C (2009) The multi-copy simultaneous search methodology: a fundamental tool for structure-based drug design. J Comput Aided Mol Des 23:475–489

100. Campbell SJ, Gold ND, Jackson RM, Westhead DR (2003) Ligand binding: functional site location, similarity and docking. Curr Opin Struct Biol 13:389–395

101. Sotriffer C, Klebe G (2002) Identification and mapping of small-molecule binding sites in proteins: computational tools for structure-based drug design. Farmaco 57:243–251

102. Landon M, Lieberman R, Hoang Q, Ju S, Caaveiro J, Orwig S, Kozakov D, Brenke R, Chuang G, Beglov D, Vajda S, Petsko G, Ringe D (2009) Detection of ligand binding hot spots on protein surfaces via fragment-based methods: application to DJ-1 and glucocerebrosidase. J Comput Aided Mol Des 23:491–500

103. Clark M, Guarnieri F, Shkurko I, Wiseman J (2006) Grand canonical Monte Carlo simulation of ligand-protein binding. J Chem Inf Model 46:231–242

104. Irwin JJ, Shoichet BK (2005) ZINC–a free database of commercially available compounds for virtual screening. J Chem Inf Model 45:177–182

105. Chen D, Ranganathan A, Ijzerman AP, Siegal G, Carlsson J (2013) Complementarity between in silico and biophysical screening approaches in fragment-based lead discovery against the A(2A) adenosine receptor. J Chem Inf Model 53:2701–2714

106. Barelier S, Eidam O, Fish I, Hollander J, Figaroa F, Nachane R, Irwin JJ, Shoichet BK, Siegal G (2014) Increasing chemical space coverage by combining empirical and computational fragment screens. ACS Chem Biol 9:1528–1535

107. Brough PA, Barril X, Borgognoni J, Chene P, Davies NG, Davis B, Drysdale MJ, Dymock B, Eccles SA, Garcia-Echeverria C, Fromont C, Hayes A, Hubbard RE, Jordan AM, Jensen MR, Massey A, Merrett A, Padfield A, Parsons R, Radimerski T, Raynaud FI, Robertson A, Roughley SD, Schoepfer J, Simmonite H, Sharp SY, Surgenor A, Valenti M, Walls S, Webb P, Wood M, Workman P, Wright L (2009) Combining hit identification strategies: fragment-based and in silico approaches to orally active 2-aminothieno[2,3-d]pyrimidine inhibitors of the Hsp90 molecular chaperone. J Med Chem 52:4794–4809

108. Nayal M, Honig B (2006) On the nature of cavities on protein surfaces: application to the identification of drug-binding sites. Proteins 63:892–906

109. Leach AR, Shoichet BK, Peishoff CE (2006) Prediction of protein-ligand interactions. Docking and scoring: successes and gaps. J Med Chem 49:5851–5855

110. Teotico DG, Babaoglu K, Rocklin GJ, Ferreira RS, Giannetti AM, Shoichet BK (2009) Docking for fragment inhibitors of AmpC beta-lactamase. Proc Natl Acad Sci U S A 106:7455–7460

111. Friesner RA, Banks JL, Murphy RB, Halgren TA, Klicic JJ, Mainz DT, Repasky MP, Knoll EH, Shelley M, Perry JK, Shaw DE, Francis P, Shenkin PS (2004) Glide: a new approach for rapid, accurate docking and scoring. 1. Method and assessment of docking accuracy. J Med Chem 47:1739–1749

112. Halgren TA, Murphy RB, Friesner RA, Beard HS, Frye LL, Pollard WT, Banks JL (2004) Glide: a new approach for rapid, accurate docking and scoring. 2. Enrichment factors in database screening. J Med Chem 47:1750–1759

113. Kawatkar S, Wang H, Czerminski R, Joseph-McCarthy D (2009) Virtual fragment screening: an exploration of various docking and scoring protocols for fragments using Glide. J Comput Aided Mol Des 23:527–539

114. Sandor M, Kiss R, Keseru GM (2010) Virtual fragment docking by Glide: a validation study on 190 protein-fragment complexes. J Chem Inf Model 50:1165–1172

115. Knehans T, Schuller A, Doan DN, Nacro K, Hill J, Guntert P, Madhusudhan MS, Weil T, Vasudevan SG (2011) Structure-guided fragment-based in silico drug design of dengue protease inhibitors. J Comput Aided Mol Des 25:263–274

116. Morris GM, Huey R, Lindstrom W, Sanner MF, Belew RK, Goodsell DS, Olson AJ (2009) AutoDock4 and AutoDockTools4: automated docking with selective receptor flexibility. J Comput Chem 30:2785–2791

117. Majeux N, Scarsi M, Caflisch A (2001) Efficient electrostatic solvation model for protein-fragment docking. Proteins 42:256–268

118. Pevzner Y, Frugier E, Schalk V, Caflisch A, Woodcock HL (2014) Fragment-based docking: development of the CHARMMing Web user interface as a platform for computer-aided drug design. J Chem Inf Model 54:2612–2620

119. Gleeson MP, Gleeson D (2009) QM/MM as a tool in fragment based drug discovery. A cross-docking, rescoring study of kinase inhibitors. J Chem Inf Model 49:1437–1448

120. Verdonk ML, Giangreco I, Hall RJ, Korb O, Mortenson PN, Murray CW (2011) Docking performance of fragments and druglike compounds. J Med Chem 54:5422–5431

121. Marcou G, Rognan D (2007) Optimizing fragment and scaffold docking by use of molecular interaction fingerprints. J Chem Inf Model 47:195–207

122. Fukunishi Y, Mashimo T, Orita M, Ohno K, Nakamura H (2009) In silico fragment screening by replica generation (FSRG) method for fragment-based drug design. J Chem Inf Model 49:925–933

123. Li H, Li C (2010) Multiple ligand simultaneous docking: orchestrated dancing of ligands in binding sites of protein. J Comput Chem 31:2014–2022

124. Li H, Liu A, Zhao Z, Xu Y, Lin J, Jou D, Li C (2011) Fragment-based drug design and drug repositioning using multiple ligand simultaneous docking (MLSD): identifying celecoxib and template compounds as novel inhibitors of signal transducer and activator of transcription 3 (STAT3). J Med Chem 54:5592–5596

125. Nabuurs SB, Wagener M, de Vlieg J (2007) A flexible approach to induced fit docking. J Med Chem 50:6507–6518

126. Totrov M, Abagyan R (2008) Flexible ligand docking to multiple receptor conformations: a practical alternative. Curr Opin Struct Biol 18:178–184

127. Meiler J, Baker D (2006) ROSETTALIGAND: protein-small molecule docking with full side-chain flexibility. Proteins 65:538–548

128. Kumar A, Zhang KY (2012) Computational fragment-based screening using RosettaLigand: the SAMPL3 challenge. J Comput Aided Mol Des 26:603–616

129. Ekonomiuk D, Su XC, Ozawa K, Bodenreider C, Lim SP, Otting G, Huang D, Caflisch A (2009) Flaviviral protease inhibitors identified by fragment-based library docking into a structure generated by molecular dynamics. J Med Chem 52:4860–4868

130. Cheney DL, Bozarth JM, Metzler WJ, Morin PE, Mueller L, Newitt JA, Nirschl AH, Rendina AR, Tamura JK, Wei A, Wen X, Wurtz NR, Seiffert DA, Wexler RR, Priestley ES (2015) Discovery of novel P1 groups for coagulation factor VIIa inhibition using fragment-based screening. J Med Chem 58:2799–2808

131. Vass M, Schmidt E, Horti F, Keseru GM (2014) Virtual fragment screening on GPCRs: a case study on dopamine D3 and histamine H4 receptors. Eur J Med Chem 77:38–46

132. Zhao H, Gartenmann L, Dong J, Spiliotopoulos D, Caflisch A (2014) Discovery of BRD4 bromodomain inhibitors by fragment-based high-throughput docking. Bioorg Med Chem Lett 24:2493–2496

133. Sarvagalla S, Singh VK, Ke YY, Shiao HY, Lin WH, Hsieh HP, Hsu JT, Coumar MS (2015) Identification of ligand efficient, fragment-like hits from an HTS library: structure-based virtual screening and docking investigations of 2H- and 3H-pyrazolo tautomers for Aurora kinase A selectivity. J Comput Aided Mol Des 29:89–100

134. Chen Y, Shoichet BK (2009) Molecular docking and ligand specificity in fragment-based inhibitor discovery. Nat Chem Biol 5:358–364

135. Bajaj M, Mamidyala SK, Zuegg J, Begg SL, Ween MP, Luo Z, Huang JX, McEwan AG, Kobe B, Paton JC, McDevitt CA, Cooper MA (2015) Discovery of novel pneumococcal surface antigen A (PsaA) inhibitors using a fragment-based drug design approach. ACS Chem Biol 10:1511–1520

136. Chen H, Knerr L, Akerud T, Hallberg K, Oster L, Rohman M, Osterlund K, Beisel HG, Olsson T, Brengdhal J, Sandmark J, Bodin C (2014) Discovery of a novel pyrazole series of group X secreted phospholipase A2 inhibitor (sPLA2X) via fragment based virtual screening. Bioorg Med Chem Lett 24:5251–5255

137. Danziger DJ, Dean PM (1989) Automated site-directed drug design: a general algorithm for knowledge acquisition about hydrogen-bonding regions at protein surfaces. Proc R Soc Lond B Biol Sci 236:101–113

138. Clark DE, Westhead DR (1996) Evolutionary algorithms in computer-aided molecular design. J Comput Aided Mol Des 10:337–358

139. Dorigo M, Di Caro G, Gambardella LM (1999) Ant algorithms for discrete optimization. Artif Life 5:137–172

140. Hiss JA, Hartenfeller M, Schneider G (2010) Concepts and applications of "natural computing" techniques in de novo drug and peptide design. Curr Pharm Des 16:1656–1665

141. DeWitt R, Shaknovich E (1996) SmoG: de novo design method based on simple, fast, and accurate free energy estimates. 1. Methodology and supporting evidence. J Am Chem Soc 118:11733–11744

142. DeWitt R, Shaknovich E (1997) SmoG: de novo design method based on simple, fast, and accurate free energy estimates. 2. Case studies on molecular design. J Am Chem Soc 119:4608–4617

143. Gillet VJ, Newell W, Mata P, Myatt G, Sike S, Zsoldos Z, Johnson AP (1994) SPROUT: recent developments in the de novo design of molecules. J Chem Inf Comput Sci 34:207–217

144. Bohacek RS, McMartin C (1994) Multiple highly diverse structures complementary to enzyme binding sites: results of extensive application of de novo design method incorporating combinatorial growth. J Am Chem Soc 116:5560–5571

145. Rotstein SH, Murcko MA (1993) Group-Build: a fragment-based method for de novo drug design. J Med Chem 36:1700–1710

146. Moon JB, Howe WJ (1991) Computer design of bioactive molecules: a method for receptor-based de novo ligand design. Proteins 11:314–328

147. Degen J, Rarey M (2006) FlexNovo: structure-based searching in large fragment spaces. ChemMedChem 1:854–868

148. Rarey M, Kramer B, Lengauer T, Klebe G (1996) A fast flexible docking method using an incremental construction algorithm. J Mol Biol 261:470–489

149. Zaliani A, Boda K, Seidel T, Herwig A, Schwab CH, Gasteiger J, Claußen H, Lemmen C, Degen J, Pärn J, Rarey M (2009) Second-generation de novo design: a view from a medicinal chemist perspective. J Comput Aided Mol Des 23:593–602

150. Boehm M, Wu TY, Claussen H, Lemmen C (2008) Similarity searching and scaffold hopping in synthetically accessible combinatorial chemistry spaces. J Med Chem 51:2468–2480

151. Parn J, Degen J, Rarey M (2007) Exploring fragment spaces under multiple physicochemical constraints. J Comput Aided Mol Des 21:327–340

152. Durrant JD, Amaro RE, McCammon JA (2009) AutoGrow: a novel algorithm for protein inhibitor design. Chem Biol Drug Des 73:168–178

153. Kutchukian PS, Lou D, Shakhnovich EI (2009) FOG: Fragment Optimized Growth algorithm for the de novo generation of molecules occupying druglike chemical space. J Chem Inf Model 49:1630–1642

154. Pearlman DA, Murcko MA (1996) CONCERTS: dynamic connection of fragments as an approach to de novo ligand design. J Med Chem 39:1651–1663

155. Bohm HJ (1992) The computer program LUDI: a new method for the de novo design of enzyme inhibitors. J Comput Aided Mol Des 6:61–78

156. Bohm HJ (1994) On the use of LUDI to search the Fine Chemicals Directory for ligands of proteins of known three-dimensional structure. J Comput Aided Mol Des 8:623–632

157. Lauri G, Bartlett PA (1994) CAVEAT: a program to facilitate the design of organic molecules. J Comput Aided Mol Des 8:51–66

158. Tschinke V, Cohen NC (1993) The NEWLEAD program: a new method for the design of candidate structures from pharmacophoric hypotheses. J Med Chem 36:3863–3870

159. Miranker A, Karplus M (1995) An automated method for dynamic ligand design. Proteins 23:472–490

160. Roe DC, Kuntz ID (1995) BUILDER v. 2: improving the chemistry of a de novo design strategy. J Comput Aided Mol Des 9:269–282

161. Stahl M, Todorov NP, James T, Mauser H, Boehm HJ, Dean PM (2002) A validation study on the practical use of automated de novo design. J Comput Aided Mol Des 16:459–478

162. Dey F, Caflisch A (2008) Fragment-based de novo ligand design by multiobjective evolutionary optimization. J Chem Inf Model 48:679–690

163. Yuan Y, Pei J, Lai L (2011) LigBuilder 2: a practical de novo drug design approach. J Chem Inf Model 51:1083–1091

164. Wang R, Gao Y, Lai L (2000) A multipurpose program for structure-based drug design. J Mol Model 6:498–516

165. Boda K, Seidel T, Gasteiger J (2007) Structure and reaction based evaluation of synthetic accessibility. J Comput Aided Mol Des 21:311–325

166. Loving K, Alberts I, Sherman W (2010) Computational approaches for fragment-based

and de novo design. Curr Top Med Chem 10:14–32

167. Massova I, Kollman PA (1999) Computational alanine scanning to probe protein-protein interactions: a novel approach to evaluate binding free energies. J Am Chem Soc 121:8133–8143

168. Still WC, Tempczyk A, Hawley RC, Hendrickson T (1990) Semianalytical treatment of solvation for molecular mechanics and dynamics. J Am Chem Soc 112:6127–6129

169. Kim JT, Hamilton AD, Bailey CM, Domaoal RA, Wang L, Anderson KS, Jorgensen WL (2006) FEP-guided selection of bicyclic heterocycles in lead optimization for non-nucleoside inhibitors of HIV-1 reverse transcriptase. J Am Chem Soc 128:15372–15373

170. Kollman PA (1993) Free energy calculations: applications to chemical and biochemical phenomena. Chem Rev 93:2395–2417

171. Oostenbrink C, van Gunsteren WF (2004) Free energies of binding of polychlorinated biphenyls to the estrogen receptor from a single simulation. Proteins 54:237–246

172. van Gunsteren WF, Berendsen HJ (1987) Thermodynamic cycle integration by computer simulation as a tool for obtaining free energy differences in molecular chemistry. J Comput Aided Mol Des 1:171–176

173. Nicolaou CA, Apostolakis J, Pattichis CS (2009) De novo drug design using multiobjective evolutionary graphs. J Chem Inf Model 49:295–307

174. Schneider G, Lee ML, Stahl M, Schneider P (2000) De novo design of molecular architectures by evolutionary assembly of drug-derived building blocks. J Comput Aided Mol Des 14:487–494

175. Vinkers HM, de Jonge MR, Daeyaert FF, Heeres J, Koymans LM, van Lenthe JH, Lewi PJ, Timmerman H, Van Aken K, Janssen PA (2003) SYNOPSIS: SYNthesize and OPtimize System in Silico. J Med Chem 46:2765–2773

176. Symyx Technology Inc., 2440 Camino Ramon, Suite 300, San Ramon, CA 94583, USA.

177. Law J, Zsoldos Z, Simon A, Reid D, Liu Y, Khew SY, Johnson AP, Major S, Wade RA, Ando HY (2009) Route designer: a retrosynthetic analysis tool utilizing automated retrosynthetic rule generation. J Chem Inf Model 49:593–602

178. Hartenfeller M (2010) Development of a computational method for reaction-driven de novo design of druglike compounds. Goethe University, Frankfurt am Main

179. Lipinski CA, Lombardo F, Dominy BW, Feeney PJ (2001) Experimental and computational approaches to estimate solubility and permeability in drug discovery and development settings. Adv Drug Deliv Rev 46:3–26

180. Hutter MC (2009) In silico prediction of drug properties. Curr Med Chem 16:189–202

181. He R, Chen D, He S (2012) Factor XI: hemostasis, thrombosis, and antithrombosis. Thromb Res 129:541–550

182. Fjellstrom O, Akkaya S, Beisel HG, Eriksson PO, Erixon K, Gustafsson D, Jurva U, Kang D, Karis D, Knecht W, Nerme V, Nilsson I, Olsson T, Redzic A, Roth R, Sandmark J, Tigerstrom A, Oster L (2015) Creating novel activated factor XI inhibitors through fragment based lead generation and structure aided drug design. PLoS One 10: e0113705

Methods in Pharmacology and Toxicology (2016): 217–255
DOI 10.1007/7653_2015_59
© Springer Science+Business Media New York 2015
Published online: 07 April 2016

# Applications of the Fragment Molecular Orbital Method to Drug Research

## Michael P. Mazanetz, Ewa Chudyk, Dmitri G. Fedorov, and Yuri Alexeev

## Abstract

The study of molecular behavior at high levels of theoretical accuracy has entered into a new age in computational drug discovery where quantum mechanical (QM) methods are becoming increasingly popular. Theoretically rigorous calculations can be prohibitively computationally expensive and time consuming. These two factors have necessitated the development of faster methods, and the fragment molecular orbital method (FMO) is one such method that has been used for efficient and accurate QM calculations in drug design. In this chapter, the use of FMO is described in detail for predicting geometry, estimating the binding energy of the ligands, conformational sampling, analysis of molecular interactions, deriving partial charges, and generating quantitative structure-activity relationship (QSAR) models.

**Keywords** QM (quantum mechanics), Quantum chemistry, FMO (fragment molecular orbitals method), CADD (computer-aided drug design), SBDD (structure-based drug design), GAMESS (general atomic and molecular electronic structure system), PIEDA (pair interaction energy decomposition analysis)

## 1 Introduction

Quantum mechanical (QM) methods provide an accurate way to compute the properties of chemical and biological systems; thus, they are appealing for use in computer-aided drug design (CADD). Historically, the use of QM methods has been viewed as too computationally expensive for routine applications in large-scale computational pipelines in CADD. However, in recent years, this obstacle has been greatly reduced owing to an increased computational power of computers and the development in QM methods. This has coincided with continued research into the applications of QM methods in CADD, including examples in docking [1], developing scoring functions [2, 3], estimating ligand energy binding [4], conformational sampling [5, 6], analysis of molecular interactions [1], deriving partial charges [7], and building quantitative structure-activity relationship (QSAR) models [1, 8, 9]. QM methods are becoming an integral part of CADD because they are regarded as the next evolutionary stage in the development of more accurate methods to assist drug design.

The theoretically less demanding alternative method to QM, widely used to study biological systems, is molecular mechanics (MM). In MM, the potential energy of the system is approximated by the sum of the individual terms describing bonded and non-bonded interactions between atoms. This is significantly less computationally expensive compared to the requirement in QM to solve the Schrödinger equation. The accuracy of MM strongly depends on the force field used, and the transferability of parameters. The standard force fields like XPLOR [10], Chemistry at HARvard Macromolecular Mechanics (CHARMM) [11, 12], or Assisted Model Building with Energy Refinement (AMBER) [13] usually provide accurate geometries of standard amino acid residues and nucleic acids [14], but struggle with more exotic molecules like ligands used in drug design, halogens, and metals (especially transition metals) [15, 16]. In addition, QM methods can compute free radicals, which often occur in the studies of radical damage in biology, and QM methods are also needed to study biochemical reactions, for example, in enzyme catalysis or when studying excited states.

In the last decade, the computer industry has undergone a significant transformation. While the clock speed of a single central processing unit (CPU) has been stagnant for years because of the limitation on the number of transistors that can be packed on a silicon chip, the advent of multicore computing is changing the computational sciences. Accelerators like graphical processing units (GPUs), Intel's many integrated core (MIC) architecture, and field-programmable gate arrays (FPGAs) offer a revolutionary potential to be harnessed. A number of MM, molecular dynamics (MD), and QM programs like NAMD [17], AMBER [18, 19], CHARMM, large-scale atomic/molecular massively parallel simulator (LAMMPS), TeraChem [20], and general atomic and molecular electronic structure system (GAMESS) [21] have been adopted for accelerators yielding an overall speedup factor of 2–7 [22]. There is also a significant interest in developing and porting drug discovery software programs on accelerators [23–28].

There has been a significant development in linear scaling approaches in recent years, which resulted in availability of a large number of linear scaling QM methods [29–31]. For example, a number of fragment-based methods have been developed over many years [32–40]. The fragment molecular orbital (FMO) method [41–45], which is discussed in this chapter, has been combined with many QM approaches. Analytic first and second derivatives have been developed for the FMO method. A concise introduction of FMO is given here and a detailed description is found elsewhere [42–45].

The FMO method is a general approach applicable to a large variety of systems: proteins, nucleotides (DNA and RNA), saccharides, molecular clusters, organic, and inorganic. Although in principle the FMO method can be applied to any system, in practice, some systems are difficult or perhaps impossible to configure to yield a successful calculation with FMO. One example of a difficult system is nanoclusters of metals. There is a continuous effort to probe the applicability of the FMO method to new kinds of systems and suggest efficient recipes for treating fragmentation issues. For example, recently, the FMO method has been applied to proteins interacting with inorganic surfaces [46, 47] which have various potential medicinal applications. The FMO method also has been used to study excited electronic states in proteins [48].

Consider the case of a large molecular system, for example, a protein. It is made of amino acid residues. These residues are polarized by the electrostatic field of the protein (and solvent), and there is some charge transfer between residues, in particular, in hydrogen bonding and salt bridges. A protein typically has many charged residues, so these effects are substantial, in particular, the polarization. The FMO method in its most commonly used two-body expansion (FMO2) has two steps. In the first step, the many-body polarization is accounted for by performing self-consistent QM fragment calculations in the electrostatic field of the protein, whereas quantum effects are accounted for at the intrafragment level. This field, denoted as the electrostatic potential (ESP), is computed from the electron densities of fragments. In the second step, fragment pair calculations are performed in the converged ESP to take into account interfragment quantum effects, such as charge transfer and exchange repulsion (the repulsion arising from the Pauli exclusion principle so that at short range electrons repel each other).

It should be clear that this approach is not exact. In other words, FMO treatment of the protein does not recover all of the QM energies. However, the difference is insignificant. The reason for the deviation lies in the neglected many-body QM effects. In FMO2, the charge transfer coupling of two hydrogen bonds between fragments $I,J$ and $J,K$ is neglected. This effect requires a fragment triple $(I,J,K)$ calculation. In other words, if some charge is transferred from $I$ to $J$, and some from $J$ to $K$, obviously, these two effects are coupled and cannot be computed independently, as is prescribed by FMO2. The three-body FMO3 does take into account this typically small effect. The error of FMO versus full QM, however, appears in the absolute total energies. If one considers energy differences, as commonly used in chemistry, for example, in the computation of binding energies, the deviations are usually very small. If the number of hydrogen bonds differs considerably between the two structures whose energies are subtracted, then the relative energies may have a noticeable error.

The issue of fragmentation in FMO has to be briefly described. Accurate FMO calculations can be performed if the electronic states of fragments are localized. For biological systems, a consequence of defining the fragmentation scheme amino acid residues across a peptide bond will result in a large error. This is because there is a strong delocalization of the electron density across a peptide bond. Therefore, in FMO, peptide bonds are left unfragmented, and instead, C–C bonds are detached (divided) between the amide carbonyl carbon and the Cα atoms, so that residue fragments differ from residues by a CO group. For nucleic acids several fragmentation schemes have been attempted [49].

Practically, graphical user interface (GUI) software such as Facio [50] can automatically fragment systems commonly appearing in biochemistry such as polypeptides, saccharides, and nucleotides, so one does not need to manually fragment these systems. However, for metal-containing enzymes, large ligands, and non-standard systems, their fragmentation will require manual intervention. The fragments in FMO are saturated by the ESP. In other words, no hydrogen caps are used. The fragmentation preserves the charge of fragments so that neutral, anionic, and cationic amino acids retain their charge as fragment residues.

As described above, FMO2 is based on calculating polarized fragments and evaluating the QM interactions between them. The basic equation is for the total energy $E$ of a system divided into $N$ fragments:

$$E^{\mathrm{FMO2}} = \sum_{I}^{N} E_I + \sum_{I>J}^{N} \left( E_{IJ} - E_I - E_J \right) \tag{1}$$

where $E_I$ are the energies of fragments, and $E_{IJ}$ are the energies of dimers. Different wave functions and basis sets can be used in the multilayer FMO approach (MFMO) [51]. Analytic first and second derivatives of this energy can be evaluated and used in geometry optimization or to simulate the IR spectra.

As described in more detail below, full geometry optimizations of all atoms have been done with FMO for several small proteins consisting of several hundreds of atoms, and a cellose nanoflake was optimized using a parametrized QM method [52]. FMO/MD because of its cost has so far found a very limited field of applications.

FMO has been implemented in several programs, among which ABINIT-MP [53], PAICS [54], and GAMESS [55] are most commonly used.

FMO is a dynamic and fast-developing method. In addition to FMO applications in CADD, a number of advancements were made to compute IR and Raman spectra with FMO [56] and accurate computation of cross section for mass spectrometry [57].

The following sections detail examples of how various CADD techniques have been approached using the FMO method [58, 59]. FMO applications are classified into two broad categories: energy computation with structure optimization and molecular properties. In the context of energy calculations, solvent models are also described. Several approaches can be taken to perform geometry optimizations with FMO, or optimization using MM can be employed to produce structures used in FMO calculations.

## 2   Energy Computation and Structure Optimization

QM methods can provide very accurate energies and geometries. The challenge in performing these calculations is in the size of the system, which for traditional QM methods scales on the order of $N^3$–$N^7$ (where $N$ is the number of atoms) depending on the level of theory. Linear scaling methods like FMO as the name suggests scale as $N$ with a large pre-factor. Thus, FMO is a more tractable approach for single-energy calculations, but it is still very expensive for geometry optimization of large systems because of the number of gradient calculations. In this section, we explain how very accurate energies and geometries can be computed with FMO. The treatment of other factors relevant for drug discovery, solvation, and entropy is also discussed.

### 2.1  Binding Energy Calculations

Prediction of binding affinities for small-molecule ligands to a target protein and correlating structure, and the function of those complexes, is one of the most challenging tasks in structure-based drug design (SBDD). From a microscopic point of view, the binding free energy ($\Delta G_{bind}$) can be calculated as a difference between the total energy of the protein-ligand complex ($\Delta G_{Protein+Ligand}$) and the sum of the energy of the protein in apo form ($\Delta G_{Protein}$) and the ligand alone ($\Delta G_{Ligand}$):

$$\Delta G_{bind} = \Delta G_{Protein+Ligand} - \left(\Delta G_{Protein} + \Delta G_{Ligand}\right) \quad (2)$$

Although this expression is quite simple, it has been proven difficult to establish those values both experimentally and computationally. Instead, in the drug discovery process, the half maximal inhibitory concentration ($IC_{50}$) values are often experimentally measured for tested inhibitors. The dependence between $IC_{50}$ and free energy of binding can be expressed as

$$\Delta G_{bind} = -RT\ln IC_{50} = \Delta H - T\Delta S \quad (3)$$

where $R$ and $T$ stand for the universal gas constant and temperature, respectively.

The second part of the equation above divides the physical effects of binding energy into enthalpy ($\Delta H$) and entropy ($\Delta S$). Depending on the inhibitor series, the roles of enthalpy and entropy in binding can be different, and ideally, both of those effects should be accounted for when performing calculations. However, due to the relatively high cost of accurate entropy calculations, it is often either simplified or completely neglected. Indeed, within a series of structurally related ligands, similar binding entropy is often assumed, and binding energy is simplified to the calculated enthalpy contribution.

FMO represents a reasonable compromise between calculation speed and accuracy for affinity prediction. Large protein systems are divided in an automatic manner along the protein backbone to include only one amino acid residue per fragment. High-level QM calculations are performed for each fragment pair and interactions include nonclassical intermolecular forces, such as cation-$\pi$, dipole-$\pi$, halogen-$\pi$, carbonyl n-$\pi^*$, and so-called nonclassical hydrogen bonds. In particular, the charge transfer and polarization effects are important for hydrogen bonding accuracy prediction. Pairwise calculations for a series of small-molecule ligands can also facilitate rationalizing structure-activity relationship (SAR) effects, directly indicating amino acids interacting stronger or weaker with ligands in the series. The physical effect, which is not usually included in the FMO calculations, is the entropy (configuration sampling), which can also play a role in some ligand series.

The FMO method was successfully applied to study the binding affinity for a series of 28 published cyclin-dependent kinase 2 (CDK2) inhibitors, based on a number of X-ray crystal structures [4]. It has been shown that the FMO-predicted gas-phase enthalpic contribution to the binding energy at MP2/6-31G* theory level correlates well with experimental $IC_{50}$ values ($r^2 = 0.68$). Further calculations on the system included the entropic correction component and solvation terms to more accurately estimate free energies of binding. The solvation energy was calculated using the relatively simple Poisson-Boltzmann equation and the solvent-accessible surface area (SASA) approach. Accounting for those two effects significantly improved the overall correlation between the calculated and predicted binding free energies (with $r^2$ values close to 0.9 for various models) [4].

In another study [74], the FMO method was used for structure optimization and binding energy for four FK506 binding protein (FKPB) complexes containing rapamycin and two synthetic ligands. The geometry optimization for those complexes was performed with the FMO-RHF method at 3-21G theory level, and then refined at FMO-MP2 theory level with a 6-31G* basis set using single-point energy calculations. For all ligands, the significant part of the total binding energy resulted from the correlation contribution, ranging between 70 and 80 % of total values. This indicated the importance of QM effects in binding affinity predictions. Similarly to the CDK2 study described above [4], solvation effects were calculated with Poisson-Boltzmann surface area method.

The FMO method has also been used to evaluate binding affinities of influenza A viral hemagglutinins (HA) [60, 61]. First, selective binding of avian and human HA subtype H3 and Neu5Acα2-3 and α2-6Gal (avian α2-3, human α2-6) was calculated at the FMO-MP2/6-31G* theory level with the polarizable continuum model (PCM) for solvent. Hydrophilic interactions between Gal-4 OH and side-chain $NH_2CO$ on Gln226 supported by the intermolecular hydrogen-bond network to the 1-COO group on Neu5Ac moiety were distinguished as a source of favorable interactions of avian H3 over the human species. Further Gln226Leu substitution in the avian H3 HA1 domain increased the binding affinity to human α2-6 due to dispersion forces. It was also found that binding between human H3 and human α2-6 was not governed by the hydrogen bond with the side chain of Ser228. This derived fragment-based knowledge improved the understanding of interactions between viral HAs and human α2-6 [60]. Binding specificity of three sialosides and HA was also estimated with FMO-MP2/PCM/6-31G(d) calculations. Binding energy calculated for those complexes was similar for all of them, suggesting that binding is not regulated by the sialoside homotropic allosteric effect [61].

Until recently, the only way to compute accurately entropy and free energies in FMO was by doing FMO/MD simulations [62]. However, they are expensive and so far have been mostly limited to chemical reactions in an explicit solvent [63, 64]. The only other example is the use of FMO-based QM/MM [54], applied to perform MD of a protein-ligand complex. Alternatively, there have been various attempts in evaluating the entropy and free energy from MM simulations [60, 61] and other modes [4].

However, with the developed analytic second derivatives of the energy, it is possible to evaluate the entropy and free energies using FMO. This is accomplished for a single minimum via the statistical mechanics. FMO has been applied to study the free energies of several chemical reactions in an explicit solvent [56, 65]. While single minimum free energies do not include conformational entropy, still it is a step forward to achieving the accuracy and reliability needed for biochemical simulations. Free energies computed from statistical mechanics for a single minimum using the FMO/frozen domain and dimers (FDD) method (*see* Section 2.3) have been reported for protein-ligand binding and enzymatic reactions [66].

**2.2  Solvation Effects**

Treatment of solvation effects is a difficult problem for atomistic methods, because solvent molecules at room temperature tend to have high entropy and the time scale required to analyze solvent behavior is large, making dynamics simulations very expensive. Water is the common solvent studied in biological systems, forming hydrogen bonds to ligands, nucleic acids, and proteins, or trapped in hydrophobic protein clefts. In addition, polar solvents such as water polarize the electronic state of the solute, and similarly the solute polarizes the solvent. Although the electrostatic component of solvent effects is relatively straightforward to take into account, many models rely on various parameters such as atomic radii or an effective dielectric constant for the solute, which often requires a manual estimation. Solvent can be considered either explicitly as atoms or implicitly via either a continuum (surface) representation; some models rely on statistical distribution functions of solvent molecules and may be considered as a separate category. Alternative mixed approaches consider explicit and implicit models, which is often resorted to by describing some strongly bound or otherwise important solvent molecules explicitly, and the rest implicitly.

Implicit solvent models have a considerable computational efficiency advantage over more accurate explicit models. The former do not require studying the dynamics of the solvent molecules. On the one hand, implicit models typically rely on parameters which have the potential of reproducing experimental results better, but on the other hand, implicit models often neglect some solvent effects, in particular, the charge transfer between solute and solvent.

Two implicit solvation methods have been interfaced with FMO: (a) polarizable continuum model (PCM) [67–70], Poisson–Boltzmann (PB) equation [71], and one statistical approach, the reference interaction site model (RISM) [72]. There are several ways to include solvent explicitly in FMO, by treating the solvent either as FMO fragments or as effective fragment potentials (EFP) [73]. The immense problem exists in the need to take into account the movement of solvent molecules.

It has been shown on many occasions [60, 74] that neglecting solvent effects results in a drastic overestimation of the binding energies, which is due to the desolvation effect [75]. Solvent also affects various electronic properties, such as pair interaction energies, which is known as the screening effects. This is described in more detail below.

## 2.3  Geometry Optimization (Ligand and Protein Enzymes)

A straightforward application of the FMO analytic gradient to geometry optimizations [76] of biochemical systems is possible for small proteins. Chignolin (PDB: 1UAO) [77], Trp-cage (1L2Y) [78], and crambin (1CRN) [79], as well as heparin oligomer [80], have been optimized in solution. However, because proteins are very flexible and take many geometry optimization steps, it is computationally too expensive to optimize larger proteins using the full approach. To accelerate geometry optimization, partial schemes have been developed in which only a part of the structure is optimized [81]: partial-energy gradient (PEG) [82] and frozen domain (FD) [66, 83–85] are two approaches.

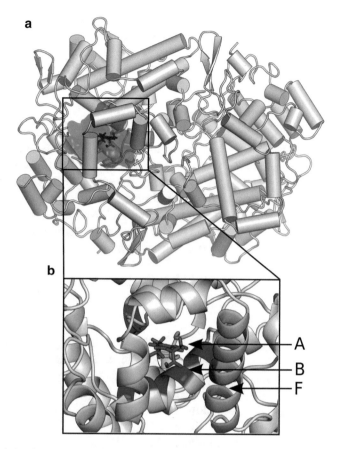

**Fig. 1** (**a**) Structure of prostaglandin H(2) synthase-1 (COX1) in complex with ibuprofen (PDB:1EQG), optimized with FMO/FDD/RHF/STO-3G:B3LYP-D/6-31G*. (**b**) Zoomed in active site with domain definition: active (**A**), polarizable buffer (**B**), and frozen (**F**) domains are colored *red*, *blue*, and *gray*, respectively

In the FMO/FD method, three domains, **A**, **B**, and **F**, are defined in a chemical system as shown in Fig. 1. The active domain, **A**, includes atoms relaxed during geometry optimization. A drug molecule is usually assigned to the domain **A**. The polarizable buffer domain, **B**, includes fragments whose electronic state is fully relaxed at each step of a geometry optimization. The domain **B** consists of the domain **A** and includes some fragments around it, typically within a distance of 3–5 Å. The frozen domain, **F**, contains all atoms not included in the domain **B**. The electronic state of the fragments in **F** is computed once at the beginning and kept fixed during geometry optimization of atoms in domain **A**. Each fragment is assigned to a domain. FMO/FD is based on the multilayer FMO, and domains **B** and **F** are assigned to layers 1 and 2, respectively.

The FMO/FD energy (detailed definitions are given elsewhere [83]) is

$$E^{\mathrm{FMO/FD}} = E^B + \Delta E^{AF} = \sum_{I \in B} E_I' + \sum_{\substack{I > J \\ I, J \in B}} \Delta E_{IJ} + \sum_{\substack{I \in A \\ J \in F}} \Delta E_{IJ}' \quad (4)$$

The computational savings come from the assumptions that the energy of fragments in **F** is constant. Thus, the gradient is zero and the energy of monomers and dimers in **F** need not be reevaluated.

An additional saving can be made if one assumes that the energy of dimers in **B** (excluding dimers containing at least one **A** fragment) is also constant. This variation of FMO/FD is called FMO/FDD (frozen domain and dimers). The energy is defined in the following way:

$$E^{\mathrm{FMO/FDD}} = E^B + \Delta E^{AF'} = \sum_{I \in B} E_I' + \sum_{\substack{I > J \\ I \in A, J \in B}} \Delta E_{IJ} + \sum_{\substack{I \in A \\ J \in F}} \Delta E_{IJ}' \quad (5)$$

FMO/FDD can considerably speed up calculations, especially if the domain **B** is large, as is the case when one includes some fragments in the binding pocket of a protein in **B**. For a short notation, both FD and FDD are denoted by FMO/FD in the general discussion below.

The FMO/FD method has some similarities with QM/MM methods, but FMO/FD is a more general and potentially more accurate approach. The **F** domain in FMO/FD is computed at a QM level only once (with FMO1), whereas in QM/MM the bulk of the system is computed with MM. Because all calculations in FMO/FD are done with QM, there is no problem with link atoms, and the active site itself can be easily resized. The polarizable buffer calculations are done using FMO efficiently because of fragmentation, compared to full QM in QM/MM.

How do you set up FMO/FD calculations? The first step is to choose the domain **A**. In drug discovery it usually includes a ligand and possibly some part of the binding pocket. A large ligand can be split into multiple FMO fragments, to determine functional group effects on binding, for example [86]. It is possible to optimize only some atoms in **A**, such as side chains. The next step is the definition of the **B** domain. This can be done automatically by including all fragments containing atoms within a certain distance, $R_B$, from **A**. Note that since all domains are defined in terms of FMO fragments, even if a single atom belongs to domain **B**, then all atoms in that fragment are included. Thus, care is required in choosing a computationally tractable $R_B$ (often about 3–5 Å, although charged fragments in **A** typically necessitate larger radii). The remainder of the system belongs to **F**. Another important issue is how to choose theories and basis sets. A high level of theory and a large basis set are usually used for the domain **B** while a low level of theory and a small basis set are used for the domain **F**, for example, RHF/STO-3G for **F** and DFT/6-31G* for **B**.

To demonstrate a ligand optimization in a large system with FMO/FDD, the solvated structure of prostaglandin H(2) synthase-1 (COX-1) in complex with the reversible competitive inhibitor ibuprofen (PDB: 1EQG) was chosen, containing 19,471 atoms total. The structures of the complex and domains are shown in Fig. 1. The ibuprofen structure inside COX-1 was optimized with FMO/FDD/RHF/STO-3G:B3LYP-D/6-31G* where **B** was treated at the B3LYP-D/6-31G* level, while **F** was described by RHF/STO-3G. The ibuprofen was assigned to **A**, while **B** was defined by an $R_B$ value of 3.9 Å. There were 25 fragments in **B**: 19 protein residues, 1 ligand, and 5 water molecules. The FMO/FDD optimization of the whole system took 31 steps computed in 32 h on 6 dual-CPU quad-core 2.83 GHz Xeon nodes. The calculations of the **F** domain took 98 min in the beginning, and each step of geometry optimization (**B**) took about 59 min [83].

Alternatively, it is possible to combine FMO with MM and optimize the coordinates of all atoms, the active-site atoms with QM (FMO), and the rest with MM. This is an attractive way to run simulations since the typical MM force fields are well parameterized in terms of accuracy when the system is composed from standard building blocks like amino acid residues in proteins or nucleotides in DNA and RNA. At the same time, MM calculations are significantly cheaper than QM calculations. The limitations of MM are often uncertain accuracy for drug molecules and the inability to deal with breaking and creating chemical bonds. There are many variations of QM/MM. One of the implementations in GAMESS interfaced with Tinker [87] is a mechanical embedding in the integrated molecular orbital (MO) molecular mechanics (IMOMM) method [88, 89] where the MO part can be a regular QM or FMO [76, 90]. The main difference with typical QM/MM is that in IMOMM there are no MM charges considered in QM calculations. Another implementation is to have QM/MM based on FMO, which has been implemented in PAICS interfaced with AMBER [54].

In FMO/MM based on the IMOMM method, the first step is to assign atoms to the FMO region, whose atoms have coordinates $R_1$, and assign the rest of the atoms to the MM region with coordinates $R_2$. The total energy and its gradient have two FMO and MM contributions:

$$E^{FMO/MM} = E^{FMO}(R_1) + E^{MM}(R_1, R_2) \qquad (6)$$

$$\frac{\partial E^{\text{FMO/MM}}}{\partial R_1} = \frac{\partial E^{\text{FMO}}}{\partial R_1} + \frac{\partial E^{\text{MM}}}{\partial R_1}$$

$$\frac{\partial E^{\text{FMO/MM}}}{\partial R_2} = \frac{\partial E^{\text{MM}}}{\partial R_2} \tag{7}$$

The interaction energy between FMO and MM is included in $E^{\text{MM}}$.

FMO/MM calculations are done in the following steps:

1. Prepare structure and assign atoms to MO and MM regions.
2. Optimize MM atoms while keeping FMO atoms fixed. Compute MM energy and gradient.
3. Compute FMO energy and gradient.
4. Compute $E^{\text{FMO/MM}}$ energy and gradient from contributions computed in previous steps.
5. If $\partial E^{\text{FMO/MM}}/\partial R_1$ is not small enough, then update the geometry and proceed to **step 2**.

An example of FMO/MM optimization has been reported in the literature [90]. FMO/MM optimization was performed on the explicitly solvated (6 Å shell) complex of CK2α and its ligand ((1-(6-[6-(cyclopentylamino)-1H-indazol-1-yl]pyrazin-2-yl)-1H-pyrrol-3-yl)-acetic acid) (PDB code: 3AT3). The FMO region ($R_1$) was defined as the ligand with all amino acid residues and water molecules within 2.0 unitless FMO distance [91] from the ligand. We assigned 667 atoms to the FMO region computed with FMO2/RHF-D/6-31G and 1980 atoms to the MM region, computed with AMBER-99 force field for protein, GAFF force field for ligand, and TIP3P model for water. The calculations were done on 112 CPU cores of Xeon 3.0 GHz. A single geometry optimization step (including one FMO gradient and MM optimization) took 36 min.

Until recently, the studies of enzymatic reactions with FMO relied on obtaining a reaction path with other approaches such as QM/MM [92–95] and a subsequent use of FMO to refine energetics (reaction energy and the barrier) via single-point FMO calculations, and also in the analysis of the contributions of residues on the catalytic activity.

Recently, two ways have been suggested to map reaction pathways with FMO/FDD. First, in constrained geometry optimizations, assuming the reaction coordinate is known a priori allows one to map a reaction path [84, 85], and second, using the intrinsic reaction coordinate (IRC). IRC requires a Hessian calculation at a transition state, and the reaction path is mapped automatically from the TS to both reactants and products [66]. Mapping a path for the reaction of phosphoglycolohydroxamic acid and the triosephosphate isomerase (PDB: 7TIM) using quantum mechanics for the whole system containing 9227 atoms took 102 h of computation time on a PC cluster.

Another way to optimize large systems is to use very fast parameterized QM methods such as the density-functional tight binding (DFTB) combined with the fragment molecular orbital method [96]. For a fullerite slab containing an impressive 1,030,440 atoms, a single-point step in the geometry optimization with FMO-DFTB took 83 min on 8 dual-CPU eight-core 2.00 GHz Xeon nodes (128 cores).

# 3 Molecular Properties

Molecular properties, which can be computed with FMO, are very diverse. They vary from multipole calculations [97] to FMO descriptors for QSAR and scoring functions. Perhaps the most important FMO application relevant to drug discovery is the analysis of molecular interactions, which is covered in great detail; other properties are reviewed briefly.

## 3.1 Molecular Interactions in FMO

Although considerable progress has been achieved with various linear-scaling QM methods, providing the total energies and gradients, it is also very desirable to be able to divide the energy into contributions corresponding to well-defined chemical constituents. This is exactly what many fragment-based methods achieve as a by-product of simulations (in addition to the total properties).

In FMO, it can be seen that the basic equation (Eq. (1)) has some form of the subsystem properties, obtained from the energies of monomers and dimers. Typically, however, Eq. (1) is rewritten separating the ESP contributions. This is convenient because in Eq. (1) the energies include the ESP contribution, which can be very large (the interaction of the electronic state with the ESP), on the order of hundreds of kcal/mol. It is more productive to use internal energies, which describe the energy of fragments polarized by the ESP, but from which the ESP energy is subtracted postfactum for the analysis (this is rather similar to the notion of the internal energy of the solute in solution in PCM).

For fragments I (and likewise for dimers IJ), the internal energy $E_I'$ is obtained from the QM energy $E_I$ by subtracting the interaction of the electronic density $\mathbf{D}^I$ with the ESP $\mathbf{V}^I$:

$$E_I' = E_I - \mathrm{Tr}(\mathbf{D}^I\mathbf{V}^I) \tag{8}$$

Using the internal energies, Eq. (1) becomes [91]

$$E^{\mathrm{FMO2}} = \sum_I^N E_I' + \sum_{I>J}^N \left(E_{IJ}' - E_I' - E_J' + \mathrm{Tr}(\Delta\mathbf{D}^{IJ}\mathbf{V}^{IJ})\right) \tag{9}$$

Here, the ESP contribution takes the form of the interaction of the density transfer matrix $\Delta\mathbf{D}^{IJ}$ in the basis of the atomic orbitals (it can also be called charge transfer) between fragments $I$ and $J$ with the ESP of dimer $IJ$.

This equation is already very useful for analysis, as it describes the energies of fragments and pair interactions (int). The latter are

$$\Delta E_{IJ}^{int} = E_{IJ}' - E_I' - E_J' + \mathrm{Tr}\left(\Delta\mathbf{D}^{IJ}\mathbf{V}^{IJ}\right) \qquad (10)$$

The values called either pair interaction energies (PIE) or interfragment interaction energies (IFIE) in FMO have been used in many applications to discuss the role of amino acid residues in binding a ligand.

The above expression has more terms in solution. In addition, it is possible to decompose the total values of PIEs into several contributions in the PIE decomposition analysis (PIEDA) [98–100]. The expression in solution (PCM) is

$$E^{FMO2/PCM} = \sum_I E_I'' + \sum_I \Delta E_I^{solv} + \sum_{I>J} \Delta E_{IJ}^{int} \qquad (11)$$

Here, the fragments are polarized by both ESP of other fragments and a potential from the solvent. The $E_I''$ term defines the internal energy of fragments in solution, $\Delta E_I^{solv}$ is the fragment solvation energy, and $\Delta E_{IJ}^{int}$ is the PIE in solution. The definitions are

$$\Delta E_I^{solv} = \Delta E_I^{cav} + \Delta E_I^{es} + \Delta E_I^{disp} + \Delta E_I^{rep} \qquad (12)$$

The $\Delta E_I^{solv}$ term in PCM is computed as the sum of the cavitation (cav) energies (the free energy loss to create the cavity in solution), to which one adds the electrostatic (es), dispersion (disp), and repulsion (rep) solvent-solute interactions:

$$\Delta E_{IJ}^{int} = \Delta E_{IJ}^{ES} + \Delta E_{IJ}^{EX} + \Delta E_{IJ}^{CT+mix} + \Delta E_{IJ}^{DI} + \Delta E_{IJ}^{SOLV} \qquad (13)$$

The PIEs $\Delta E_{IJ}^{int}$ in solution are decomposed into the electrostatic (ES: note that this is the solute-solute electrostatic interaction; do not confuse it with the solute-solvent (es) interaction), exchange repulsion (EX), charge transfer, and higher order mix terms (CT + mix), dispersion (DI), and solvent screening (SOLV):

$$\Delta E_{IJ}^{SOLV} = \Delta E_{IJ}^{es2} + \Delta E_{IJ}^{es3} + \Delta E_{IJ}^{disp} + \Delta E_{IJ}^{rep} \qquad (14)$$

The solvent screening $\Delta E_{IJ}^{SOLV}$ is the direct solvent contribution to PIEs (indirectly, solvent affects other components as well, because the solute is polarized by the solvent). It is computed as the sum of the electrostatic screening (es2), describing the interaction of the induced solvent charges with the solute (a counterforce to the strong electrostatic solute-solute ES interactions), the coupling of the solute density transfer $\Delta\mathbf{D}^{IJ}$ with the solute potential (es3), as well as the non-electrostatic contributions to the solvent screening: dispersion (disp) and repulsion (rep). The latter two describe non-electrostatic components for the interaction of the solvent molecules with the solute, counteracting the solute-solute interactions of DISP and EX, respectively. Note that in PCM there is no explicit solute-solvent charge transfer, so there is no solute-solvent counterpart to CT + mix. The dominant part of $\Delta E_{IJ}^{SOLV}$ is typically the $\Delta E_{IJ}^{es2}$ component.

The interaction energies in solution $\Delta E_{IJ}^{int}$ include the solvent screening and commonly their values are smaller than PIEs in a vacuum. It should be noted that the "perfect" screening, i.e., the reduction of the electrostatic interaction by the factor of the dielectric constant, $\varepsilon$, is observed only for the interaction of two-point charges. Indeed, this picture is observed in the interaction of two solvated ions at a relatively long distance computed with PIEDA/PCM.

The question is however what is the physical nature of the electrostatic solvent screening. PIEDA/PCM gives a simple answer to this as the cross-interaction of the induced solvent charges with the solute. Consider a cation, $Q_1^+$, and an anion, $Q_2^-$. Between them there is a very strong attractive interaction $Q_1^+ Q_2^- / R_{12}$ where $R_{12}$ is the separation. The screening in solvent arises because around each ion there is an induced solvent charge of the opposite charge, $q_1^-$ and $q_2^+$. The interaction between the two charges $Q_1^+$ and $Q_2^-$ in solution has an additional interaction between the induced charges and ions, $\left(Q_1^+ q_2^- + q_1^- Q_2^-\right)/(2R_{12})$. The screening is thus directly related to the induced charges. The cross-interaction is so called because it is the interaction between one ion and the induced solvent charge of the other ion, and vice versa. Finally, it can be noted that the induced charge in the stand-alone case (when ions are infinitely separated) is given by $q_1^- = -(\varepsilon - 1)Q_1^+/\varepsilon$, which gives the expression that in solution the interaction between the two ions is $Q_1^+ Q_2^-/(\varepsilon R_{12})$ (*see* reference [98] for full derivation).

The actual electronic structure and the solvent-induced charge distribution are much more complex. For example, let us consider a protein. If there are only two charged residues in the whole protein, and these two residues are quite far from each other (so that there is little charge transfer between them), then the above picture of the electrostatic interaction between them (ES) being reduced by the factor of $\varepsilon$ so that $\Delta E_{IJ}^{ES}/\left(\Delta E_{IJ}^{ES} + \Delta E_{IJ}^{SOLV}\right) \approx \varepsilon$ can be expected to hold approximately. This is because the solvent charges (which determine the solvent screening) around each of the two ions are determined to a good approximation by each ion independently. Now imagine that there are three ions, two cations $Q_1^+$ and $Q_2^+$, and one anion $Q_3^-$, and the interaction of $Q_1^+$ and $Q_3^-$ is to be determined, with $Q_2^+$ lying near $Q_3^-$. In this case, the solvent charges around the anion are now determined by both the anion itself and the other cation $(Q_2^+)$. This leads to the so-called charge quenching effect [98] where the induced charges are reduced (quenched) because of the addition of the solvent potentials due to both $Q_3^-$ and $Q_2^+$, which determine the induced solvent charge around $Q_3^-$. In this case, the potentials of the opposite ions have the opposite sign. Thus, the total potential, the induced charge, and the screening are reduced.

Summarizing, the presence of a third ion affects (reduces or increases) the induced charges on the other two ions, and the screening effect is now determined not only by the two ions themselves, but also by the third ion. Thus, in proteins with many-charge residues, various kinds of screenings can be observed. In fact, FMO provides a way of defining local dielectric constants either for the fragments themselves or for individual pairs. Three types of the effective screening are the regular screening $\varepsilon > 1$, negative screening $\varepsilon < 0$, and anti-screening $0 < \varepsilon < 1$. In the regular screening, the strong electrostatic ES interaction between two fragments is reduced by the solvent, in the anti-screening screening it is enhanced, and in the negative screening the sign of the interaction changes. This complex picture arises because of the many-body effects (e.g., the coupling of the solute potential of three charged residues).

An alternative to PCM, which has its own strong and weak points, is to use explicit solvent. One way is to describe the solvent with effective fragment potentials (EFP) [101]. For the FMO/EFP method, there is an analysis somewhat analogous to, but in other ways different from, PIEDA, called interaction energy analysis (IEA). It has been applied to analyze the solvent effects on the protein-ligand binding [102]. While such explicit solvent treatment in principle is ultimately superior to continuum treatment, there remains the issue of having to average solvent configurations, potentially requiring calculations to be performed in combination with MD.

To improve the reliability of PIEs, the counterpoise correction for the basis set superposition error (BSSE) can be applied to PIEs [103, 104]. Also, a contraction of many-body effects in FMO3 and FMO4 can be accomplished producing a formal two-body PIE [90, 105]. It has been argued that this is useful for drug design as amino acid residues can be subdivided into more than one fragment, thereby producing a more detailed interaction picture. Basis set superposition error (BSSE) corrections have been suggested for pair interactions only [103, 104]. Alternatively, one can use the complete basis set limit (CBS) in the FMO integrated into our own $n$-layered integrated molecular orbital and molecular mechanics (ONIOM) [106].

A further aspect for consideration is the amount of configurational contribution to the PIE. There are two ways to address this: either to compute PIEs along an MD trajectory [103] or to use a classical model describing the temperature effects on PIEs [107].

In understanding the interactions involved in biochemical systems, the details of fragment-fragment interactions are often required beyond just the bulk information. For example, a ligand can have two functional groups, and the contribution of each group to the protein-ligand binding may be of interest. In the context of FMO, this can make use of the configuration analysis for fragment interaction (CAFI) [108] or a fragment interaction analysis based on local MP2 (FILM) [109]. The former focuses on providing polarization and charge transfer components, while the latter focuses on the dispersion; both divide the total PIE into MO-based contributions, and the MOs can be associated with a functional group by looking at its space distribution.

## 3.2 Molecular Interaction Applications

One of the goals of structure-based drug discovery is to design ligands, which can exploit favorable protein-ligand interactions, and to minimize unfavorable interactions toward the protein target of interest. The FMO method facilitates this process by making the analysis of protein-ligand interactions possible from the output of PIE and PIEDA calculations. These calculations provide both the total energy of a ligand-protein interaction and the decomposed energy components which can include electrostatics, exchange repulsion, charge transfer, and higher order mix terms, dispersion, and solvent screening. In addition, the reduced computational expense of this linear scaling method allows for satisfactory throughput of ligands for routine visual inspection of the results. FMO therefore lends itself to many useful applications which exploit molecular interactions, including:

- During structure- and fragment-based drug discovery when there is a requirement to rationalize an SAR

- Investigating the thermodynamic profile of an X-ray crystal fragment hit

- Ranking and prioritizing virtual screening hits, ligand-binding poses, and results derived from scaffold-hopping studies

- Decomposing a ligand into fragments to study the structural contributions to binding free energy

- Protein structure and stability studies

This section reviews examples of these applications in more detail.

An SAR can be analyzed and the design of new molecules can be driven using the FMO methodology. This process is optimal when the initial starting points for the calculations are derived from

X-ray crystal structures. Other researchers have opted to take a random sample [110] from the production run of an MD simulation, an averaged structure sampled from an MD trajectory [111], or representative structures following clustering of the simulation outputs [112]. Another approach would be to sample multiple MD runs [47]. Often MD simulations can be fairly time consuming, and thus, an assumption is made that the conformation of the X-ray crystal structure is likely to contribute significantly to the Boltzmann-averaged potentials for the free-energy estimation. Performing a single-point calculation in FMO with this starting point is more likely to be a good representation of the system than one from which the phase space is poorly sampled. This method has been used previously to generate poses for FMO calculations [4].

For protein-ligand interactions, particularly in the context of drug discovery and guiding medicinal chemistry, the most important pairwise fragment interactions are those between the ligand and the protein fragments. Subtle changes in ligand substituents can be studied using FMO in a congeneric series of compounds. Here an assumption is made that the ligand changes do not affect protein-heavy atom positions, thereby reducing the need to re-optimize the entire system. This has been demonstrated through the analysis of 14 X-ray structures taken from the literature of CDK2 inhibitors [4]. Here, the sum of the PIE for the 14 inhibitors correlated well ($r^2 = 0.68$) with the free energy of binding as calculated from the measured potencies. Using PIEDA, the quantum mechanical component of ligand binding can be observed and understood (Fig. 2). Compound **18** differs from **17** by a di-fluoro substitution on the phenyl ring. The two fluorines have an additive favorable influence in the charge transfer between the Lys33 and the Asp145 residues of CDK2, as seen in Fig. 2a. There is an increase in the total favorable interaction energy between **17** and **18**, −7.1 kcal/mol and −25.3 kcal/mol, respectively, and a similar increase in charge transfer, as seen in Fig. 2b. This QM effect, in addition to potential solvation and entropic ligand conformation effects, results in an increase in potency from 140 nM for **17** to 3 nM for **18**.

The Facio software allows for a graphical representation of the data [50, 113]. Single FMO PIEDA results are best viewed as histogram plots whilst comparisons between a larger number of ligands can be viewed as heat maps, as shown in Fig. 2. Amari et al. developed a visualized cluster analysis of protein-ligand interactions (VISCANA) which measures the squared Euclidean distance between two ligands by their amino acid fragment—ligand interaction energy patterns (fingerprints)—and clusters the ligands based on the dissimilarity measure (Eq. (15)) [1]:

$$d_{IJ} = \sum_{K=1} \left( \Delta E_{IK} - \Delta E_{JK} \right)^2 \tag{15}$$

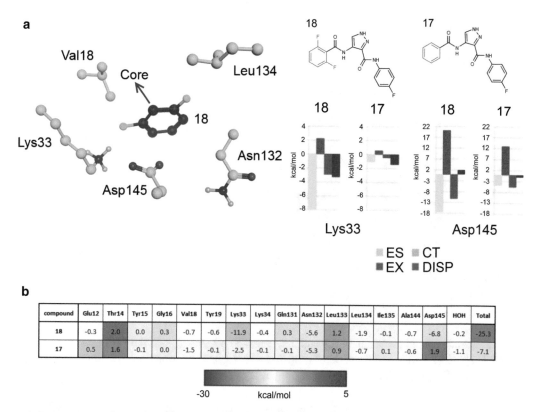

**Fig. 2** (**a**) *Left:* Truncated X-ray structure of PDB ID 2VTP and the aryl moiety (in *blue*) on which the calculation was based. *Right:* Structures of compounds **17** (PDB ID: 2VTO) and **18** (PDB ID: 2VTP) with the aryl moiety used in the FMO calculation (*blue*) taken from [98] and the associated PIEDA plots for interactions with Lys33 and Asp145. (**b**) Heatmap showing the PIE for the aryl moieties from compounds **17** and **18**

This method is sufficiently computationally efficient at the FMO-HF/STO-3G level that it has been applied to the analysis of VS hits where 100 ligand-protein complexes can be calculated in less than a day on a 60-processor cluster [1].

Recently, Kurauchi et al. have extended this work to incorporate the MACCS structural keys [114] of the ligand molecules into the clustering and they also utilized self-organizing maps (SOM) [115] and multidimensional scaling (MDS) [116] techniques to assist in the visual interpretation of the clustering [117]. These extensions were aimed at identifying false-positive ligands more efficiently and in potentially identifying structural changes to improve weaker binders or remove false-negative ligands.

The above procedures can also be used on multiple conformations of a single molecule, as derived from a molecular docking experiment, for example. This enables a refinement of free energy of binding predictions over those derived from the docking algorithm, which traditionally has been cited as being better at generating poses as opposed to the accurate prediction of binding free energies [118].

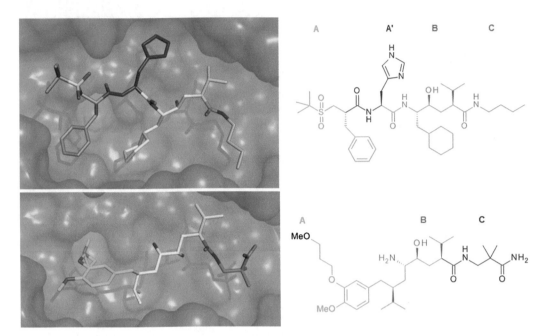

**Fig. 3** X-ray structures of peptidomimetics and fragmentation scheme used in the FMO analysis. *Left*: *Top*: CGP 38'560 (PDB ID: 1RNE); *bottom*: Aliskiren (PDB ID: 2V0Z). *Right*: The corresponding fragmentation scheme used during the FMO calculations

Figure 3 demonstrates that examination of a functional group of ligands molecules can give an insight into the effect of ligand binding within the local environment and the contribution that the fragment has the total enthalpic free energy of binding of the whole ligand. This can be quantified into a molecular metric, the fragment efficiency ($FE_{PIE}$) calculated by dividing the fragment PIE by the fragment heavy atom count [86]:

$$FE_{PIE} = \text{Fragment pair interaction energy/heavy atom count}$$

(16)

As an example with the protein renin, the peptidomimetic inhibitor CGP38'560 and Aliskiren were fragmented to demonstrate the ability of the method to illustrate the size and efficiency of different molecular interactions. The derived PIE was divided by heavy atom count to give a theoretical $FE_{PIE}$, as seen in Table 1. As a result, the ligand fragments have differing $FE_{PIE}$ values. The higher $FE_{PIE}$ values contribute more to the enthalpic component of binding than the lower $FE_{PIE}$ fragments. In particular, FMO illustrates the opportunities to further optimize ligand functional groups to have further gains in protein-ligand interactions.

An elaboration of this method is to apply FMO in a combinatorial fashion to study the expansion of fragment- and lead-like hits, to explore fragment merging, functional group replacements, and

**Table 1**
**Fragment efficiency (FE$_{PIE}$)**

| Compound | Activity (nM) | Total PIE (kcal/mol) | Fragment[a] | PIE (kcal/mol) | FE$_{PIE}$ |
|---|---|---|---|---|---|
| CGP 38'560 | 1 | −177 | A | −27.40 | −1.71 |
| | | | A′ | −28.43 | −2.84 |
| | | | B | −85.98 | −4.78 |
| | | | C | −34.84 | −4.98 |
| Aliskiren | 0.6 | −191 | A | −51.47 | −3.43 |
| | | | B | −83.95 | −6.00 |
| | | | C | −55.69 | −5.57 |

Examination of the fragment contributions to the total pair interaction energies (PIE) for the peptidomimetic inhibitor CGP 38'560 and Aliskiren. Showing the activity in nM, the total PI, and the fragment contributions to PIE and FE$_{PIE}$
[a]*See* Fig. 3 for the fragmentation scheme

scaffold hopping via multiple calculations based around a single-crystal structure. Fragment linking strategies can also be realized in circumstances where there are multiple distinct neighboring binding pockets on a protein surface and there are fragments which occupy one or a number of these sites taken from one or more crystal structures [119]. The ideal fragment-linking process will produce positive cooperativity [120] between binding partners, which is where a compound has additive potency gains through combining the individual fragments. A recent review identified several examples of fragment linking in the literature [4]. This has been demonstrated in the fragment linking of two Hsp90 fragments, **1** (IC$_{50}$ = 1500 μM) and **2** (IC$_{50}$ = 1000 μM), to yield the more potent inhibitor **3** (IC$_{50}$ = 1.5 μM) [121], *see* Fig. 4.

These results were supported by FMO analysis using MP2 and the 6-31G* basis set in combination with the PCM implicit solvation model to generate PIE values (Fig. 5). The linking of fragments **1** (−8.87 kcal/mol) and **2** (−9.03 kcal/mol) using a propyl linker to afforded inhibitor **3** (−41.3 kcal/mol) was confirmed in the measured potency [121]. In successful fragment linking strategies, the maintenance of the thermodynamic profile of the linking partners is observed. Fragments which are stabilized through electrostatic dominant forces, like H-bonds, are predominantly enthalpic in nature to the receptor and in addition they can accommodate a degree of substitution. Thus, they are attractive starting points for fragment expansion [122]. However fragments, which have an entropic thermodynamic signature, are bound through more hydrophobic interactions, such as in π-π stacking of aryl rings. This entropic signature is associated with the hydrophobic effect of fragment binding. An important consideration in ligand binding is the contribution of hydration to the thermodynamics [123, 124]. Here, the removal of high-energy (unstable) water molecules from the binding site upon ligand association has a major entropic

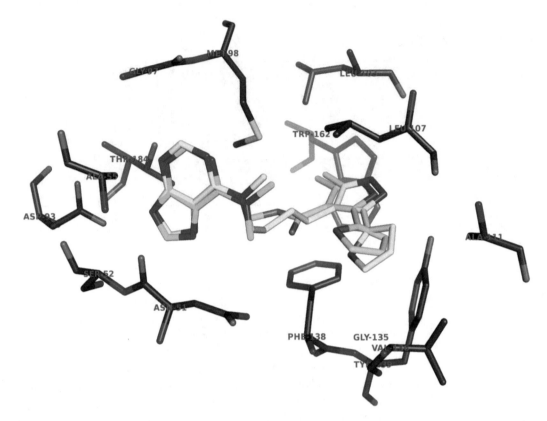

**Fig. 4** The complex of fragments **1** (*green*) and **2** (*cyan*) bound together in Hsp90 (PDB ID: 3HZ1) aligned to the crystal structure (PDB ID: 3HZ5) of the Hsp90 inhibitor **3** (*yellow*)

energetic contribution to the hydrophobic effect. We believe that the ligand-binding sites with dominant dispersion interaction terms identified by PIEDA are more likely to be associated with the presence of these high-energy waters. Hydrogen bonds have a large electrostatic energy term, whereas the dispersion energy term is the dominant attractive component in hydrophobic interactions. The ratio of the electrostatic and dispersion energy terms to the sum of the PIE results is a useful metric to measure the suitability of a fragment for hit expansion (*see* Fig. 5).

PIEDA [99] allows these terms to be extracted from the FMO calculation, as shown in Fig. 5. Fragment **1** has a much larger electrostatic component than fragment **2**, which is dominant over the dispersion energy contribution (ES/(DI + CT) = 1.48) (*see* Fig. 5). Hydrogen bonds are highly directional and when they are optimally formed between a fragment and a receptor, they anchor the fragment in place. This is in stark contrast with fragments which bind through dispersion forces where there is increased entropy and multiple binding poses are often possible, as was observed for fragment **2** where two crystal structures gave two different binding poses [121]. Fragment **2** has a reduced ES/(DI + CT) (*see* Fig. 5).

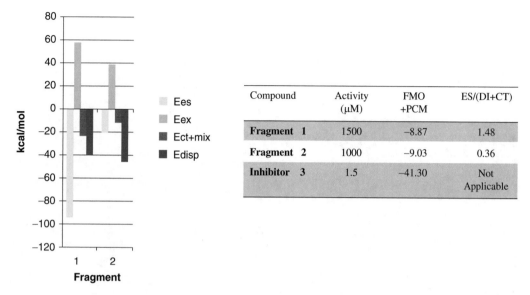

**Fig. 5** *Left*: PIEDA for fragments **1** and **2**. Showing the electrostatic term (Ees = $\Delta E_{IJ}^{ES}$), the exchange repulsion term (Eex = $\Delta E_{IJ}^{EX}$), the CT and mixing terms (Ect + mix = $\Delta E_{IJ}^{CT+mix}$), and the dispersion term (Edisp = $\Delta E_{IJ}^{DI}$), energies are in kcal/mol. *Right*: Table showing the activity in (μM) of fragments **1** and **2** and inhibitor **3**; FMO + PCM, the total sum of the PIE in addition a PCM-calculated desolvation penalty; ES/(DI + CT), ratio of the electrostatic term over the sum of the dispersion and CT terms extracted from the PIEDA

Capturing the thermodynamic nature of fragment binding in a simple metric like ES/(DI + CT) is useful information in fragment linking, and also particularly important in the selection of fragment hits for further fragment expansion and evolution studies.

As well as studying the nature of fragment binding during a fragment-based drug discovery project, functional groups can also be considered as fragments that are modified during hit and lead optimization. Here, a virtual library of compounds can be built around a functional group which is to be replaced or modified. This is known as scaffold replacement [86]. An X-ray crystal structure is routinely used as a starting point to explore chemical modification to a ligand, and the use of an FMO in a predictive fashion to measure the PIE changes can be performed. In this procedure, the size of the system to be calculated is kept at a minimum. Typically, the ligand and only the surrounding amino acid residues are within 5 Å, to ensure reasonable throughput. This technique is often used for initial fragment-hit expansion or for optimization of a congeneric series of compounds and it is particularly effective for solvent-inaccessible rigid-binding pockets as most of the energetic terms not accounted for by the FMO method tend to cancel out. We have termed this procedure "SAR-by-FMO" and an example of this is reproduced below [58].

**Table 2**
**SAR-by-FMO**

| Compound | $\Delta$PIE (kcal/mol) | A | R1 | R2 |
|---|---|---|---|---|
| 1 | 0 | N | Cl | $NH_2$ |
| 2 | 1.31 | N | F | $NH_2$ |
| 3 | 1.21 | N | H | $NH_2$ |
| 4 | 1.44 | C | H | $NH_2$ |
| 5 | 0.37 | C | $CH_3$ | $NH_2$ |
| 6 | −1.09 | N | Cl | H |
| 7 | 0.12 | N | H | H |
| 8 | 0.31 | N | Cl | $OCH_3$ |
| 9 | −2.76 | N | Cl | $NHCOCH_3$ |
| 10 | −2.62 | | | |
| 11 | 0.34 | C | Cl | $NH_2$ |
| 12 | 0.38 | N | $CH_3$ | $NH_2$ |
| 13 | −1.59 | N | Cl | NHPh |

Fragment analysis using FMO to calculate the relative values of pair interaction energies ($\Delta$PIE), using 1WCC as a reference (PIE = −21.44 kcal/mol) for a series of fragment replacements of 1WCC

Work at Astex during a fragment-based drug design campaign against CDK2 identified a number of fragment hits, which were then crystallized [125]. One of the resolved structures was the fragment hit (PDB ID: 1WCC) [126], entry 1 in Table 2.

This fragment has low activity of 64 % inhibition at 1 mM. In spite of this, the fragment forms a number of good enthalpic hydrogen bonds with the backbone of the CDK2 Hinge region including residues Glu81, Phe82, and Leu83. 1WCC thus is an ideal fragment as it acts as a potential anchoring point for further modification from some useful vectors off the molecule and it has a good $FE_{PIE}$ value of −2.68. These are depicted in Fig. 6, and following the FMO convention of fragmentation are labeled

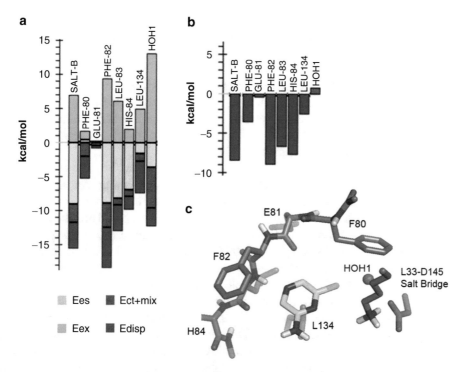

**Fig. 6** FMO analysis of 1WCC. (**a**) PIEDA for entry 1 Table 2 (PDB ID: 1WCC) showing the electrostatic term (Ees = $\Delta E_{IJ}^{ES}$), the exchange repulsion term (Eex = $\Delta E_{IJ}^{EX}$), the CT and mixing terms (Ect + mix = $\Delta E_{IJ}^{CT+mix}$), and the dispersion term (Edisp = $\Delta E_{IJ}^{DI}$), energies are in kcal/mol. (**b**) PIE for each of the amino acids neighboring the fragment, showing attractive and repulsive energy contributions in kcal/mol. (**c**) Depiction of the fragment within the CDK2 binding pocket, taken from the PDB ID: 1WCC [126]

Phe-82, Leu-83, and His-84, respectively. An examination of the PIEDA histogram plot reveals some important interactions, which have recently become better understood in the field of medicinal chemistry. An interaction that was not thoroughly examined in the literature is that formed between the chloro substituent and the gatekeeper Phe80 residue, which contributes favorably to about 3 kcal/mol of energy, Fig. 6b.

At the MP2/6-31G* level of theory the interaction can be observed as being a combination of dispersion and CT energy terms, Fig. 6a. This is likely as the chloro group has a positively charged σ hole which is likely to interact with the electron-rich π-system of Phe-80 [127]. Halogen-π bonds have traditionally been poorly represented in MM force fields and the nature of the interaction has been misunderstood. Although it is also reasonable to assume that the chlorine atom may be replacing a high-energy solvating water molecule, which might exist in this part of the binding pocket, the contribution from this type of halogen-π interaction cannot be ignored. Further examination of the PIEDA plots shows that there is a pattern to the contributions that the energy terms make to the individual residue-fragment interactions.

This pattern seen for Phe-82, Leu-83, and His-84 is a typical hydrogen-bond energy contribution. What we observe from the X-ray structure is that only the Phe-82 NH forms a classical hydrogen bond to the ring N or 1WCC. Two additional hydrogen bonds are formed to the carbonyl O of Glu81 and Leu83 and they are nonclassical in nature. A good example of the usefulness of CH-$\pi$ interactions in understanding protein-ligand interactions is in the work of Ozawa et al. in their study of the $\beta$-2 adrenergic G-protein-coupled receptor [128].

The SAR-by-FMO approach can be demonstrated using 1WCC as a starting point, and performing simple modifications to 1WCC, such that any induced fitting to the protein is reduced. A small virtual library is designed, often based around easily sourced commercial analogues. Their FMO interaction energies are calculated (Table 2) so that the effect of substituent changes on the binding free energy can be predicted. Replacing the chloro in 1WCC (entry 1 Table 2) for a fluoro (entry 2), proton (entry 3), or methyl group (entry 12) all result in a loss in binding energy (and an increase in $\Delta$PIE). This is the same for entries 4, 5, and 7. This suggests that the chloro is necessary for activity. Further changes to the ring system, chaining a ring N to a C, pyrazine to pyridine (entry 11, Table 2), could be demonstrated by FMO to create less favorable changes. However, substituent changes to the amino group could offer further gains in potency. The authors went on to prepare compound 13 (Table 2), which had reasonable activity ($IC_{50} = 7$ µM). This SAR-by-FMO analysis reveals that there are other scaffolds that could have also been interesting fragment hits for further investigation, including entries 6, 9, and 10 (Table 2), all of which have increased binding interactions to the receptor compared to the initial 1WCC fragment hit. This SAR-by-FMO is equally applicable during hit-to-lead and in ligand-optimization phases of drug design where the impact of small substituent changes to a ligand is being examined.

The fragment replacement and the calculation of PIE are applicable to proteins as well as to ligands. It is particularly useful in the analysis of the robustness of homology models or to assess the impact of single-point mutations in protein design to determine protein stability for X-ray crystallography. An example of mutation studies is the work in the area of the influenza virus. Recently, there has been research performed to quantify, through the use of FMO calculations, the mutations from the avian to the human hemagglutinin protein in strengthening the binding affinity of human hemagglutinin to the human receptor [129]. Other researchers have explored efforts to predict putative mutations in the hemagglutinin protein [130].

### 3.3 FMO-Derived Partial Charges

Receptor-specific scoring functions can offer significant improvements in ligand-binding affinity predictions. This can be useful, especially when predicting electrostatic interactions, which in most of the current non-polarizable force fields (such as AMBER94) are based on partial charges assigned to each atom. FMO-derived charges were proven to give equally good or improved correlations with experimental values when compared to classical force field charges [7, 131–133].

It has been shown that partial charges derived from FMO calculations in the pairwise manner agree well with those determined from the conventional molecular orbital method [131]. Three different methods were employed for charge comparison, including charges from electrostatic potentials using the grid-based method (CHELPG), the electrostatic potential fitting with Merz-Kollman scheme (MK), and the restrained electrostatic potential (RESP) fitting. The observed error between FMO and the conventional molecular orbital systems was within 1 %. The dependency of charges on the structural variation of the glycine trimer and the reproducibility of the electrostatic potential on the surface of the ligand-binding pocket of the estrogen receptor were also analyzed. This has proven that the adverse effect of fragmentation on charge derivation was rather minor, and results were consistent with the conventional molecular orbital calculations. Also, the MK and the RESP charges derived from FMO calculations showed good reproducibility of electrostatic potential on the molecular surface [131].

It has been proposed that the classical electrostatic model can be improved by introducing partial charges derived from high-level quantum chemical calculations using relatively fast FMO calculations [7]. Those parameters have been used to characterize docking results for estrogen receptor subtype $\alpha$ (ER$\alpha$) and the retinoic acid receptor of isotype $\gamma$ (RAR$\gamma$). A set of quantum mechanically characterized ligands have been docked into the ER$\alpha$ and RAR$\gamma$ receptors, which were characterized with both the force field and the quantum-based scoring functions. For the ER$\alpha$ binding, the affinity predictions were significantly improved when QM-based partial charges were used, reaching $R^2$ values of 0.81 and 0.54 for QM and the classical electrostatic description, respectively. The RAR$\gamma$ experimental and computational predictions were almost equally good, with $R^2$ values in excess of 0.9 for both the classical and quantum-derived scoring functions [7].

In another study, receptor-specific FMO charges derived with the optimally weighted RESP method were used to improve force field system descriptions during MD simulations [132]. The reliability of the FMO charges was proven based on a comparison with the well-established AMBER94 force field. The MD simulation performed on the crambin protein system also showed electrostatic reproducibility within short time scale calculations. However, a more significant variation of the structure during MD simulation might lead to a less accurate electrostatic description. It is due to the fact that FMO charges were based on a single-point structure, and they were not redistributed for the transient structures. For that reason, FMO-derived charges were found to be the most effective when dealing with short time scale MD simulations or receptor-ligand docking, where the reproducibility of the electrostatic interactions is the most important [132].

Recently, protein-specific force field charges were used to improve protein-ligand binding affinity calculations [133]. Both FMO protein-specific charges and AMBER94 charges were applied to study two protein systems, dodecin and hen egg-white lysozyme, and their ligands. The molecular mechanics Poisson–Boltzmann surface area (MM-PBSA) method was used to calculate binding free energies for considered complexes. For the FMO-RESP charges, the accuracy of the binding free energy was improved for five ligands that were interacting with the dodecin receptor due to the electrostatic energy, compared to the AMBER94 performance. Although the magnitude difference between the partial charges obtained with the FMO-specific force field and the AMBER94 force field was relatively small, a better correlation with the experimental values was achieved with the former. For the hen egg-white lysozyme system, the binding affinity correlation was equally good for both charge sets [133].

### 3.4 FMO-Based Molecular Descriptors in QSAR, Scoring Functions

There are two 3D-QSAR methods that have been used extensively in CADD, comparative molecular field analysis (CoMFA) [134], and comparative molecular similarity indices analysis (CoMSIA) [135]. In a typical setup, partial least squares (PLS) is computed to correlate molecular structure and connectivity of atoms to the desired properties of the system. Both methods rely on molecular interaction fields (MIFs) that are usually calculated by using classical force fields. Thus, CoMFA and CoMSIA suffer from all of the drawbacks and weaknesses associated with the force fields. At the same time, the QM methods are inherently more accurate than the force fields and they can be a feasible alternative. The common complaint is that the QM methods are too expensive, but this issue can be partially addressed by using semiempirical or linearly scaling methods like FMO. FMO has been used in CoMFA [136, 137] and the use of FMO in CoMSIA methods has been discussed.

A key problem in QSAR is the choice of an accurate descriptor. There are, for example, a few types of the molecular descriptors available such as molecular weight, graph-based connectivity of atoms, and charges of atoms. Using QM methods, including FMO, allows computing arguably more useful and sophisticated descriptors, like dipole moment, mean polarizability, partial charge, and the highest occupied and the lowest unoccupied orbital energies. In addition to these descriptors, FMO can provide new valuable types of descriptors. These descriptors take advantage of the fragmented nature of FMO, which allows extracting information about interactions between fragments where fragments are defined as ligand and amino acids in the protein. Chuman et al. [8, 9, 111, 138–142] have used protein-ligand-binding energies and pair interaction energies from FMO calculations as descriptors in QSAR. The ligand-binding energy is defined as

$$\Delta E_{\text{ligand}} = E(\text{complex}) - [E(\text{protein}) + E(\text{ligand})] \tag{17}$$

where each energy term is estimated with FMO. These energy calculations can include a dispersion calculation (empirical dispersion or from MP2) and a solvation energy estimate by using, for example, PCM. In other words, the enthalpy of ligand-binding energy can be estimated very accurately. Once $\Delta E_{\text{ligand}}$ is computed, it can be used as any other descriptor in QSAR calculations. But, by using FMO, it is possible to narrow down exactly which amino acid-residue ligand interactions contributed mostly to the ligand-binding energy. Moreover, these interaction energies can be analyzed by type, for example, electrostatic, dispersion, or charge transfer internal energies. These internal energies can be used as descriptors by themselves as shown in the work of Chuman et al. [138].

### 3.5 Molecular Electrostatic Potential

The molecular electrostatic potential (MEP) is a useful tool to analyze intermolecular electrostatic interactions and the properties of the system. It is an especially important tool for CADD where understanding electrostatic and topographic complementarity in a receptor-ligand complex is key for rational SBDD. This tool is used to predict ligand specificity, for example, the polarity in the active site of a receptor, as a part of the docking routine.

MEP allows the visualization of the charge distribution of the molecule on a molecular surface. The first requirement is to determine how to define the surface. One approach is to use van der Waals molecular surface—a union of spherical atom surfaces—where each atom surface is defined by the van der Waals radius. These radii are derived for non-bonded atoms and as such they provide an approximation of the surface. A more accurate way to compute the surface is by computing the electron density of the molecule with a QM method and extracting the electron density isosurface. The commonly accepted electron density cutoff value is 0.002, which captures almost all of the electron density. The second step is to compute the electrostatic potential. A widespread model for computing electrostatic properties is the Poisson–Boltzmann (PBE) equation:

$$-\nabla \cdot \varepsilon(x) \nabla \phi(x) + \bar{k}^2(x) \sinh \phi(x) = f(x) \tag{18}$$

where $\phi$ is the electrostatic potential, $\varepsilon$ is the dielectric constant of solute and solvent, $\bar{k}^2$ is related to the ionic strength of the solution and the accessibility of ions to the solute interior, and $f$ describes the distribution of atomic partial charges of solute. An efficient PBE solver for computing MEP is implemented in the popular package APBS [143] as well as in the package DelPhi [144]. A more accurate way to compute electrostatic potential is with a QM method. Using Hartree-Fock or DFT, MEP can be computed as

$$\varphi(\mathbf{r}) = \sum_{A}^{\text{atoms}} \frac{Z_A}{|\mathbf{r} - \mathbf{R}_A|} - \sum_{\mu\nu} D_{\mu\nu} \int \chi_{\mu}^{*}(\mathbf{r}') \frac{1}{|\mathbf{r} - \mathbf{r}'|} \chi_{\nu}(\mathbf{r}') d\mathbf{r}' \quad (19)$$

where $Z_A$ is the nuclear charge of atom $A$, $\mu$ and $\nu$ are atomic orbital basis functions, and $D_{\mu\nu}$ is the one-electron density matrix.

Many QM programs including GAMESS are capable of computing MEP. It is also possible to compute MEP for very large systems by using the FMO method [145]. Watanabe et al. have shown how dimerization changes the MEP for the estrogen receptor affecting its association with DNA [145]. To demonstrate MEP computed with FMO implemented in GAMESS, we chose a small Trp-cage miniprotein (PDB: 1L2Y) docked with deprotonated *o*-phenolic acid. The electron density and MEP are computed at the FMO2-RHF level of theory with STO-3G basis set. The cutoff value is 0.002. The 1L2Y MEP with ligand is shown in Fig. 7.

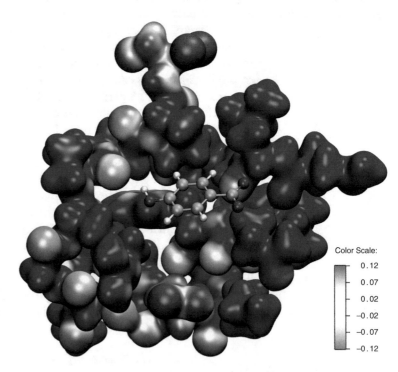

Color Scale:
| 0.12
| 0.07
| 0.02
| −0.02
| −0.07
| −0.12

**Fig. 7** Electrostatic potential of Trp-cage protein (PDB: 1L2Y) docked with deprotonated *o*-phenolic acid shown in the *balls*-and-*sticks* representation. The 1LY2 MEP is shown on the electron density isosurface computed with the cutoff value 0.002. *Red* signifies a negative charge while *blue* shows a positive charge

## 4   Conclusions and Outlook

There have been significant advancements in the field of QM applications for drug research in recent years. On the methodological side, a large number of promising linearly scaling QM methods have been developed. Some of these methods, like FMO, have proven to be invaluable tools in drug design. At the same time, new computer technologies like GPUs, MIC architecture, and FPGAs provide the ability to significantly speed up calculations at a fraction of the cost. Some of the assumptions (for example, fragmentation of the system) made in the linear scaling methods often allow efficient parallelization of the code. The combination of these three factors drove the cost of QM calculations significantly down on the commodity hardware like PC clusters. For example, at the time of the publication, authors routinely run 1000–10,000 atom simulations on PC clusters. However, QM calculations are still too expensive for large-scale ligand screening. Other problematic QM areas are entropy, solvation, and dynamics. But these areas can be effectively addressed by using classical MD with force fields. In the future, we expect that there will be more widespread use of both approaches for drug design.

In this chapter, we discussed in detail the use of FMO. Next, we will summarize why the FMO method is well fitted for CADD:

1. It is a computationally inexpensive method compared to traditional QM methods.

2. An analysis of interactions between fragments can be done. Thus, a wealth of information can be learned about the way a drug interacts with amino acids in the active site. Therefore, SBDD is a natural fit for FMO.

3. FMO can be applied for predicting geometry, estimating binding energy of the ligands, completing conformational sampling, analyzing molecular interactions, deriving partial charges, and generating QSAR models.

4. FMO is well suited to run in parallel on PC clusters [146] and supercomputers [147], making it possible to run large-scale simulations in a reasonable time. As a result, large-scale screening of ligands is possible on supercomputers.

5. Due to the availability of GUI [50, 113], setting up FMO calculations and visualizing the results can be done almost automatically, provided that a preliminary structure refinement is performed (the structures available in PDB need to be protonated and usually optimized in some way), facilitating a routine use of FMO in drug research.

FMO is an efficient and accurate QM method, which is well suited for CADD. It is our hope that FMO will become a standard and widely used tool in CADD.

## Acknowledgments

Dmitri G. Fedorov has been supported by the Next Generation Super Computing Project, Nanoscience Program (MEXT, Japan) and Computational Materials Science Initiative (CMSI, Japan). This research used resources of the Argonne Leadership Computing Facility, which is a DOE Office of Science User Facility supported under Contract DE-AC02-06CH11357.

The submitted manuscript has been created by UChicago Argonne, LLC, Operator of Argonne National Laboratory ("Argonne"). Argonne, a US Department of Energy Office of Science laboratory, is operated under Contract No. DE-AC02-06CH11357. The US Government retains for itself, and others acting on its behalf, a paid-up nonexclusive, irrevocable worldwide license in said article to reproduce, prepare derivative works, distribute copies to the public, and perform publicly and display publicly, by or on behalf of the government.

## Glossary

| | |
|---|---|
| **AMBER** | Assisted Model Building with Energy Refinement |
| **CADD** | Computer-Aided Drug Design |
| **CHARMM** | Chemistry at HARvard Macromolecular Mechanics |
| **EFP** | Effective Fragment Potential |
| **ESP** | Electrostatic Potential |
| **FD** | Frozen Domain |
| **FDD** | Frozen Domain and Dimers |
| **FMO** | Fragment Molecular Orbital |
| **GAMESS** | General Atomic and Molecular Electronic Structure System |
| **LAMMPS** | Large-scale Atomic/Molecular Massively Parallel Simulator |
| **MD** | Molecular Dynamics |
| **MM** | Molecular Mechanics |
| **PB** | Poisson–Boltzmann |
| **PCM** | Polarizable Continuum Model |
| **PIE** | Pair Interaction Energy |
| **PIEDA** | PIE Decomposition Analysis |
| **QM** | Quantum Mechanical |
| **QSAR** | Quantitative SAR |
| **SAR** | Structure-Activity Relationship |
| **SBDD** | Structure Based Drug Design |

# References

1. Amari S, Aizawa M, Zhang J, Fukuzawa K, Mochizuki Y, Iwasawa Y, Nakata K, Chuman H, Nakano T (2006) VISCANA: visualized cluster analysis of protein-ligand interaction based on the ab initio fragment molecular orbital method for virtual ligand screening. J Chem Inf Model 46(1):221–230

2. Raha K, Merz KM (2004) A quantum mechanics-based scoring function: study of zinc ion-mediated ligand binding. J Am Chem Soc 126(4):1020–1021

3. Raha K, Merz KM (2005) Large-scale validation of a quantum mechanics based scoring function: predicting the binding affinity and the binding mode of a diverse set of protein-ligand complexes. J Med Chem 48 (14):4558–4575

4. Mazanetz MP, Ichihara O, Law RJ, Whittaker M (2011) Prediction of cyclin-dependent kinase 2 inhibitor potency using the fragment molecular orbital method. J Cheminform 3 (1):2

5. He X, Fusti-Molnar L, Cui G, Merz KM (2009) Importance of dispersion and electron correlation in ab initio protein folding. J Phys Chem B 113(15):5290–5300

6. Faver JC, Zheng Z, Merz KM (2011) Model for the fast estimation of basis set superposition error in biomolecular systems. J Chem Phys 135:144110

7. Fischer B, Fukuzawa K, Wenzel W (2008) Receptor-specific scoring functions derived from quantum chemical models improve affinity estimates for in-silico drug discovery. Proteins 70(4):1264–1273

8. Yoshida T, Fujita T, Chuman H (2009) Novel quantitative structure-activity studies of HIV-1 protease inhibitors of the cyclic urea type using descriptors derived from molecular dynamics and molecular orbital calculations. Curr Comput Aided Drug Des 5(1):38–55

9. Hitaoka S, Matoba H, Harada M, Yoshida T, Tsuji D, Hirokawa T, Itoh K, Chuman H (2011) Correlation analyses on binding affinity of sialic acid analogues and antiinfluenza drugs with human neuraminidase using ab Initio MO calculations on their complex structures-LERE-QSAR analysis (IV). J Chem Inf Model 51:2706–2716

10. Brunger AT, Adams PD (2002) Molecular dynamics applied to X-ray structure refinement. Acc Chem Res 35(6):404–412

11. Brooks BR, Brooks C, Mackerell A, Nilsson L, Petrella R, Roux B, Won Y, Archontis G, Bartels C, Boresch S, Caflisch A, Caves L, Cui Q, Dinner AR, Feig M, Fischer S, Gao J, Hodoscek M, Im W, Kuczera K, Lazaridis T, Ma J, Ovchinnikov V, Paci E, Pastor RW, Post CB, Pu JZ, Schaefer M, Tidor B, Venable RM, Woodcock HL, Wu X, Yang W, York DM, Karplus M (2009) CHARMM: the biomolecular simulation program. J Comput Chem 30 (10):1545–1614

12. Vanommeslaeghe K, Hatcher E, Acharya C, Kundu S, Zhong S, Shim J, Darian E, Guvench O, Lopes P, Vorobyov I, Mackerell ADJ (2010) CHARMM general force field: a force field for drug-like molecules compatible with the CHARMM all-atom additive biological force fields. J Comput Chem 31 (4):671–690

13. Pearlman DA, Case DA, Caldwell JW, Ross WS, Cheatham TE, DeBolt S, Ferguson D, Seibel G, Kollman P (1995) AMBER, a package of computer programs for applying molecular mechanics, normal mode analysis, molecular dynamics and free energy calculations to simulate the structural and energetic properties of molecules. Comput Phys Commun 91(1):1–41

14. Engh RA, Huber R (1991) Accurate bond and angle parameters for X-ray protein structure refinement. Acta Crystallogr A 47 (4):392–400

15. Ryde U (2007) Accurate metal-site structures in proteins obtained by combining experimental data and quantum chemistry. Dalton Trans 6:607–625

16. Cramer CJ (2004) Essentials of computational chemistry: theories and models, 2nd edn. John Wiley & Sons Inc, Chichester

17. Stone JE, Phillips JC, Freddolino PL, Hardy DJ, Trabuco LG, Schulten K (2007) Accelerating molecular modeling applications with graphics processors. J Comput Chem 28 (16):2618–2640

18. Götz AW, Williamson MJ, Xu D, Poole D, Le Grand S, Walker RC (2012) Routine microsecond molecular dynamics simulations with AMBER on GPUs. 1. Generalized born. J Chem Theory Comput 8(5):1542–1555

19. Salomon-Ferrer R, Götz AW, Poole D, Le Grand S, Walker RC (2013) Routine microsecond molecular dynamics simulations with AMBER on GPUs. 2. Explicit solvent particle mesh Ewald. J Chem Theory Comput 9 (9):3878–3888

20. Luehr N, Ufimtsev IS, Martínez TJ (2011) Dynamic precision for electron repulsion integral evaluation on graphical processing units

(GPUs). J Chem Theory Comput 7 (4):949–954

21. Asadchev A, Gordon MS (2012) New multi-threaded hybrid CPU/GPU approach to Hartree–Fock. J Chem Theory Comput 8 (11):4166–4176

22. Stone JE, Hardy DJ, Ufimtsev IS, Schulten K (2010) GPU-accelerated molecular modeling coming of age. J Mol Graph Model 29 (2):116–125

23. Kozakov D, Brenke R, Comeau SR, Vajda S (2006) PIPER: an FFT-based protein docking program with pairwise potentials. Proteins 65 (2):392–406

24. Kantardjiev AA (2012) Quantum. Ligand. Dock: protein–ligand docking with quantum entanglement refinement on a GPU system. Nucleic Acids Res 40(W1):W415–W422

25. Korb O, Stützle T, Exner TE (2011) Accelerating molecular docking calculations using graphics processing units. J Chem Inf Model 51(4):865–876

26. Zhang X, Wong SE, Lightstone FC (2013) Message passing interface and multithreading hybrid for parallel molecular docking of large databases on petascale high performance computing machines. J Comput Chem 34 (11):915–927

27. Hagiwara Y, Ohno K, Orita M, Koga R, Endo T, Akiyama Y, Sekijima M (2013) Accelerating quantum chemistry calculations with graphical processing units-toward in high-density (HD) silico drug discovery. Curr Comput Aided Drug Des 9(3):396–401

28. Ilatovskiy AV, Abagyan R, Kufareva I (2013) Quantum mechanics approaches to drug research in the era of structural chemogenomics. Int J Quantum Chem 113 (12):1669–1675

29. Scuseria GE (1999) Linear scaling density functional calculations with Gaussian orbitals. J Phys Chem A 103(25):4782–4790

30. Zalesny R, Papadopoulos MG, Mezey PG, Leszczynski J (eds) (2011) Linear-scaling techniques in computational chemistry and physics: methods and applications, vol 13. Springer Science & Business Media, Berlin

31. Reimers JR (ed) (2011) Computational methods for large systems: electronic structure approaches for biotechnology and nanotechnology. John Wiley & Sons, New York, NY

32. Otto P, Ladik J (1975) Investigation of the interaction between molecules at medium distances: I. SCF LCAO MO supermolecule, perturbational and mutually consistent calculations for two interacting HF and $CH2O$ molecules. J Chem Phys 8 (1):192–200

33. Gao J (1997) Toward a molecular orbital derived empirical potential for liquid simulations. J Phys Chem B 101(4):657–663

34. Gordon MS, Pruitt SR, Fedorov DG, Slipchenko LV (2012) Fragmentation methods: a route to accurate calculations on large systems. Chem Rev 112(1):632–672

35. Pruitt SR, Bertoni C, Brorsen KR, Gordon MS (2014) Efficient and accurate fragmentation methods. Acc Chem Res 47 (9):2786–2794

36. Wang B, Yang KR, Xu X, Isegawa M, Leverentz HR, Truhlar DG (2014) Quantum mechanical fragment methods based on partitioning atoms or partitioning coordinates. Acc Chem Res 47(9):2731–2738

37. He X, Zhu T, Wang X, Liu J, Zhang JZ (2014) Fragment quantum mechanical calculation of proteins and its applications. Acc Chem Res 47(9):2748–2757

38. Raghavachari K, Saha A (2015) Accurate composite and fragment-based quantum chemical models for large molecules. Chem Rev 115(12):5643–5677

39. Collins MA, Bettens RP (2015) Energy-based molecular fragmentation methods. Chem Rev 115(12):5607–5642

40. Akimov AV, Prezhdo OV (2015) Large-scale computations in chemistry: a bird's eye view of a vibrant field. Chem Rev 115 (12):5797–5890

41. Kitaura K, Ikeo E, Asada T, Nakano T, Uebayasi M (1999) Fragment molecular orbital method: an approximate computational method for large molecules. Chem Phys Lett 313(3-4):701–706

42. Fedorov DG, Kitaura K (2007) Extending the power of quantum chemistry to large systems with the fragment molecular orbital method. J Phys Chem A 111(30):6904–6914

43. Fedorov D, Kitaura K (eds) (2009) The fragment molecular orbital method: practical applications to large molecular systems. CRC Press, Boca Raton, FL

44. Fedorov DG, Nagata T, Kitaura K (2012) Exploring chemistry with the fragment molecular orbital method. Phys Chem Chem Phys 14:7562–7577

45. Tanaka S, Mochizuki Y, Komeiji Y, Okiyama Y, Fukuzawa K (2014) Electron-correlated fragment-molecular-orbital calculations for biomolecular and nano systems. Phys Chem Chem Phys 16(22):10310–10344

46. Okiyama Y, Tsukamoto T, Watanabe C, Fukuzawa K, Tanaka S, Mochizuki Y (2013) Modeling of peptide–silica interaction based on four-body corrected fragment molecular orbital (FMO4) calculations. Chem Phys Lett 566:25–31

47. Kato K, Fukuzawa K, Mochizuki Y (2015) Modeling of hydroxyapatite-peptide interaction based on fragment molecular orbital method. Chem Phys Lett 629:58–64

48. Taguchi N, Mochizuki Y, Nakano T, Amari S, Fukuzawa K, Ishikawa T, Sakurai M, Tanaka S (2009) Fragment molecular orbital calculations on red fluorescent proteins (DsRed and mFruits). J Phys Chem B 113 (4):1153–1161

49. Fukuzawa K, Watanabe C, Kurisaki I, Taguchi N, Mochizuki Y, Nakano T, Tanaka S, Komeiji Y (2014) Accuracy of the fragment molecular orbital (FMO) calculations for DNA: total energy, molecular orbital, and inter-fragment interaction energy. Comput Theor Chem 1034:7–16

50. Suenaga M (2008) Development of GUI for GAMESS/FMO calculation. J Comput Chem Jpn 7:33–53

51. Fedorov DG, Ishida T, Kitaura K (2005) Multilayer formulation of the fragment molecular orbital method (FMO). J Phys Chem A 109 (11):2638–2646

52. Nishimoto Y, Fedorov DG, Irle S (2015) Third-order density-functional tight-binding combined with the fragment molecular orbital method. Chem Phys Lett 636:90–96

53. Nakano T, Mochizuki Y, Fukuzawa K, Amari S, Tanaka S (2006) Developments and applications of ABINIT-MP software based on the fragment molecular orbital method. In: Starikov EB, Lewis JP, Tanaka S (eds) Modern methods for theoretical physical chemistry of biopolymers. Elsevier, Amsterdam, pp 39–52

54. Okamoto T, Ishikawa T, Koyano Y, Yamamoto N, Kuwata K, Nagaoka M (2013) A minimal implementation of the AMBER-PAICS interface for ab initio FMO-QM/MM-MD simulation. Bull Chem Soc Jpn 86 (2):210–222

55. Schmidt MW, Baldridge KK, Boatz JA, Elbert ST, Gordon MS, Jensen JH, Koseki S, Matsunaga N, Nguyen KA, Su S, Windus TL, Dupuis M, Montgomery JAJ (1993) General atomic and molecular electronic structure system. J Comput Chem 14(11):1347–1363. doi:10.1002/jcc.540141112

56. Nakata H, Nagata T, Fedorov DG, Yokojima S, Kitaura K, Nakamura S (2013) Analytic second derivatives of the energy in the fragment molecular orbital method. J Chem Phys 138(16):164103

57. Alexeev Y, Fedorov DG, Shvartsburg AA (2014) Effective ion mobility calculations for macromolecules by scattering on electron clouds. J Phys Chem A 118(34):6763–6772. doi:10.1021/jp505012c

58. Alexeev Y, Mazanetz M, Ichihara O, Fedorov DG (2012) GAMESS as a free quantum-mechanical platform for drug research. Curr Top Med Chem 12(18):2013–2033

59. Mazanetz MP (2013) Quantum mechanical applications in drug discovery. In: In silico drug discovery and design. Future Science Ltd., London, pp 64–79. doi:10.4155/9781909453012

60. Sawada T, Fedorov DG, Kitaura K (2010) Role of the key mutation in the selective binding of avian and human influenza hemagglutinin to sialosides revealed by quantum-mechanical calculations. J Am Chem Soc 132:16862–16872

61. Sawada T, Fedorov DG, Kitaura K (2010) Binding of influenza A virus hemagglutinin to the sialoside receptor Is not controlled by the homotropic allosteric effect. J Phys Chem B 114:15700–15705

62. Komeiji Y, Mori H, Nakano T, Mochizuki Y (2012) Recent advances in fragment molecular orbital-based molecular dynamics (FMO-MD) simulations. In: Wang L (ed) Molecular dynamics - theoretical developments and applications in nanotechnology and energy. Rijeka, Croatia: INTECH, pp 3–24

63. Sato M, Yamataka H, Komeiji Y, Mochizuki Y, Ishikawa T, Nakano T (2008) How does an SN2 reaction take place in solution? Full ab initio MD simulations for the hydrolysis of the methyl diazonium ion. J Am Chem Soc 130(8):2396–2397

64. Sato M, Yamataka H, Komeiji Y, Mochizuki Y (2012) FMO-MD simulations on the hydration of formaldehyde in water solution with constraint dynamics. Chemistry 18 (31):9714–9721

65. Nakata H, Fedorov DG, Zahariev F, Schmidt MW, Kitaura K, Gordon MS, Nakamura S (2015) Analytic second derivative of the energy for density functional theory based on the three-body fragment molecular orbital method. J Chem Phys 142(12):124101

66. Nakata H, Fedorov DG, Nagata T, Kitaura K, Nakamura S (2015) Simulations of chemical reactions with the frozen domain formulation of the fragment molecular orbital method. J Chem Theory Comput 11(7):3053–3064. doi:10.1021/acs.jctc.5b00277

67. Fedorov DG, Kitaura K, Li H, Jensen JH, Gordon MS (2006) The polarizable continuum model (PCM) interfaced with the fragment molecular orbital method (FMO). J Comput Chem 27(8):976–985

68. Li H, Fedorov DG, Nagata T, Kitaura K, Jensen JH, Gordon MS (2010) Energy gradients in combined fragment molecular orbital and polarizable continuum model (FMO/PCM) calculation. J Comput Chem 31(4):778–790

69. Nagata T, Fedorov D, Li H, Kitaura K (2012) Analytic gradient for second order Møller-Plesset perturbation theory with the Polarizable Continuum Model based on the Fragment molecular Orbital method. J Chem Phys 136:204112

70. Nakata H, Fedorov DG, Kitaura K, Nakamura S (2015) Extension of the fragment molecular orbital method to treat large open-shell systems in solution. Chem Phys Lett 635:86–92

71. Watanabe H, Okiyama Y, Nakano T, Tanaka S (2010) Incorporation of solvation effects into the fragment molecular orbital calculations with the Poisson–Boltzmann equation. Chem Phys Lett 500(1):116–119

72. Yoshida N (2014) Efficient implementation of the three-dimensional reference interaction site model method in the fragment molecular orbital method. J Chem Phys 140(21):214118

73. Nagata T, Fedorov DG, Kitaura K, Gordon MS (2009) A combined effective fragment potential–fragment molecular orbital method. I. The energy expression and initial applications. J Chem Phys 131:024101

74. Nakanishi I, Fedorov DG, Kitaura K (2007) Molecular recognition mechanism of FK506 binding protein: an all-electron fragment molecular orbital study. Proteins 68(1):145–158

75. Murata K, Fedorov DG, Nakanishi I, Kitaura K (2009) Cluster hydration model for binding energy calculations of protein–ligand complexes. J Phys Chem B 113(3):809–817

76. Fedorov DG, Ishida T, Uebayasi M, Kitaura K (2007) The fragment molecular orbital method for geometry optimizations of polypeptides and proteins. J Phys Chem A 111(14):2722–2732

77. Fedorov DG, Kitaura K (2014) Use of an auxiliary basis set to describe the polarization in the fragment molecular orbital method. Chem Phys Lett 597:99–105

78. Nagata T, Fedorov DG, Ishimura K, Kitaura K (2011) Analytic energy gradient for second-order Møller-Plesset perturbation theory based on the fragment molecular orbital method. J Chem Phys 135:044110

79. Nakata H, Fedorov DG, Yokojima S, Kitaura K, Nakamura S (2014) Simulations of Raman spectra using the fragment molecular orbital method. J Chem Theory Comput 10(9):3689–3698

80. Sawada T, Fedorov DG, Kitaura K (2009) Structural and interaction analysis of helical heparin oligosaccharides with the fragment molecular orbital method. Int J Quantum Chem 109(9):2033–2045

81. Tsukamoto T, Mochizuki Y, Watanabe N, Fukuzawa K, Nakano T (2012) Partial geometry optimization with FMO-MP2 gradient: application to TrpCage. Chem Phys Lett 535:157–162

82. Ishikawa T, Yamamoto N, Kuwata K (2010) Partial energy gradient based on the fragment molecular orbital method: application to geometry optimization. Chem Phys Lett 500(1):149–154

83. Fedorov DG, Alexeev Y, Kitaura K (2011) Geometry optimization of the active site of a large system with the fragment molecular orbital method. J Phys Chem Lett 2(4):282–288. doi:10.1021/jz1016894

84. Steinmann C, Fedorov DG, Jensen JH (2013) Mapping enzymatic catalysis using the effective fragment molecular orbital method: towards all ab initio biochemistry. PLoS One 8(4):e60602

85. Christensen AS, Steinmann C, Fedorov DG, Jensen JH (2014) Hybrid RHF/MP2 geometry optimizations with the effective fragment molecular orbital method. PLoS One 9(2):e88800

86. Mazanetz M, Law R, Whittaker M (2013) Hit and Lead Identification from fragments. In: Schneider G (ed) De novo molecular design. Wiley-VCH Verlag GmbH & Co. KGaA, Weinheim, pp 143–200. doi:10.1002/9783527677016.ch6

87. Ponder JW, Richards FM (1987) An efficient Newton-like method for molecular mechanics energy minimization of large molecules. J Comput Chem 8(7):1016–1024

88. Maseras F, Morokuma K (1995) IMOMM: a new integrated ab initio molecular mechanics geometry optimization scheme of equilibrium structures and transition states. J Comput Chem 16(9):1170–1179

89. Shoemaker JR, Burggraf LW, Gordon MS (1999) SIMOMM: an integrated molecular orbital/molecular mechanics optimization scheme for surfaces. J Phys Chem A 103(17):3245–3251

90. Fedorov DG, Asada N, Nakanishi I, Kitaura K (2014) The use of many-body expansions and geometry optimizations in fragment-based methods. Acc Chem Res 47(9):2846–2856

91. Nakano T, Kaminuma T, Sato T, Fukuzawa K, Akiyama Y, Uebayasi M, Kitaura K (2002) Fragment molecular orbital method: use of approximate electrostatic potential. Chem Phys Lett 351(5-6):475–480

92. Ishida T, Fedorov DG, Kitaura K (2006) All electron quantum chemical calculation of the entire enzyme system confirms a collective catalytic device in the chorismate mutase reaction. J Phys Chem B 110(3):1457–1463

93. Jensen JH, Willemoës M, Winther JR, De Vico L (2014) In silico prediction of mutant HIV-1 proteases cleaving a target sequence. PLoS One 9(5):e95833

94. Ito M, Brinck T (2014) Novel approach for identifying key residues in enzymatic reactions: proton abstraction in ketosteroid isomerase. J Phys Chem B 118(46):13050–13058

95. Hediger MR, Steinmann C, De Vico L, Jensen JH (2013) A computational method for the systematic screening of reaction barriers in enzymes: searching for Bacillus circulans xylanase mutants with greater activity towards a synthetic substrate. PeerJ 1:e111

96. Nishimoto Y, Fedorov DG, Irle S (2014) Density-functional tight-binding combined with the fragment molecular orbital method. J Chem Theory Comput 10(11):4801–4812

97. Sugiki SI, Kurita N, Sengoku Y, Sekino H (2003) Fragment molecular orbital method with density functional theory and DIIS convergence acceleration. Chem Phys Lett 382 (5):611–617

98. Fedorov DG, Kitaura K (2012) Energy decomposition analysis in solution based on the fragment molecular orbital method. J Phys Chem A 116:704–719

99. Fedorov DG, Kitaura K (2007) Pair interaction energy decomposition analysis. J Comput Chem 28(1):222–237

100. Green MC, Fedorov DG, Kitaura K, Francisco JS, Slipchenko LV (2013) Open-shell pair interaction energy decomposition analysis (PIEDA): formulation and application to the hydrogen abstraction in tripeptides. J Chem Phys 138(7):074111

101. Bandyopadhyay P, Gordon MS, Mennucci B, Tomasi J (2002) An integrated effective fragment - polarizable continuum approach to solvation: theory and application to glycine. J Chem Phys 116:5023

102. Nagata T, Fedorov DG, Sawada T, Kitaura K (2012) Analysis of solute–solvent interactions in the fragment molecular orbital method interfaced with effective fragment potentials: theory and application to a solvated griffith-sin–carbohydrate complex. J Phys Chem A 116(36):9088–9099

103. Ishikawa T, Ishikura T, Kuwata K (2009) Theoretical study of the prion protein based on the fragment molecular orbital method. J Comput Chem 30(16):2594–2601

104. Okiyama Y, Fukuzawa K, Yamada H, Mochizuki Y, Nakano T, Tanaka S (2011) Counterpoise-corrected interaction energy analysis based on the fragment molecular orbital scheme. Chem Phys Lett 509 (1):67–71

105. Watanabe C, Fukuzawa K, Okiyama Y, Tsukamoto T, Kato A, Tanaka S, Mochizuki Y, Nakano T (2013) Three-and four-body corrected fragment molecular orbital calculations with a novel subdividing fragmentation method applicable to structure-based drug design. J Mol Graph Model 41:31–42

106. Asada N, Fedorov DG, Kitaura K, Nakanishi I, Merz KM Jr (2012) An efficient method to evaluate intermolecular interaction energies in large systems using overlapping multicenter ONIOM and the fragment molecular orbital method. J Phys Chem Lett 3 (18):2604–2610

107. Tanaka S, Watanabe C, Okiyama Y (2013) Statistical correction to effective interactions in the fragment molecular orbital method. Chem Phys Lett 556:272–277

108. Mochizuki Y, Fukuzawa K, Kato A, Tanaka S, Kitaura K, Nakano T (2005) A configuration analysis for fragment interaction. Chem Phys Lett 410(4):247–253

109. Ishikawa T, Mochizuki Y, Amari S, Nakano T, Tokiwa H, Tanaka S, Tanaka K (2007) Fragment interaction analysis based on local MP2. Theor Chem Acc 118(5-6):937–945

110. Ishikawa T, Kuwata K (2009) Interaction analysis of the native structure of prion protein with quantum chemical calculations. J Chem Theory Comput 6(2):538–547

111. Hitaoka S, Harada M, Yoshida T, Chuman H (2010) Correlation analyses on binding affinity of sialic acid analogues with influenza virus Neuraminidase-1 using ab Initio MO calculations on their complex structures. J Chem Inf Model 50(10):1796–1805

112. Dedachi K, Hirakawa T, Fujita S, Khan MTH, Sylte I, Kurita N (2011) Specific interactions and binding free energies between thermolysin and dipeptides: molecular simulations combined with Ab initio molecular orbital and classical vibrational analysis. J Comput Chem 32(14):3047–3057

113. Suenaga M (2005) Facio: new computational chemistry environment for PC GAMESS. J Comput Chem Jpn 4(1):25–32

114. Durant JL, Leland BA, Henry DR, Nourse JG (2002) Reoptimization of MDL keys for use in drug discovery. J Chem Inf Comput Sci 42 (6):1273–1280

115. Kohonen T (2001) Self-organizing maps, vol 30, 3rd edn, Information sciences. Springer, Berlin

116. Hefner R (1959) Book review: Warren S. Torgerson, Theory and methods of scaling. New York: John Wiley and Sons, Inc. 1958. Syst Res Behav Sci 4(3):245–247

117. Kurauchi R, Watanabe C, Fukuzawa K, Tanaka S (2015) Novel type of virtual ligand screening on the basis of quantum-chemical calculations for protein–ligand complexes and extended clustering techniques. Comput Theor Chem 1061:12–22

118. Verkhivker GM, Bouzida D, Gehlhaar DK, Rejto PA, Arthurs S, Colson AB, Freer ST, Larson V, Luty BA, Marrone T (2000) Deciphering common failures in molecular docking of ligand-protein complexes. J Comput Aided Mol Des 14(8):731–751

119. Neumann L, Von König K, Ullmann D (2011) HTS reporter displacement assay for fragment screening and fragment evolution toward leads with optimized binding kinetics, binding selectivity, and thermodynamic signature. Methods Enzymol 493:299–320

120. Williams DH, Stephens E, O'Brien DP, Zhou M (2004) Understanding noncovalent interactions: ligand binding energy and catalytic efficiency from ligand-induced reductions in motion within receptors and enzymes. Angew Chem Int Ed 43(48):6596–6616

121. Barker JJ, Barker O, Courtney SM, Gardiner M, Hesterkamp T, Ichihara O, Mather O, Montalbetti CAGN, Müller A, Varasi M (2010) Discovery of a novel Hsp90 inhibitor by fragment linking. ChemMedChem 5 (10):1697–1700

122. Ferenczy GG, Keseru GM (2012) Thermodynamics of fragment binding. J Chem Inf Model 52(4):1039–1045

123. Abel R, Young T, Farid R, Berne BJ, Friesner RA (2008) Role of the active-site solvent in the thermodynamics of factor Xa ligand binding. J Am Chem Soc 130(9):2817–2831

124. Huggins DJ, Sherman W, Tidor B (2012) Rational approaches to improving selectivity in drug design. J Med Chem 55(4):1424–1444

125. Wyatt PG, Woodhead AJ, Berdini V, Boulstridge JA, Carr MG, Cross DM, Davis DJ, Devine LA, Early TR, Feltell RE (2008) Identification of N-(4-piperidinyl)-4-(2, 6-dichlorobenzoylamino)-1 H-pyrazole-3-carboxamide (AT7519), a novel cyclin dependent kinase inhibitor using fragment-based X-Ray crystallography and structure based drug design. J Med Chem 51 (16):4986–4999

126. Hartshorn MJ, Murray CW, Cleasby A, Frederickson M, Tickle IJ, Jhoti H (2005) Fragment-based lead discovery using X-ray crystallography. J Med Chem 48(2):403–413

127. Imai YN, Inoue Y, Nakanishi I, Kitaura K (2009) Cl–π Interactions in protein–ligand complexes. QSAR Comb Sci 28(8):869–873

128. Ozawa T, Okazaki K (2008) CH/π hydrogen bonds determine the selectivity of the Src homology 2 domain to tyrosine phosphotyrosyl peptides: an ab initio fragment molecular orbital study. J Comput Chem 29 (16):2656–2666

129. Anzaki S, Watanabe C, Fukuzawa K, Mochizuki Y, Tanaka S (2014) Interaction energy analysis on specific binding of influenza virus hemagglutinin to avian and human sialosaccharide receptors: importance of mutation-induced structural change. J Mol Graph Model 53:48–58

130. Yoshioka A, Fukuzawa K, Mochizuki Y, Yamashita K, Nakano T, Okiyama Y, Nobusawa E, Nakajima K, Tanaka S (2011) Prediction of probable mutations in influenza virus hemagglutinin protein based on large-scale ab initio fragment molecular orbital calculations. J Mol Graph Model 30:110–119

131. Okiyama Y, Watanabe H, Fukuzawa K, Nakano T, Mochizuki Y, Ishikawa T, Tanaka S, Ebina K (2007) Application of the fragment molecular orbital method for determination of atomic charges on polypeptides. Chem Phys Lett 449(4):329–335

132. Okiyama Y, Watanabe H, Fukuzawa K, Nakano T, Mochizuki Y, Ishikawa T, Ebina K, Tanaka S (2009) Application of the fragment molecular orbital method for determination of atomic charges on polypeptides. II. Towards an improvement of force fields used for classical molecular dynamics simulations. Chem Phys Lett 467(4):417–423

133. Chang L, Ishikawa T, Kuwata K, Takada S (2013) Protein-specific force field derived from the fragment molecular orbital method can improve protein–ligand binding interactions. J Comput Chem 34(14):1251–1257

134. Cramer RD, Patterson DE, Bunce JD (1988) Comparative molecular field analysis (CoMFA). 1. Effect of shape on binding of steroids to carrier proteins. J Am Chem Soc 110(18):5959–5967

135. Klebe G, Abraham U, Mietzner T (1994) Molecular similarity indices in a comparative analysis (CoMSIA) of drug molecules to correlate and predict their biological activity. J Med Chem 37(24):4130–4146

136. Zhang Q, Yang J, Liang K, Feng L, Li S, Wan J, Xu X, Yang G, Liu D, Yang S (2008) Binding interaction analysis of the active site and its inhibitors for neuraminidase (N1 subtype) of human influenza virus by the integration of molecular docking, FMO calculation and 3D-QSAR CoMFA modeling. J Chem Inf Model 48(9):1802–1812

137. Zhang Q, Yu C, Min J, Wang Y, He J, Yu Z (2011) Rational questing for potential novel inhibitors of FabK from Streptococcus pneumoniae by combining FMO calculation, CoMFA 3D-QSAR modeling and virtual screening. J Mol Model 17(6):1483–1492

138. Yoshida T, Yamagishi K, Chuman H (2008) QSAR study of cyclic urea type HIV-1 PR inhibitors using ab initio MO calculation of their complex structures with HIV-1 PR. QSAR Comb Sci 27(6):694–703

139. Yoshida T, Munei Y, Hitaoka S, Chuman H (2010) Correlation analyses on binding affinity of substituted benzenesulfonamides with carbonic anhydrase using ab initio MO calculations on their complex structures. J Chem Inf Model 50(5):850–860

140. Munei Y, Shimamoto K, Harada M, Yoshida T, Chuman H (2011) Correlation analyses on binding affinity of substituted benzenesulfonamides with carbonic anhydrase using ab initio MO calculations on their complex structures (II). Bioorg Med Chem Lett 21 (1):141–144

141. Mashima A, Kurahashi M, Sasahara K, Yoshida T, Chuman H (2014) Connecting classical QSAR and LERE analyses using modern molecular calculations, LERE-QSAR (VI): hydrolysis of substituted hippuric acid phenyl esters by trypsin. Mol Inform 33 (11-12):802–814

142. Hitaoka S, Chuman H, Yoshizawa K (2015) A QSAR study on the inhibition mechanism of matrix metalloproteinase-12 by arylsulfone analogs based on molecular orbital calculations. Org Biomol Chem 13(3):793–806

143. Baker NA, Sept D, Joseph S, Holst MJ, McCammon JA (2001) Electrostatics of nanosystems: application to microtubules and the ribosome. Proc Natl Acad Sci U S A 98(18):10037–10041

144. Li L, Li C, Sarkar S, Zhang J, Witham S, Zhang Z, Wang L, Smith N, Petukh M, Alexov E (2012) DelPhi: a comprehensive suite for DelPhi software and associated resources. BMC Biophys 5(1):9

145. Watanabe T, Inadomi Y, Fukuzawa K, Nakano T, Tanaka S, Nilsson L, Nagashima U (2007) DNA and estrogen receptor interaction revealed by fragment molecular orbital calculations. J Phys Chem B 111 (32):9621–9627

146. Fedorov DG, Olson RM, Kitaura K, Gordon MS, Koseki S (2004) A new hierarchical parallelization scheme: generalized distributed data interface (GDDI), and an application to the fragment molecular orbital method (FMO). J Comput Chem 25(6):872–880

147. Alexeev Y, Mahajan A, Leyffer S, Fletcher GD, Fedorov DG Heuristic static load-balancing algorithm applied to the Fragment Molecular Orbital method. In: Proceedings of the ACM/IEEE Supercomputing 2012 Conference, Salt Lake City, 2012. IEEE, pp 1–13

Methods in Pharmacology and Toxicology (2016): 257–296
DOI 10.1007/7653_2014_35
© Springer Science+Business Media New York 2014
Published online: 22 January 2015

# Recent Advances in the Open Access Cheminformatics Toolkits, Software Tools, Workflow Environments, and Databases

## Pravin Ambure, Rahul Balasaheb Aher, and Kunal Roy

## Abstract

Cheminformatics utilizes various computational techniques to solve a wide variety of drug discovery problems, including drug design and predictive toxicology. These computational exercises employ various toolkits/libraries, workflows, databases, etc. for their applications in lead optimization, virtual screening, chemical database mining, structure-activity/toxicity studies, etc. It is therefore important for such techniques to be freely available. Open-access resources permit free use and redistribution of a product via a free license, while open-source resources also provide source code that can be utilized to modify the product. In order to extract the knowledge from enormous amount of data that accumulates at a staggering rate, open-access or open-source cheminformatics packages also need to be efficient and user-friendly. In this chapter, we record the recent advances in freely available (including both open access and open source) cheminformatics toolkits, software (stand-alone and online applications), workflow environment, and databases. The objective of this chapter is to get the readers acquainted with the freely available resources, so that they can utilize those tools for solving different drug discovery challenges. We will start with the toolkit/libraries such as Chemistry Development Kit (CDK), Open Babel, RDKit, ChemmineR, Indigo, chem$^f$, etc., which provide various functionalities that can aid researchers to develop their own cheminformatics software/ applications. Next we will discuss various cheminformatics software tools, including iDrug, PharmDock, DecoyFinder, DemQSAR, Chembench, etc. which have recently been developed with a wide variety of applications. We will further discuss workflow environments, including Konstanz Information Miner (KNIME), Taverna, recent combinations, i.e., CDK-KNIME or CDK-Taverna and their contributions in the cheminformatics field. At the end, we will briefly touch various recent databases, such as QSAR DataBank, VAMMPIRE, CREDO, PubChem3D, MMsINC, etc., and their applications. The open-access resources covered in this chapter would enable the medicinal chemists and cheminformaticians to solve various problems encountered during their research.

**Key words** Open source, Open access, Cheminformatics, Tool kits, Software, Databases, Stand-alone tools, Online tools, Workflows

# 1 Introduction

Cheminformatics is an applied field of chemistry that involves the use of different computational resources for solving a variety of problems arising in chemical, pharmaceutical, and allied industries. This field is a combination of chemistry, computer science, and information science that aids in transforming huge raw data into information and this information into knowledge. Cheminformatics has revolutionized various areas including pharmaceutical and chemical research, in taking faster decisions, cutting cost, and hence increasing efficiency.

The availability of cheminformatics resources is based on the provider/source that are commonly categorized into commercially available, open access, or open source. Commercial resources are normally well developed but expensive; thus, their users are limited to those who can afford such costly services. Open-source resources, on the other hand, are freely available (i.e., open access), and their source code is openly accessible for modification or distribution. To best support the majority of the scientific community in resolving the different problems arising in multifarious areas of chemistry, it is essential that cheminformatics resources are openly accessible, which is not only important for resolving problems but also critical for bringing new amendments to overcome shortcomings of current resources and for exploring innovative concept/ideas associated with cheminformatics resources. Developing and managing such freely available cheminformatics resources is often "community driven" and an outcome of a teamwork from numerous contributors. In this chapter, we highlight the advances made in a variety of freely available (both open access and open source) cheminformatics resources, i.e., toolkits, software, workflow, and databases.

## 2    Cheminformatics Toolkits

Cheminformatics toolkits are a set of libraries comprising of source codes for various algorithms/functions that allow the cheminformaticians to develop their own software applications for possible use in structural similarity searching, virtual screening, database mining, structure-activity relationship analysis, etc. The development of open-source cheminformatics toolkits has started more than a decade ago, and so far many highly functional toolkits have been developed. Some toolkits were developed from the scratch, e.g., Chemistry Development Kit (CDK) [1] and Open Babel [2], while others, such as RDKit [3] and Indigo [4] toolkits, were made open source by donating *in-house* source code under liberal licenses. The development of such cheminformatics toolkits became a part of the Blue Obelisk movement [5, 6] established in 2005 as a response to the lack of Open Data, Open Standards and Open source (ODOSOS) in chemistry.

The main reason that these toolkits are so essential is that their availability aids the development of a next generation of cheminformatics software like Bioclipse [7], Avogadro [8], CDK Descriptor Calculator GUI [9], etc., where there is no need to concern about the low-level details of manipulating and/or handling various algorithms; thus one can focus on providing additional functionality and/or ease of use [6].

In this section, we describe various cheminformatics toolkits (*see* Table 1 for a brief summary) and their recent progress.

### 2.1 Chemistry Development Kit (CDK)

The CDK is an open-source Java library for structural cheminformatics and bioinformatics. This project was initiated in 2000 by Christoph Steinbeck, Egon Willighagen, and Dan Gezelter, the developers of Jmol [20] and JChemPaint [21]. Till date, it is one of the most active open-source cheminformatics projects that are being carried out with wide support from the scientific community. The number of contributors to this project has increased to 89 in 2014 [22].

CDK toolkit provides many functionalities for developing new software in the cheminformatics field such as various chemical input/output (I/O) file formats, including simplified molecular-input line-entry system (SMILES), Chemical Markup Language (CML), and MIT Design Language (MDL); structure generators; 2D diagram editing and generation; 3D geometry generation; substructure search using exact structures and Smiles ARbitrary Target Specification (SMARTS)-*like* queries; molecular descriptor calculation for quantitative structure-activity relationship (QSAR) study; fingerprint calculation; International Chemical Identifier (InChI) support (via JNI-InChI); etc., and in bioinformatics field, the functionalities include cognate ligand detection, metabolite identification, etc. [1, 23, 24].

At present, the CDK is the source for a number of software projects including JChemPaint [21], SENECA [25], NMRShiftDB [26], PaDEL-Descriptor [27], Jmol [20], JOELib, Nomen, Safe-Base, and many more [28]. The functionality of CDK can also be freely accessed through workflow system, such as KNIME and Taverna, which are discussed in the workflow section of this chapter.

The CDK developers regularly perform unit testing, code quality checking, bug fixing, and proper versioning of CDK library. Information about the library functionality, core classes, inheritance hierarchy, and the dependencies among the fundamental classes of the CDK are well described in the literature [1, 10].

CDK is available for Windows, UNIX, and Mac OS and is freely distributed under the GNU Lesser General Public License (LGPL) version 2.0 (v2). In contrast to the more common GNU General Public License (GPL), the LGPL allows the use of the CDK in proprietary software packages.

### 2.2 RDKit

The RDKit was developed and employed at Rational Discovery during 2000–2006, for building predictive models for absorption, distribution, metabolism, elimination, toxicity, and biological activity. In June 2006, Rational Discovery was shut down, but the

**Table 1**
**Summary of cheminformatics toolkits**

| Sr. No. | Name | Link | Programming language (wrapper, if any) | Operating system(s) | License | Reference No. |
|---|---|---|---|---|---|---|
| 1 | Chemistry Development Kit (CDK) | http://sourceforge.net/projects/cdk/ | Java | Platform independent | LGPL | [1, 10] |
| 2 | RDKit | http://www.rdkit.org/ | C++ (Python, Java and C# wrapper) | Mac, Windows, and Linux | BSD | [3] |
| 3 | Open Babel | http://openbabel.org/ | C++ (Java, .NET platform, Perl, Python, and Ruby wrapper) | Windows, Mac OS X, Linux | GPL | [2] |
| 4 | Cinfony | https://code.google.com/p/cinfony/ https://github.com/cinfony/cinfony | Python, Jython | Platform independent | BSD | [11] |
| 5 | Small Molecule Subgraph Detector (SMSD) | http://www.ebi.ac.uk/thornton-srv/software/SMSD/ | Java | Platform independent | Creative Commons (CC) | [12] |
| 6 | Biochemical Algorithms Library (BALL) | http://www.ball-project.org | C++ | Windows, Linux, and Mac OS X | LPGL and GPL | [13] |

| 7 | Indigo | http://www.ggasoftware.com/opensource/indigo | C++ (Python, Java, and C# wrappers available) | Windows, Linux, and Mac OS X | GPL | [4] |
|---|---|---|---|---|---|---|
| 8 | jCompoundMapper | http://jcompoundmapper.sourceforge.net/ | Java | Platform independent | LPGL | [14] |
| 9 | chem[f] | https://github.com/stefan-hoeck/chemf http://www.scala-lang.org/ | Scala (runs on Java platform) | Platform independent | GPL | [15] |
| 10 | Cheminformatics in Python (ChemoPy) | https://code.google.com/p/pychem/downloads/list | Python | Linux and Windows | – | [16] |
| 11 | ChemmineR | http://www.bioconductor.org/packages/release/bioc/html/ChemmineR.html | Statistical programming environment "R" | Windows and Mac OS X | Artistic 2.0 | [17] |
| 12 | Compound-Protein Interaction with R (Rcpi) | http://bioconductor.org/packages/release/bioc/html/Rcpi.html | Statistical programming environment "R" | Windows and Mac OS X | Artistic 2.0 | [18] |
| 13 | Chemkit | http://wiki.chemkit.org/Main_Page | C++ | Windows, Mac, and Linux | BSD | [19] |

toolkit was released as open source under BSD license. At present, the open-source development of RDKit is actively contributed by Novartis, which includes the source code donated by Novartis [29].

RDKit offers various functionalities such as different chemical I/O formats, including SMILES/SMARTS, structure data format (SDF), Thor data tree (TDT), Sybyl line notation (SLN), Corina mol2, and Protein Data Bank (PDB); substructure searching; canonical SMILES; chirality support (i.e., R/S or E/Z labeling); chemical transformations (e.g., remove matching substructures); chemical reactions; molecular serialization; similarity/diversity selection; 2D pharmacophores; Gasteiger-Marsili charges; hierarchical subgraph/fragment analysis; Bemis and Murcko scaffold determination; retrosynthetic combinatorial analysis procedure (RECAP) and BRICS implementations; multi-molecule maximum common substructure; feature maps; shape-based similarity; RMSD-based molecule-molecule alignment; shape-based alignment; unsupervised molecule-molecule alignment using Open3-DALIGN algorithm; integration with PyMOL for 3D visualization; functional group filtering; salt stripping; molecular descriptor library; similarity maps; machine learning; etc.

The *Contrib* directory [30] is a part of the standard RDKit distribution that includes source code that has been contributed by the community members, for instance, Local Environment Fingerprints (LEF), a Python source code; plane of best fit (PBF), a C++ source code; matched molecular pair algorithm (mmpa), a Python source code and sample data; a fragment indexing algorithm; and synthetic accessibility (SA) score, a Python source code.

RDKit has an official website, i.e., http://www.rdkit.org/, for online documentation, recent news, Wiki link, and other related information. The core data structures and algorithms are written in C++ programming language, but Python wrapper (generated using Boost.Python) and Java and C# wrapper (generated using SWIG) are also available. Here, wrapper or binding means a thin layer of code that converts a library's existing interface into a user's compatible interface, so that one can use the library in other programming languages. RDKit is supported by Mac, Windows, and Linux operating system [31].

### 2.3 Open Babel

Open Babel is an open-source chemical toolbox intended to be a cross-platform library that is built to support interconversion between various file formats used in cheminformatics, molecular modeling, and related areas. In addition to the complete, extensible toolkit/libraries, it also offers ready-to-use applications for the development of cheminformatics software [2].

Open Babel 2.3 can perform reading, writing, and interconversion of over 111 chemical file formats that includes reading and writing of 82 and 85 file formats, respectively. These encompass common formats used in cheminformatics (SMILES, InChI,

MOL, MOL2), I/O files from a variety of computational chemistry packages (GAMESS, Gaussian, MOPAC), crystallographic file formats (CIF, ShelX), reaction formats (MDL RXN), file formats used by molecular dynamics simulation (Amber) and docking packages (AutoDock), formats used by 2D drawing packages (ChemDraw), 3D viewers (Chem3D, Molden), chemical kinetics, and thermodynamics (ChemKin, Thermo). It supports filtering and searching molecule files using Daylight SMARTS pattern matching and computes group contribution descriptors such as LogP, polar surface area (PSA). and molar refractivity (MR). It also provides extensible molecular fingerprinting and molecular mechanics functions.

File formats are employed as "plug-ins" which aid users to contribute new file formats. Further, depending on the file format, Open Babel can extract additional information besides molecular structure. For instance, property fields can be read from SDF files, unit cell information can be extracted from CIF files, and vibrational frequencies can be extracted from computational chemistry log files. For each file format, multiple choices/options can be chosen to read or write in a particular format.

Open Babel has its origin in a version of OELib, which was released as open-source software by OpenEye Scientific under the GNU GPL v2. In 2001, OpenEye decided to rewrite OELib *in-house* as the proprietary OEChem library, and the existing code from OELib was released as the new Open Babel project. Since then, Open Babel has been developed and substantially extended as an open-source project with extensive international collaborations. Up to November 2014, it has over 324,780 downloads [32] and more than 476 citations [33] and has been utilized by over 40 software projects. While the majority of the Open Babel library is written in C++, its bindings have been developed for other programming languages, including Java, .NET platform, Perl, Python, and Ruby. These can be automatically generated from the C++ header files using the SWIG tool. Open Babel supports a wide variety of C++ compilers (MSVC, GCC, Intel Compiler, MinGW, Clang), operating systems (Windows, Mac OS X, Linux), and platforms (32-bit, 64-bit). OpenEye scientific has also provided a set of cheminformatics and modeling toolkits [34] that are freely accessible under the free public domain research license [35].

In summary, Open Babel offers a solution to deal with the growing number of chemical file formats along with various functionalities like conformer searching, 2D depiction, filtering, batch conversion, and substructure and similarity search. For software developers, it can be used as a library to handle data in ample of areas such as organic chemistry, drug design, molecular modeling, and computational chemistry [2, 36].

Scripting languages like Python are highly popular since they allow rapid writing of scripts within a few lines of code and are well suited for common programming tasks in cheminformatics. For the same reason, a Python wrapper for Open Babel called Pybel [37] has been made available. It is an open-source, cross-platform Python module that provides the functionality of the Open Babel toolkit to Python programmers.

### 2.4 Cinfony

In the present scenario, the most active open-source cheminformatics toolkits under development comprise of Open Babel, the CDK, and the RDKit. All of these toolkits share the same core functionality although the implementation details and the chemical model employed may differ. However, these toolkits are independently developed, and therefore, each has certain specific functionalities, e.g., these toolkit support different sets of file formats and force fields and represent various molecular fingerprints and descriptors in different ways. There are also features in each of the toolkits that are not shared by the others.

To this end, Cinfony is a Python module which provides a common interface for Open Babel, RDKit, and CDK through a simple and robust method to pass the chemical models among these toolkits. It is an extension of Pybel (*discussed above*), a Python module that only provides access to Open Babel. It allows interoperability at the application programming interface (API) level, which has the advantage of not requiring any changes to the existing software. It is platform independent and hence supported by all operating systems such as Mac, Windows, and Linux operating system and is released as open source under the BSD license. The details about the barriers, interoperability, implementation, and performance are well discussed in the literature [11].

### 2.5 Small Molecule Subgraph Detector (SMSD)

The chemical similarity determination between molecules is widely used to compute chemical diversity and for clustering analysis of similar molecules. This is a highly useful concept in cases like discovering new *drug-like* molecules. Maximum common subgraph (MCS) is one of the recent methods that overcome nearly all the shortcomings posed by descriptor- or fragment-based similarity searches. All of the early MCS algorithms lacked chemical knowledge to rank the MCS solutions, which led to the development of SMSD toolkit [12].

SMSD is a chemically sensitive and robust tool, which uses a combination of various graph-matching algorithms (i.e., CDKMCS, MCS+, and VF+ Lib [12]) for finding the MCS among small molecules. It can generate bond-sensitive and bond-insensitive MCS and ranks the solutions according to minimal fragments, bond breaking energy, and stereochemical matches. It also overcomes the disadvantages of MCS algorithm coded in the CDK toolkit (CDKMCS) by first using the atom and bond count filter to discriminate between two dissimilar structures before performing the MCS search and, secondly, by using the VF+ Lib and MCS+ method. The reported disadvantages of CDKMCS include: (a) it may treat two chemically nonidentical molecules as identical because it works on the maximum common induced subgraph (MCIS) principle, and (b) the runtime is high if two graphs are large with few dissimilar edges.

SMSD is a combination of various algorithms (i.e., CDKMCS, MCS+, and VF+ Lib). The choice of using which algorithm is completely based on the complexity of the input molecules. CDKMCS is used first for molecules whose bond count and atom count are not equal. If the solution is not computed within a limited set time, then it is passed to the MCS+ algorithm, which starts the search from the scratch. If the $d$-edge count (those edges that do not share similar bond types) is greater than 99,999, then VF+ Lib is used to find MCS, which is very efficient in handling medium- to large-sized graphs. The MCS solutions are then passed to the chemical post-filters, which ranks the solutions in a chemically meaningful way. The three filters are applied in the following orders: (a) specific matching of the chemical functional groups, bond types, and stereochemistry of molecules are identified and matched; (b) the resulting solutions are sorted in ascending order of the total bond breaking energy required by this MCS match (i.e., lowest energy is highest ranked); and (c) the top solutions are selected based on the above two steps (in the case that the matched part of the molecule is detached from the reference structure, the solutions are sorted again in decreasing order based on the number of fragments generated). In such a way, one can get chemically relevant MCS solutions computed in polynomial time.

SMSD can be applied in a variety of bioinformatics and cheminformatics areas for exhaustive MCS matching. For example, it can be employed to analyze metabolic networks by matching the reactants with the products of the reactions. It can also be used to detect the MCS/substructure in small molecules reported by metabolomics experiments, as well as to screen for *drug-like* compounds with similar substructures.

SMSD is a Java-based toolkit, which is platform independent and is released under Creative Commons (CC) license [38]. This toolkit is freely available at www.ebi.ac.uk [12].

### 2.6 Biochemical Algorithms Library (BALL) 1.3

BALL is written in C++ with a specific purpose of significantly reducing the development time of building derived computational applications while ensuring stability and errorless implementation in the computational biology and molecular modeling field. It provides an extensive set of data structures along with classes for molecular mechanics (MM), file I/O, comparison and analysis of protein structures, advanced solvation methods, and visualization. BALL has been designed to be robust, easy to use, and also simply extensible due to its object-oriented programming background. In 2010, a new version, i.e., BALL 1.3, was released, and this version showed significant improvements in functionality compared to the previous version that had been released in 1999 [13].

BALL handles a variety of molecular structure formats. The previously published version only supported the PDB and MOL2 molecular file formats, while version 1.3 additionally reads and writes MOL, HIN, XYZ, KCF, and SD files. It also supports a variety of other data sources, such as DCD, DSN6, GAMESS, JCAMP, SCWRL, and TRR. Along with this, the new version also offers functionality for generating and editing molecules. For proteins, DNA, and RNA, BALL 1.3 can automatically deduce much of the missing information such as connectivity or bond order or missing hydrogen from an extensible fragment database. Both fragment database and rotamer library have been significantly improved in the latest version. A rotamer library allows the user to easily determine the most likely side-chain conformation of a protein residue or to switch between various rotameric states. The new features also include a kekulizer (an aromaticity processor), a secondary structure predictor, and hydrogen bond detection.

The previous version of BALL has provided two force field classes, i.e., CHARMM and AMBER. In the 1.3 version, an implementation of the Merck Molecular Force Field (MMFF94) has been included that allows handling of almost all types of organic compounds. The energy minimization functions have been extended via providing standard methods like steepest descent and conjugate gradient and the well-known methods, i.e., L-BFGS and shifted L-VMM algorithms [13].

BALL is freely available and supported by all major operating systems, including Linux, Windows, and Mac OS X. Previously, BALL was distributed as a commercial product, but now it is released open source under the GNU Lesser General Public License (LGPL), and parts of the code are released under the GNU GPL. The source code and binary packages are available from the project website at http://www.ball-project.org [13].

### 2.7  Indigo

In 2009, GGA software services released a toolkit titled "Indigo" and related software under the terms of GNU GPL. It includes some unique algorithms developed by GGA, along with some standard well-known algorithms.

The main features of Indigo are:

- Supports commonly used and popular chemistry formats: mol-files/Rxnfiles v2000 and v3000, SDF, RDF, SMILES, SMARTS, and SMIRKS

- Supports tetrahedral and *cis-trans* stereochemistry

- Molecule and reaction rendering to PNG, SVG, and PDF files

- Molecule and reaction depiction

- Aromatization and kekulization

- Canonical (isomeric) SMILES computation
- Exact and substructure matching for molecules and reactions
- Support matching and highlighting
- Matching of tautomers and resonance structures
- Computing molecule and reaction fingerprints
- Similarity search
- Maximum common substructure (MCS) algorithm
- R-group deconvolution and scaffold detection

It is a C++ language-based library, majorly focused on performance and essential chemical features. The high-level wrappers or bindings are built around it for Python, Java, and C# language. This library also allows multi-threaded use. All binaries are supported by all the essential operating systems, i.e., Windows, Linux, and Mac OS X, both 32-bit and 64-bit [39]. The JAVA GUI utilities, command-line utilities, KNIME nodes, and documentation material are available on their official website [4]. A commercial license version is also available for receiving ongoing support and maintenance and for clients who like to include Indigo as a component in their proprietary software product [4].

### 2.8  jCompoundMapper

jCompoundMapper [14] is an open-source Java library for the encoding of chemical graphs as fingerprints. It offers a variety of topological (e.g., radial atom environments, extended connectivity fingerprints, depth-first search fingerprints, or autocorrelation vectors) and geometrical (e.g., 2-point and 3-point encodings or geometrical atom environments) fingerprints. It is based on CDK, which offers the basic functionality for parsing, typing, and graph algorithms for molecular data and also provides several fingerprint functionalities. But unlike CDK, jCompoundMapper focuses on exact definition of its encoding and provides functionality to export the fingerprints or pairwise similarity matrices to formats of popular machine learning toolboxes such as comma-separated value (*csv*) format, LIBSVM format (sparse and matrix), and WEKA ARFF. Hence, various data mining libraries can be directly applied on the output files.

This library is built from various implementations of literature fingerprints and descriptors used in comparison studies, and its algorithms can be parameterized with various options to adapt the encodings, for instance, by applying a custom labeling function; adjusting the search depth, the distance cutoff, or the geometrical scaling factor; etc.

jCompoundMapper is platform independent and is released under the LPGL license. It features a command-line interface but can also be used as a Java application programming interface (API). The access via the API or the binary using the command-line interface enables the user to utilize the library for batch processing. The source code and an executable library are available at SourceForge [40].

**2.9 chem$^f$**

Chem$^f$ is a chemistry toolkit, a first of its kind being built using a functional programming language named "*Scala*" [15]. *Scala* is a modern multi-paradigm open-source programming language that is fully object-oriented with a strong support for typical concepts from functional programming such as higher-order functions, type inference, and pattern matching. It has one of the most expressive type systems [41].

Most of the freely available and widely used cheminformatics toolkits, such as the CDK or Open Babel, are written in object-oriented languages using typical imperative concepts such as mutable data structures and opaque methods to implement chemical entities and algorithms. The developers of the Chem$^f$ toolkit have discussed the advantages of functional programming compared to the imperative programming languages and reported an example for justification, i.e., the comparison between CDK's and Chem$^f$'s SMILES parser [15].

Functional programming languages were designed with referential transparency in mind, and they encourage a more declarative style of programming without the control statements and value assignments that are typically found in imperative languages. An expression in a program is called referentially transparent when it performs calculation of the result just from its input parameters. Functional programming significantly facilitates writing referentially transparent functions and using immutable data structures. The methods and objects written in most of the languages (other than functional languages) are a priori unsafe to be used in parallel computations (i.e., multi-threaded operations) unless their documentation explicitly states differently. More detailed information about the functional programming, *Scala* language, and some examples illustrating its basic syntax and comparison with other open-source toolkits are provided in the freely accessible literature [15].

In summary, chem$^f$ is an open-source toolkit written in Scala language and is released under GNU GPL and is currently under development [42].

**2.10 Cheminformatics in Python (ChemoPy)**

ChemoPy is an open-source package for computing the commonly used structural and physicochemical features. It depends on several other packages that are Pybel, RDKit, Open Babel, and MOPAC, in order to provide its complete functionalities. It calculates about 16 feature groups composed of 19 various features that in all comprises of around 1,135 descriptors. Additionally, it offers seven types of molecular fingerprint systems that include topological fingerprints, electro-topological state fingerprints,

MACCS keys, FP4 keys, atom-pair fingerprints, topological torsion fingerprints, and Morgan/circular fingerprints. Some of these features and fingerprints are derived using Open Babel and RDKit. Using MOPAC, ChemoPy computes a large number of 3D molecular descriptors. Interestingly, ChemoPy is reported as the first open-source package computing a large number of molecular features based on the MOPAC optimization.

The ChemoPy toolkit encloses several modules and functions manipulating drug molecules. For instance, to obtain the molecular structures easily, ChemoPy provides a downloadable module to get molecular structures from four databases (i.e., KEGG, PubChem, DrugBank, and CAS). Further, ChemoPy can compute a large number of 2D and 3D descriptors and offers two ways to calculate these molecular descriptors. One way is to utilize the built-in modules, which consist of 19 modules responding to the calculation of descriptors from 16 feature groups, and the second way is to call the PyChem2d or PyChem3d class by importing the pychem module [43], which encapsulates commonly used descriptor calculation methods. Here, PyChem2d and PyChem3d are responsible for the calculation of 2D and 3D molecular descriptors, respectively.

The developers of ChemoPy have recommended utilizing this toolkit to analyze and represent the drugs or ligand molecules under investigation and suggested that this package will be helpful when exploring questions concerning drug activity, ADME/T, and drug-target interactions [16].

ChemoPy is written solemnly in Python language. It is supported by Linux and Windows operating systems. New extensions or functionalities can be implemented easily without cumbersome or time-consuming modifications in the source code because of the modular structure of ChemoPy [16].

## 2.11  ChemmineR

ChemmineR is a cheminformatics package for analyzing drug-like small molecule data in the popular statistical programming environment R. The first version of this package was published in 2008 [17]. It comprised of functions for 2D structural similarity comparisons between compounds, similarity searching against compound databases, functions for clustering entire compound libraries, and visualizing the clustering results.

The recent version of ChemmineR released in 2013 has additional utilities and add-on packages, including functions for efficient processing of large numbers of small molecules, physicochemical/structural property predictions, structural similarity searching, classification, and clustering of compound libraries with a wide spectrum of algorithms, including mismatch tolerant MCS search algorithm [44] used for pairwise compound comparisons. Accelerated compound similarity searching is now enabled with *eiR* add-on package [45]. The current version of ChemmineR also integrates a subset of cheminformatics functionalities implemented in the Open Babel C++ library. These utilities can be enabled by installing the ChemmineOB package and the Open Babel software. ChemmineR can automatically detect ChemmineOB and make use of its additional utilities. Streaming functionality allows processing of millions of molecules using *sdfStream* function. The recent addition also includes fast and memory-efficient fingerprint search, which supports the use of atom pair or PubChem fingerprints, and improved SMILES support via new SMIset object class and SMILES import/export functions.

ChemmineR is freely available from the Bioconductor official website (http://www.bioconductor.org/packages/release/bioc/html/ChemmineR.html). It is distributed under Artistic 2.0 license and is available for both Windows and Mac OS X operating systems [17].

### 2.12 Compound-Protein Interaction with R (Rcpi)

Rcpi toolkit provides a freely available R/Bioconductor package focusing on integrating bioinformatics and cheminformatics into a molecular informatics platform for drug discovery. It aims at providing a complete toolkit for complex molecular representation from small molecules and proteins and more complex interactions, including protein-protein and compound-protein interactions [18].

The functionalities provided by Rcpi toolkit can be divided into four groups as follows:

(a) For small molecules:
- It calculates more than 300 molecular descriptors, including constitutional, topological, geometrical, electronic, hybrid, and molecular property descriptors.
- It calculates ten types of molecular fingerprints, including standard and extended Daylight fingerprints, graph fingerprints based on simple connectivity, hybridization fingerprints only based on hybridization state, FP4 keys, E-state fingerprints, MACCS keys, PubChem fingerprints, KR fingerprints defined by Klekota and Roth, short path fingerprints, etc.
- It can compute parallelized pairwise similarity derived by fingerprints and five types of similarity measures within a list of small molecules.
- It also perform parallelized chemical similarity search with selected similarity metrics and MCS search between a query molecule and a molecular database.

(b) For protein sequences:

- It computes a large number of commonly used structural and physicochemical descriptors, such as amino acid composition descriptors; autocorrelation descriptors; composition, transition, and distribution descriptors; conjoint triad descriptors; quasi-sequence-order descriptors; and pseudo amino acid composition descriptors; etc.

- It calculates six types of generalized scale-based descriptors for proteochemometric (PCM) modeling, such as generalized scale-based descriptors derived by principal component analysis, amino acid properties, molecular descriptors, factor analysis, and multidimensional scaling, and generalized BLOSUM/PAM matrix-derived descriptors.

- It computes profile-based protein features based on position-specific scoring matrix (PSSM).

- It also performs parallelized similarity derived by protein sequence alignment and Gene Ontology (GO) semantic similarity measures between a list of protein sequences/ GO terms/Entrez Gene IDs.

(c) For interaction data:

By combining various types of descriptors for drugs and proteins, interaction descriptors representing protein-protein or compound-protein interactions could be conveniently generated with Rcpi, including:
- Two types of compound-protein interaction descriptors
- Three types of protein-protein interaction descriptors

(d) Several useful secondary utilities are also included in Rcpi that are as follows:
- Parallelized molecule and protein sequence retrieval from several online databases, such as PubChem, ChEMBL, KEGG, DrugBank, UniProt, RCSB PDB, etc.

- Molecular reading/writing in SMILES/SDF formats for small molecules and FASTA/PDB formats for proteins

- Molecular format conversion between around 140 types of molecular file formats defined by Open Babel

It is recommended to use Rcpi to analyze and represent various complex molecular data under study as well as to explore various queries concerning structure, functions, and interactions of such molecules in system biology perspective. Rcpi is freely available from the Bioconductor official website (http://bioconductor. org/packages/release/bioc/html/Rcpi.html) and is released under Artistic 2.0 license. It is available for Windows and Mac OS

X operating systems. Users can conveniently apply various statistical machine learning methods in R to solve various problems in drug discovery and computational biology [18].

*2.13  Chemkit*

Chemkit is an open-source library developed by Kyle Lutz [19], which supports molecular modeling, cheminformatics, and visualization functionalities. The key features provided by Chemkit include I/O chemical file formats (pdb, cml, cjson, cube, fhz, fps, inchi, mol, mol2, sdf, smi, etc.), access to the Web resources (e.g., Protein Data Bank, PubChem), calculation of various molecular descriptors, automatic atom typing and topology building, and visualization based on OpenGL.

The Chemkit library is written in C++ language, and it uses Qt framework for graphics. It is released under the BSD license. It is a cross platform library and is supported by Windows, Mac, and Linux operating systems.

Other toolkits that are not recently updated and/or not actively maintained but are worth mentioning include Chemfp 1.1 (http:// chemfp.com/; Python Library), Chemical Descriptor Library (http://cdelib.sourceforge.net/doc/index.html; a C++ library), PerlMol–Perl Modules for Molecular Chemistry (http://www.per lmol.org/; collection of Perl scripts), MayaChemTools (http:// www.mayachemtools.org/; collection of Perl scripts), JOELib/ JOELib2 (http://sourceforge.net/projects/joelib/; Java library), and mx-Java (https://code.google.com/p/mx-Java/; Java Library).

# 3   Cheminformatics Software

Software is a set of machine-readable instructions that directs a computer's processor to perform specific functions. It is usually written in high-level programming languages that are easier and more efficient for humans to understand and employ than the machine language. Cheminformatics software provides various ready-to-use cheminformatics functionalities like virtual screening, chemical structural editor, QSAR model development, molecular dynamics packages, etc. that are most often user-friendly tools comprising of graphical user interface (GUI).

Software can be commercial, open access, or open source. They can be developed with or without the use of external libraries/ toolkits. Existing libraries/toolkits may help reduce the software development time because source codes for various algorithms are already well defined in terms of efficiency and are ready to use. However, in many cases, the developers prefer not to use external toolkits to avoid the usage of inefficient or time-consuming algorithms, but to develop their own more efficient algorithms.

In this section, we have divided the cheminformatics software tools into two parts: stand-alone software and online tools.

The stand-alone software is a tool/application that can work offline and does not require another software package to run. The online tool means a Web-based platform-independent software tool that runs online, making the facilities available to users over the Internet. Here, both open-access and open-source software are discussed, including computer as well as mobile applications. The brief summary of cheminformatics software and their home page, supporting operating system, and programming languages are listed in Table 2.

### 3.1 Stand-Alone Software Tools

#### 3.1.1 Molpher

Molpher [46] is an open-source software framework for the systematic exploration of the chemical space. When a source/target molecular pair is given as an input entry, Molpher identifies the structural neighborhood through a process known as molecular morphing. The molecular morphing process produces a path in the chemical space by an iterative application of morphing operators, which represent a structural change such as the addition or removal of an atom or a bond. This path consisting of molecules called as morphs and its surroundings constitutes a virtual chemical library focused on a mechanistic class of compounds given by the characteristics of the source/target pair. Although Molpher is written in C++ language, it uses Boost C++ libraries [47] for standard tasks and employs open-source cheminformatics RDKit [3] for chemical functionalities. It could be easily incorporated into any computational drug design pipeline and thus is highly useful for either discovery of novel drugs or as new tool for chemical biology [46].

#### 3.1.2 PharmDock

PharmDock [48] is a pharmacophore-based docking program that combines pose sampling and ranking, which are based on optimized protein-based pharmacophore models, with local optimization using an empirical scoring function. The testing of PharmDock for ligand pose prediction, binding affinity estimation, compound ranking, and virtual screening yielded comparable or better performance as compared to other existing and widely used docking programs [49, 50]. This docking program comes with an easy-to-use GUI within PyMOL [48].

#### 3.1.3 VHELIBS

VHELIBS (validation helper for ligands and binding sites) is a software tool for assessing the quality of ligands and binding sites in the crystallographic models from the PDB/PDB_REDO for the non-crystallographers (i.e., users with little or no crystallography knowledge). It allows the users to check how the ligand and binding site coordinates fit to the electron density map (ED) and to validate the protein structures prior their use for the drug discovery purposes [51].

#### 3.1.4 MOLE 2.0

MOLE 2.0 [52] is an advanced software tool for analyzing the molecular channel and pores of the biomolecular surface. MOLE 2 also estimates the physicochemical properties of the identified

**Table 2**
**Summary of cheminformatics software**

| Sr. No. | Stand-alone software/online tools | Project home page | Operating system(s) | Programming language |
|---|---|---|---|---|
| A | *Stand-alone software* | | | |
| 1 | *Molpher* | http://siret.cz/molpher/ | MS Windows (client and server), Linux (server) | C++ |
| 2 | *PharmDock* | http://people.pharmacy.purdue.edu/~mlill/software/pharmdock | Linux | C, Python |
| 3 | *VHELIBS* | http://urvnutrigenomica-ctns.github.com/VHELIBS/ | Platform independent, Linux (server) | Python, Java |
| 4 | *MOLE 2.0* | http://mole.chemi.muni.cz | Mac OS, Linux, Windows | C# |
| 5 | *FragVLib* | http://www.unc.edu/~raed/FragVLib.zip | MS Windows, Linux | C++ |
| 6 | *TB Mobile (iOS)* | https://itunes.apple.com/us/app/tbmobile/id567461644?mt=8 | iOS | Objective-C programming |
| 7 | *TB Mobile (Android)* | http://play.google.com/store/apps/details?id=com.mmi.android.tbmobile | Android | Java |
| 8 | *JSME* | http://peter-ertl.com/jsme/ | Platform independent | JavaScript |
| 9 | *CheS-Mapper* | http://ches-mapper.org | Cross-platform | Java with Java Web Start support (can be started from a Web browser) |
| 10 | *ScreeningAssistant2 (SA2)* | http://sa2.sourceforge.net/ | Platform independent | JAVA/SQL |
| 11 | *LipidMapsTool* | www.lipidmaps.org/downloads/ | Platform independent | Perl |
| 12 | *DecoyFinder* | http://urvnutrigenomica-ctns.github.io/DecoyFinder/ | Linux, Windows | Python |

| | | | | |
|---|---|---|---|---|
| 13 | *Open Molecule Generator (OMG)* | http://sourceforge.net/p/openmg | Linux 64 bits, Linux 32 bits, Mac OS X | Java, C |
| 14 | *mol2chemfig* | http://chimpsky.uwaterloo.ca/mol2chemfig/ | Linux, Windows, Mac | Python 2.7 |
| 15 | *LICSS* | http://code.google.com/p/excel-cdk/ | Windows (XP, Vista or Windows7); Microsoft Excel for Windows (1997–2010) | VBA, Java, C++ |
| 16 | *Avogadro* | http://avogadro.openmolecules.net/ | Cross-platform | C++, Python |
| 17 | *MyChemise* | http://www.knalltundstinkt.de/englische%20Version/knalltundstinktE.html | Web based, Windows | Java |
| 18 | *Open3DALIGN* | http://open3dalign.org/ | Windows 32/64-bit, Linux 32/64-bit, Solaris x86 32/64-bit, FreeBSD 32/64-bit, Intel Mac OS X 32/64-bit | C, BLAS and LAPACK libraries |
| 19 | *mpAD4* | http://autodock.scripps.edu/downloads/multilevel-parallel-autodock4.2 | Platform independent | C++ |
| 20 | *DemQSAR* | http://agknapp.chemie.fu-berlin.de/dempred/ | Platform-independent | Java |
| 21 | *Shape* | http://sourceforge.net/projects/shapega | Linux | Java 1.5 or higher |
| 22 | *OrChem* | http://orchem.sourceforge.net/ | Platform independent | Java 1.5 or higher; *Database system:* Oracle 11 g (with JRE 1.5) |
| 23 | *PaDEL-Descriptor* | http://padel.nus.edu.sg/software/padeldescriptor/ | Platform independent | Java |
| 24 | *QSARINS and QSARINS-Chem* | http://www.qsar.it/ | Windows 2000 or more recent version | C++ |

(continued)

**Table 2**
(continued)

| Sr. No. | Stand-alone software/online tools | Project home page | Operating system(s) | Programming language |
|---|---|---|---|---|
| 25 | *VEGANIC* | http://www.vega-qsar.eu/download.html | Platform independent | Java |
| 26 | *OECD QSAR toolbox* | http://www.oecd.org/chemicalsafety/risk-assessment/theoecdqsartoolbox.htm | Windows XP | – |
| 27 | *ChemAxon Software tools* | http://www.chemaxon.com/free-software/ | Platform independent | Java |
| 28 | *DTC-Lab Software tools* | http://teqip.jdvu.ac.in/QSAR_Tools/ | Platform independent | Java |
| B | *Online tools* | | | |
| 1 | *iDrug* | http://lilab.ecust.edu.cn/idrug | Web-based platform independent | Java, Python |
| 2 | *OCHEM* | http://ochem.eu | Web-based platform independent | Java |
| 3 | *Chembench* | http://chembench.mml.unc.edu | Web-based platform independent | Java |
| 4 | *Spectral Game* | http://spectralgame.com | Web-based platform independent | HTML, PHP, JavaScript, JAVA (JSpecView) |
| 5 | *ACD/I-Lab tool* | http://www.acdlabs.com/resources/ilab/ | Web-based platform independent | – |

channels, i.e., hydropathy, hydrophobicity, polarity, charge, and mutability; this feature was absent in the previously developed related software tools, such as MOL 1.x [53], MolAxis [54, 55], and CAVER 3.0 [56]. The estimated physicochemical properties of the identified channels in the selected biomacromolecules corresponded well with the known functions of the respective channels. Thus, the predicted physicochemical properties by MOLE 2.0 provide useful information about the potential functions of identified channels [52].

*3.1.5 FragVLib*

FragVLib is a free database mining software for performing similarity search across database(s) of ligand-receptor complexes for identifying binding pockets which are similar to that of a target receptor. The methodology employed relies on the graph representation of interfacial atoms for the ligand-receptor complex. The interfacial atoms are defined as nodes, and the distances between them are represented by edges connecting these nodes. The search is based on 3D geometric and chemical similarity of the atoms forming the binding pocket. For each match identified, the ligand fragments corresponding to that binding pocket are extracted, and thus the formed virtual library of fragments (FragVLib) is useful to the structure-based drug design [57].

*3.1.6 TB Mobile*

TB Mobile is a mobile application (app) that provides the useful functionality for viewing and manipulating data about the antitubercular compounds with activity against *Mycobacterium tuberculosis* (Mtb), their targets, pathways, and other related information available in the Collaborative Drug Discovery (CDD) database. The app enables the similarity searching to identify the potential targets and to retrieve the active compounds. The molecules can be copied to the clipboard, opened with other apps, and bookmarked and exported. TB Mobile may assist the researchers as part of their workflow in identifying the potential targets for hits generated from phenotypic screenings and in hit prioritizations. The TB Mobile app is freely available from the Apple iTunes App Store and Google Play [58].

*3.1.7 JSME*

JSME is the free molecular editor (JSME) written in the JavaScript. The actual molecule editing Java code of the JME editor was translated into a JavaScript with the help of the Google Web Toolkit compiler and a custom library that emulates a subset of the GUI features of the Java runtime environment (JRE). In this process, the editor performance was enhanced by the additional functionalities of a substituent menu; copy/paste, drag and drop, and undo/redo capabilities; and an integrated help as compared to the previously available JME applet. The editor supports a molecule editing on the touch devices, such as iPhone, iPad, Android phones, and tablets in addition to the desktop computers. This new editor is easy to use and easy to be incorporated into the Web pages [59].

*3.1.8   CheS-Mapper*

CheS-Mapper (Chemical Space Mapper) is a 3D molecular viewer software tool to visualize and explore the chemical datasets. It divides a large dataset into clusters of similar compounds and consequently arranges them in the 3D space, such that their spatial proximity reflects their similarity. The tool detects the subgroups (clusters) within the data and can be employed to analyze the data to find the possible structure-activity relationship (SAR) information. This tool also calculates different kind of features, such as structural fragments as well as quantitative chemical descriptors [60].

*3.1.9*
*ScreeningAssistant2 (SA2)*

ScreeningAssistant2 (SA2) is an open-source Java software dedicated to the storage and analysis of small to very large chemical libraries. SA2 stores the unique molecules in a MySQL database and encapsulates several cheminformatics methods such as provider's management, interactive visualization, scaffold analysis, diverse subset creation, descriptors calculation, substructure/ SMART search, similarity search, and filtering. It facilitates the management of chemical libraries through an intuitive and interactive graphical interface and provides a set of advanced methods to analyze and exploit their content. Thus, it is useful for removing a variety of classes of compounds that are likely to be characterized as false positives in biochemical screening [61].

*3.1.10   LipidMapsTool*

LipidMapsTool is a software package for the template-based combinatorial enumeration of virtual compound libraries for lipids. A set of command-line scripts is used to enumerate all possible structures corresponding to the specified lipid abbreviations without any additional input requirements from the user. The virtual libraries are enumerated for the specified lipid abbreviations by using matching lists of predefined templates and chain abbreviations, instead of core scaffolds and lists of R-groups provided by the user. This tool is capable of generating large virtual compound libraries for lipids with minimal input from the user [62].

*3.1.11   DecoyFinder*

DecoyFinder [63] is a Python-based GUI application for the building of target-specific decoy sets. It selects a set of decoys for a target from a compound database based on a given collection of active ligands. The algorithm for decoy selection implemented in Decoy-Finder is similar to that used to construct the DUD database [64, 65] and other benchmarks [66]. The MACCS fingerprints [67] and five physical descriptors are calculated for each active and potential decoy molecule using the Open Babel toolbox [2]. The Decoys are selected if they are similar to the active ligands according to five physical descriptors (molecular weight, number of rotational bonds, total hydrogen bond donors, total hydrogen bond acceptors, and the octanol-water partition coefficient) without being chemically similar to any of the active ligands used as an input (according to the Tanimoto coefficient between MACCS fingerprints). This is the first application designed to build the target-specific decoy sets [63].

### 3.1.12 Open Molecule Generator (OMG)

OMG is the first open-source structure generator, which produces all the non-isomorphic chemical structures that match with a given elemental composition. Also, this structure generator accepts additional input as one or multiple nonoverlapping prescribed substructures to drastically reduce the number of possible chemical structures. OMG relies on a modified version of the Canonical Augmentation Path approach, which grows intermediate chemical structures by adding bonds and checks that at each step only unique molecules are produced. When OMG was compared with the commercially available structure generator such as MOLGEN [68], the results obtained, i.e., the number of molecules generated, were identical for elemental compositions having only C, O, and H. The major advantage of OMG is that it is an open-source software; thus, the user can understand the functioning of software and also can customize the software according to his/her requirements. This structure generator would be useful to many fields, especially to the metabolomics area, where identifying the unknown metabolites is still a major bottleneck [69].

### 3.1.13 mol2chemfig

This tool is written in the Python language to convert a large number of structures in molfile or SMILES format into the LATEX source code. Its output is written in the syntax defined by the chemfig TEX package, which allows for flexible and concise description of chemical structures and reaction mechanisms. The program is freely available through a Web interface. It also can be locally installed on the user's computer, and the source code is accessible from the home page [70].

### 3.1.14 LICSS

LICSS is the lightweight Excel-based chemical spreadsheet (open-source software) which stores structures as SMILES strings. Chemical operations are carried out by calling Java code modules, which uses the CDK, JChemPaint, and OPSIN libraries to provide the cheminformatics functionality. The compounds in the sheets may be visualized (individually or combined), and the sheets may be searched by substructure or similarity. The descriptors available in CDK may also be calculated for all the compounds, and various cheminformatics operations such as fingerprint calculation, Sammon mapping, clustering, and R-group table creation may be carried out. It can be used suitably on a sheet containing thousands of compounds without compromising the normal performance of Microsoft Excel [71].

*3.1.15   Avogadro*

The Avogadro library is an advanced semantic chemical editor, visualization, and analysis platform. This framework provides a code library and application programming interface (API) with the three-dimensional visualization capabilities and has direct applications for research and education in the fields of chemistry, physics, materials science, and biology. Moreover, this application also provides a rich graphical interface using dynamically loaded plug-in through the library itself. The application and library can be extended by implementing a plug-in module in C++ or Python to explore different visualization techniques, build/manipulate molecular structures, and interact with the other programs [8].

*3.1.16   MyChemise*

My Chemical Structure Editor (MyChemise) is a new 2D structure editor designed as a Java applet, which enables the direct creation of structures in the Internet using a Web browser. It has a morphing module, which allows the creation of different types of presentation for dynamic visualization, for example, clear and simple illustration of molecule vibrations and reaction sequences. Thus, this new 2D drawing program has a versatile way of creating structural images [72].

*3.1.17   Open3DALIGN*

Open3DALIGN is an open-source software tool which is capable of carrying out conformational searches and multi-conformational, unsupervised rigid-body alignment of 3D molecular structures. The multiple alignment paradigms (i.e., atom-based, pharmacophore-based and mixed) are implemented in the methodology. The mixed and atom-based superposition algorithms give rise to the most consistent and well-ordered alignments, which are particularly suitable for the 3D-QSAR techniques. The high computational performance, the unsupervised nature of the alignment algorithms, and its scriptable interface make Open3DALIGN an ideal component of automated cheminformatics workflows. The Open3DALIGN tool is written in C language and linked to high-performance BLAS and LAPACK libraries with parallel algorithms implemented for high computational performance using the multiprocessor architectures [73].

*3.1.18   mpAD4*

Norgan et al. [74] reported the multilevel parallelized AutoDock 4.2 (mpAD4) software which was built using system-level (MPI) and node-level (OpenMP) parallelization to facilitate the application of this docking software on MPI-enabled systems and multi-thread the execution of individual docking jobs. The multi-threading of AutoDock's Lamarkian Genetic Algorithm with OpenMP increases the speed of individual docking jobs; when combined with MPI parallelization, it can significantly reduce the execution time of virtual screenings. This multilevel parallelized AutoDock 4.2 software speeds up the execution of certain molecular docking workloads and allows the user to optimize the degree of system-level (MPI) and node-level (OpenMP) parallelization to best fit both the workloads and the computational resources.

### 3.1.19 DemQSAR

DemQSAR is a stand-alone Java application tool that can be used to predict the human volume of distribution ($VD_{ss}$) and human clearance (CL). DemQSAR integrates the open-source CDK library to compute various molecular descriptors and fingerprints, and thus the QSAR models can be built without any additional software. DemQSAR incorporates two state-of-the-art feature selection strategies: embedded Lasso and recursive feature elimination (RFE). The appropriate quality measures are computed automatically depending upon whether the analysis being performed is classification based or regression based. In addition to the predicted $VD_{ss}$ and CL values, 2D images, SMILES codes, molecular formula, and molecular weights are also computed for the uploaded compounds. Due to its fully automated approach and good predictive power, DemQSAR is an attractive tool for many QSAR/QSPR tasks [75].

### 3.1.20 Shape

Shape software package is used for predicting 3D conformation of carbohydrates up to a considerable size, which covers most of the known biologically active oligosaccharide compounds. Because detailed experimental three-dimensional structures of carbohydrates are often difficult to acquire, software, such as Shape, is an alternative and attractive method for the prediction of oligosaccharide conformations. The predictions of Shape agreed well with experimental data as well as with other published conformation prediction studies [76].

### 3.1.21 OrChem

OrChem is an open-source extension of the Oracle 11G database platform. It added the registration and indexing of chemical structures functions to support the fast substructure and similarity searching. Its cheminformatics functionality is provided by the CDK toolkit. OrChem provides similarity searching with response times in the order of seconds for databases with millions of compounds, depending on a given similarity cutoff [77].

### 3.1.22 PaDEL-Descriptor

PaDEL-Descriptor is a free and open-source software for calculating the molecular descriptors and fingerprints. This software calculates 797 descriptors (663 1D and 2D descriptors, 134 3D descriptors) and ten types of fingerprints. It has both graphical user interface and command-line interface that function on all major platforms (Windows, Linux, MacOS). PaDEL-Descriptor supports more than 90 different molecular file formats and is multi-threaded [27].

*3.1.23  QSARINS and QSARINS-Chem*

QSARINS (QSAR-INSUBRIA) is a free software for the development, analysis, validation, and application of QSAR MLR models according to the OECD principles. The updated version of QSARINS, i.e., QSARINS-Chem, comprises several datasets of environmental pollutants and their corresponding endpoints (i.e., physicochemical properties and biological activities). Those chemicals can be accessed by querying CAS number, SMILES string, compound names, etc., and the developed models can be downloaded in the QSAR model reporting format (QMRF) [78].

*3.1.24  VEGA Non-Interactive Client (VEGANIC)*

VEGA [79] (**V**irtual models for property **E**valuation of chemicals within a **G**lobal **A**rchitecture) is an open-source platform that provides the valid QSAR models to be used especially under the European legislation for chemical substances (REACH). VEGANIC is a software under VEGA platform in which one can execute all the VEGA models on the local machine without sending any information to the server. It is freely available for download from the VEGA website [79], and the endpoints and properties such as BCF (bioconcentration factor), mutagenicity, carcinogenicity, developmental toxicity, skin sensitization, $LC_{50}$ aquatic toxicity, biodegradability, and LogP can be determined.

*3.1.25  OECD QSAR Toolbox*

OECD QSAR toolbox [80] is a software application intended to be used by governments, chemical industries, and other stakeholders in filling the gaps in (eco)toxicity data needed for assessing the hazards of chemicals. The key features of this toolbox include identification of relevant structural characteristics and potential mechanism or mode of action of a target chemical, identification of other chemicals that have the same structural characteristics and/or mechanism or mode of action, filling the data gap(s), using existing experimental data, and systematically grouping of chemicals into categories according to the presence or potency of a particular effect for all members of the category.

*3.1.26  ChemAxon Software Tools*

ChemAxon is a software company specializing in developing programming interfaces and end-user applications for cheminformatics and life science research. It provides some of the noncommercial and academic free version tools such as MarvinSketch, MarvinView, MarvinSpace, Marvin JS, JChem Base/JChem Cartridge, MolConverter, and JChem for Excel applications [81].

*3.1.27  DTC Lab Software Tools*

The Drug Theoretics and Cheminformatics laboratory (DTC Lab., Jadavpur University, India) has developed several open-access cheminformatics tools, mostly dealing with QSAR studies. All the stand-alone tools are built using Java language and can be freely downloaded from the official website [82]. These basic QSAR tools such as MLR plus Validation (*for performing MLR and computing all validation parameters*), dataset division GUI (*dataset division into training and test sets using various algorithms*), data pretreat-ment GUI (*to remove constant and intercorrelated descriptors prior to model development*), modified K-medoid (*clustering method*), AD-MDI and Euclidean (*to define applicability domain*), genetic algorithm, stepwise MLR and MLR best subset selection (*variable selection methods*), etc., are very helpful when performing QSAR studies; manuals and sample input files of these software tools are also provided.

### 3.2   Online Tools

#### 3.2.1   iDrug

*i*Drug is a versatile Web-based server for pharmacophore and similarity-based virtual screening and target identification to facili-tate computational drug discovery. It provides ready-to-access compounds and pharmacophore target databases (such as ZINC, NCI, PharmTargetDB) for virtual screening and target identifica-tion. Different modules such as Cavity (detects and scores potential binding sites of a protein), Pocket v.2 (derives pharmacophore models based on a given receptor of complex structure), Pharm-Mapper (pharmacophore mapping), SHAFTS (3D similarity calcu-lation), Cyndi (molecular conformation generation), and Pybel (Python wrapper for the Open Babel cheminformatics toolkit) have been incorporated and can work together as a pipeline. Differ-ent molecular design processing tasks can be submitted and visua-lized simply in one browser without installing locally any stand-alone modeling software. It provides a novel, fast, and reliable tool for conducting drug design experiments [83].

#### 3.2.2   OCHEM

OCHEM is a Web-based platform that provides the tools for automation of typical steps necessary to create a predictive QSAR/QSPR model. The platform consists of two major subsys-tems: a database of experimental measurements and a modeling framework. The database contains almost 10,000 data points for the density, bubble point, and azeotropic behavior of binary mix-tures. The OCHEM has the features that allow the reading and uploading of data for binary nonadditive mixtures, creating special descriptors for mixtures, and validating models. It is a useful Web-based tool for the modeling and prediction of mixtures of chemical compounds [84].

#### 3.2.3   Chembench

Chembench [85] is a Web-based tool for analyzing the experimen-tal chemical structure-activity data (QSAR modeling and predic-tion). It provides a broad range of tools for data visualization and embeds a rigorous workflow for creating and validating the predic-tive QSAR models and using them for virtual screening of chemical libraries to prioritize the compound selection for drug discovery and/or chemical safety assessment. It supports model building with kNN [86] and random forest [87] techniques. User may predict a specific activity or a spectrum of activities for a virtual chemical library or a single compound (available libraries include NCI diversity set (http://dtp.nci.nih.gov/branches/dscb/diversity_explanation.html), DrugBank [88], ChEMBL (http://www.ebi.ac.uk/chembldb/), and Wombat [89]); user may also upload his own library [85].

*3.2.4  Spectral Game*    Spectral Game is a Web-based game where players try to match molecules to various forms of interactive spectra, including 1D/2D NMR, mass spectra, and infrared spectra. Player earns one point for every correct answer, and the play continues until player supplies the incorrect answer. The game is usually played by using a Web browser interface. The spectra are uploaded as Open Data to ChemSpider in JCAMP-DX format and are used for the problem sets together with structures extracted from the website. The spectra are displayed using JSpecView, an open-source spectrum viewing applet, which affords zooming and integration. The application of the game is also utilized for the teaching of proton NMR spectroscopy [90].

*3.2.5  ACD/I-Lab Tool*    ACD/I-Lab [91] is a Web-based prediction engine which provides structure-based predictions of the following properties: free basic physicochemical properties and IUPAC naming capabilities for structures containing 50 atoms or less, advanced physicochemical properties (absolve, boiling point/vapor pressure, adsorption coefficient/BCF, Log$P$, log$D$, p$K_a$, solubility, etc.), ADME characteristics (bioavailability, absorption, active transport, plasma binding, Vd, Pgp inhibitors, and Pgp substrates), toxicity hazards (AMES test, genotoxicity, aquatic toxicity, health effects, endocrine disruption, MRDD), NMR spectra and chemical shifts for $^{13}$C, and systematic chemical nomenclature and structure generation (IUPAC, index names). Several of these predictions are free, while others require licenses.

# 4  Workflows

Workflow systems in various fields including cheminformatics allow users/scientists to define, manage, and execute time-consuming processes in succession and/or to perform recurring task effectively. A workflow process is logically carried out using a GUI (*see* Fig. 1) where various types of nodes or software components are available for connection through edges or pipes that define the workflow process. Here, nodes are defined by three parameters, i.e., (1) input metadata, (2) algorithms or user-defined parameters or rules, and (3) output metadata. Further, nodes can be connected together only if the output of the previous node represents the mandatory input requirements of the subsequent node. Edges or pipes are the visual representation that provides information about

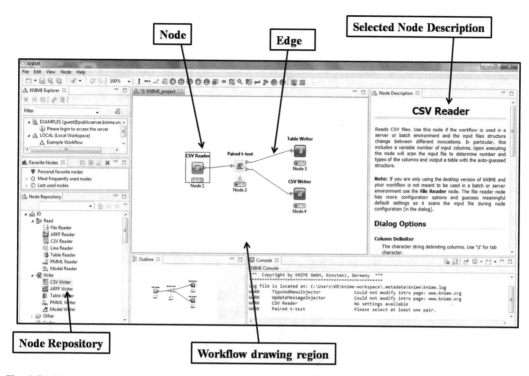

**Fig. 1** Basic components of a workflow system (a snapshot of KNIME workflow was taken for demonstration)

the direction of execution process and are also used for dividing the workflow process [92].

Workflows are increasingly employed and are very useful in cheminformatics since numerous recurring tasks can be automated, which in many cases significantly reduces the manual attention for time-consuming multiple step processes, such as virtual screening via various filters, docking of huge libraries, QSAR studies, etc. There are several commercially well-established workflow systems that are developed for the cheminformatics field such as Pipeline Pilot [93] from Accelrys (*now BIOVIA Pipeline Pilot*) and the InforSense Knowledge Discovery Environment (KDE) from Infor-Sense [94]. Initially, Pipeline Pilot was mainly employed in the cheminformatics field but later extended its functionality to other scientific fields such as next-generation sequencing and imaging. In 2009, the InforSense organization was acquired by IDBS and the KDE has further made progress in the translational medicine field since then [95].

**4.1 Open-Source Workflows**

In the open-source community, Konstanz Information Miner (KNIME) and Taverna have made a significant impact and offer a wide applicable domain. Cancer Grid (CaGrid) [96] is another open-source workflow system which is an extension of Taverna. *myExperiment* [97] is a collaborative environment where scientists can safely publish their workflows and is the largest freely accessible public repository of scientific workflows. Many examples of KNIME and Taverna workflows that are highly useful for various cheminformatics tasks can be found in the repository.

In this section, we will discuss in detail the recent developments in the above mentioned open-source workflows, especially the new functionalities/plug-in added in these workflow systems.

*4.1.1 Taverna*

Taverna workflow management system was created by myGrid team (http://www.mygrid.org.uk/) and is currently funded through FP7 projects BioVeL (http://www.biovel.eu/), SCAPE (http://www.scape-project.eu/), and Wf4Ever (http://www.wf4ever-project.org/). It is licensed under the Lesser General Public License (LGPL) Version 2.1. Taverna was initially used in bioinformatics but is now employed in other fields too, including cheminformatics. Recently, the CDK toolkit was combined to Taverna workflow system [98] to improve the handling of various cheminformatics functionalities.

*CDK-Taverna*: The integration of CDK with Taverna was started in 2005 to extend the functionalities of Taverna in the cheminformatics domain. Both the CDK and Taverna, as well as combined technology, are open source.

The CDK-Taverna 1.0 plug-in provides 164 different workers (note that in case of Taverna, nodes are called workers). These include workers for I/O of various chemical files and line notation formats, databases I/O, and clustering methods and for computing descriptors for atoms, bonds, and molecules. The miscellaneous workers comprise of a substructure filter, a reaction enumerator, an aromaticity detector, etc. The complete list of workers with short description is provided at http://cdk.sourceforge.net/cdk-taverna/workers.html. The architecture of Taverna does not allow the "*loop*" function to control huge data entries to process them one by one. Combining Taverna with CDK allowed workers to act like loops and permit workflows to process large datasets using Taverna's iteration-and-retry mechanism. To allow storage and fast retrieval of up to a million molecules without running into memory limitations, the CDK-Taverna 1.0 supports database system using the PostgreSQL relational database management system (RDBMS) with the open-source Pgchem::tigress extension [98].

The version 2.0 of CDK-Taverna was further developed to extend its usability and strength; CDK-Taverna 2.0 not only made improvements in all workers but also major improvements to the whole platform through a complete setup on the basis of Taverna 2.2 and CDK 1.3.5. This improved version now provides 192 different workers and supports 64-bit computing and multi-core usages by paralleled threads allowing fast in-memory processing and analysis of huge number of molecules, which benefits workers associated with molecular descriptor calculation or machine learning.

The data analysis abilities are also extended with newly added workers that offer access to the open-source WEKA library for clustering and machine learning in addition to dataset division into training and test sets. CDK-Taverna 1.0 offered basic functions for combinatorial chemistry-related reaction enumeration; it supported the use of only two reactants, a single product and one generic group per reactant. As a comparison, the advanced reaction enumeration options employed by CDK-Taverna 2.0 incorporated significant improvements including multi-match detection, no limitation for number of reactants, products or generic groups, and variable R-groups, ring sizes, and atom definitions. This version also provided two groups of workers to compute natural product (NP)-*likeness* core for small molecules.

The CDK-Taverna 2.0 plug-in is built in Java (platform independent) and supported by Windows, Linux, and Mac OS/X (32- and 64-bit). It is released under the GNU LGPL. For its installation, it takes advantage of the plug-in detection manager of Taverna. The plug-in is available at http://www.cdk-taverna.de/plug-in/ and the user can select the desired version. The CDK-Taverna plug-in uses Maven 2 as a build system. It also uses other open-source components such as Bioclipse for visualization of workflow results and Pgchem::tigress as an interface to the database back end for storage of large datasets. A Wiki page is available for this version, which provides general information about the project, documentation, and installation procedure [99, 100].

*CaGrid*: Cancer Grid (CaGrid) is a workflow system, which prefers to employ and extend Taverna due to a number of benefits including integration with the Web services technology, plug-in architecture which provides an easy integration of third party extensions, and a wide scientific community base. CaGrid is the underlying infrastructure of Cancer Biomedical Informatics Grid (caBIG) and is built on the Globus Toolkit Grid middleware. CaGrid consists of Web services as virtualized access points of data and analytical resources related to cancer detection, diagnosis, treatment, and prevention [96].

*Biological Data Interactive Clustering Explorer (BioDICE) Taverna Plug-In*: BioDICE is a recent Taverna plug-in [101] that offers clustering analysis capacity and provides visualization of multidimensional biological datasets. The Self-organizing map (SOM) is a well-known unsupervised method for data visualization and clustering. The core algorithm in BioDICE is a fast learning SOM (FLSOM), an improved version of the SOM algorithm that belongs to the category of the emergent self-organizing maps (ESOM). BioDICE is the first Taverna component performing SOM clustering with U-Matrix visualization. Other Taverna plug-ins, i.e., CDK or RapidMiner, were lacking these functionalities; hence BioDICE filled such a gap. The BioDICE plug-in and its documentation, tutorial, workflow, and dataset examples are available at http://biolab.pa.icar.cnr.it/biodice.html.

*4.1.2 KNIME*

KNIME was developed by a team of software engineers led by Michael Berthold at the University of Konstanz, Germany. It is licensed under GNU GPL. Initially, KNIME entered the market as a data mining tool but rapidly gained popularity in the cheminformatics community. Further combination of KNIME with CDK [102] extended a large amount of cheminformatics functionalities.

*KNIME-CDK*: The KNIME workflow platform supports a wide range of functionality and has a large number of active users in the cheminformatics community. Thus, CDK is combined with KNIME to wrap the CDK's core functionality and released to the users. This KNIME-CDK plug-in, similar to the CDK-Taverna plug-in, is open source and community driven.

KNIME-CDK [102] consists of various functions which include molecule conversion to/from commonly used formats, generation of signatures, fingerprints, and molecular properties. The plug-in recognizes molecules in CML, SDFile, MDL Mol, InChI, and SMILES formats via the *Molecule to CDK* node and can write SDFiles via the *CDK to Molecule* node. All other operations are performed on the internal CDK molecule representation that includes generation of coordinates, hydrogen manipulator, structure sketcher, atom signatures, common fingerprints (e.g., MACCS and Pubchem), 2D and 3D descriptor values (e.g., XLogP and Lipinski's rule of five), chemical name lookup via OPSIN, and substructure search. It can also be utilized in the management and analysis of chemical libraries through descriptors, conformer analysis via RMSD, and NMR spectra prediction. The KNIME preference page contains a CDK tab to set global visualization preferences, and a renderer is provided to draw the molecules using the JChemPaint library. The different routes employed in the workflow can be run in parallel and the nodes are always run multi-threaded.

KNIME-CDK plug-in has been developed in Java (platform independent) and installed via the KNIME update mechanism. It is build under GNU LGPL license.

# 5 Databases

A database is a collection of systematically organized or structured repository of indexed information that allows easy retrieval, updating, analysis, and output of data. Freely accessible cheminformatics databases include the databases of chemical structures, proteins, QSAR models, drugs, biological targets, bioactive molecules, etc. The widely used cheminformatics databases, their official links, and a brief description about each database are illustrated in Table 3. Each of these tabulated databases has its own application in specific areas.

**Table 3**

**List of cheminformatics databases, their links and brief description for each database**

| Sr. No. | Name of database | Database link | Description (reference) |
|---|---|---|---|
| 1 | QSAR DataBank | http://qsardb.org/repository/ | QSAR DataBank [103] |
| 2 | VAMMPIRE | http://vammpire.pharmchem.uni-frankfurt.de/vammpire/ | Structure-based drug design and optimization [104] |
| 3 | PubChem3D | https://pubchem.ncbi.nlm.nih.gov/ | Open repository for small molecules and their experimental biological activity [105] |
| 4 | MMsINC | http://mms.dsfarm.unipd.it/MMsINC/search/ | Chemical structures database [106] |
| 5 | CREDO | http://marid.bioc.cam.ac.uk/credo | Protein–ligand interaction database [107] |
| 6 | ChemBank | http://chembank.broadinstitute.org/ | Small molecule database [108] |
| 7 | DrugBank | http://www.drugbank.ca/ | Drugs and target information [88] |
| 8 | ChemDB | http://cdb.ics.uci.edu | Small molecule database [109] |
| 9 | ChemMine | http://chemminedb.ucr.edu/ | Compound mining database for chemical genomics [110] |
| 10 | National Cancer Institute (NCI) 3D database | http://www.cancer.gov/cancertopics/pdq/cancerdatabase | Anticancer drug database |
| 11 | ZINC | http://zinc.docking.org | A free database of commercially available small molecules [113] |
| 12 | ChEMBL | https://www.ebi.ac.uk/chembl/ | Bioactive molecules with drug-like properties |
| 13 | Therapeutic Target Database (TTD) | http://xin.cz3.nus.edu.sg/group/ttd/ttd.asp | Drug database |

(continued)

**Table 3**
**(continued)**

| Sr. No. | Name of database | Database link | Description (reference) |
|---------|------------------|---------------|--------------------------|
| 14 | PharmGKB | http://www.pharmgkb.org/ | Pharmacogenomics knowledge resource |
| 15 | STITCH (search tool for interactions of chemicals) | http://stitch.embl.de/ | Resource to explore known and predicted interactions of chemicals and proteins |
| 16 | SuperTarget | http://bioinf-apache.charite.de/supertarget_v2/ | Drugs and target proteins database |
| 17 | ChemSpider | http://www.chemspider.com/About.aspx | Chemical structure database [112] |

The **QsarDB** [103] could be used to solve everyday QSAR and predictive modeling problems, including applications in the field of predictive toxicology. The utility and benefit of QsarDB can also be applied to a wide variety of other endpoints.

**VAMMPIRE** [104], a matched molecular pair database, provides valuable information for structure-based lead optimization and for fundamental studies such as understanding protein-ligand interactions.

**PubChem3D** [105], an addition to the existing contents of PubChem, provides a new dimension to its ability to search, subset, export, visualize, and analyze chemical structures and associated biological data.

**MMsINC** [106] is a database of nonredundant, richly annotated, and biomedically relevant chemical structures. It has been created to support chemo-centric approach to relate protein pharmacology by ligand chemistry.

**CREDO** [107] is a novel and comprehensive publicly available database of protein-ligand interactions, which uses contacts as structural interaction fingerprints, implements novel features, and is completely scriptable through its application programming interface.

**ChemBank** [108] consists of freely available data derived from small molecules and small molecule screens, which can be used to guide chemists in synthesizing novel compounds or libraries and aid biologists in identifying small molecules that block the specific biological pathways of the target protein.

The **DrugBank** database [88] contains the information of both the drug (i.e., chemical, pharmacological, and pharmaceutical compound) and drug targets (i.e., sequence, structure, and pathway). The different categories of drugs include FDA-approved small molecule drugs, FDA-approved biotech (protein/peptide) drugs, nutraceuticals, and experimental drugs.

**ChemDB** [109] and **ChemMine** [110] are public databases of small molecules and for chemical genomics, respectively. The ChemMine database, a compound mining database, facilitates drug and agrochemical discovery and chemical genomics screening.

The **NCI DIS** 3D database [111] is a collection of 3D structures of drugs. It was built and maintained by the Developmental Therapeutics Program, Division of Cancer Treatment and Diagnosis, National Cancer Institute, Rockville, USA. This 3D database is being used for identifying 3D pharmacophoric features in order to discover novel active anticancer molecules.

**ChemSpider** [112] is a free online chemical structure database owned by Royal Society of Chemistry. It provides fast access to over 32 million structures, properties, and associated information. By combining and integrating compounds from varied data sources, ChemSpider facilitates the discovery of chemical data from a single online search. It offers both text and structure search for the query compound and provides a unique service to improve this information by curation and annotation.

In summary, the information associated with all these databases is a valuable resource of small molecules/drugs/proteins for medicinal chemists, biologists, cheminformaticians, and bioinformaticians for their exploitation in their respective researches.

# 6    Conclusion

This chapter highlights freely available cheminformatics resources including toolkits, software, workflow, and databases. The readers will get acquainted to the functionalities as well as the recent advances of these open-source toolkits, workflow systems, ready-to-use software, and freely accessible databases. The information provided would assist the cheminformaticians, including programmers/developers, to explore and utilize these freely available resources to resolve different computational challenges in the cheminformatics field and further contribute in new advancement for the next-generation cheminformatics resources.

## References

1. Steinbeck C, Han Y, Kuhn S, Horlacher O, Luttmann E, Willighagen E (2003) The Chemistry Development Kit (CDK): an open-source Java library for chemo- and bioinformatics. J Chem Inf Comput Sci 43:493–500

2. O'boyle NM, Banck M, James CA, Morley C, Vandermeersch T, Hutchison GR (2011) Open Babel: an open chemical toolbox. J Cheminform 3:33

3. Landrum G (2013) RDKit: cheminformatics and machine learning software. rdkit.org

4. http://ggasoftware.com/opensource/indigo

5. Guha R, Howard MT, Hutchison GR, Murray-Rust P, Rzepa H, Steinbeck C, Wegner J, Willighagen EL (2006) The blue obelisk interoperability in chemical informatics. J Chem Inf Model 46:991–998

6. O'Boyle NM, Guha R, Willighagen EL, Adams SE, Alvarsson J, Bradley J-C, Filippov IV, Hanson RM, Hanwell MD, Hutchison GR (2011) Open data, open source and open standards in chemistry: the Blue Obelisk five years on. J Cheminform 3:37

7. Spjuth O, Helmus T, Willighagen EL, Kuhn S, Eklund M, Wagener J, Murray-Rust P, Steinbeck C, Wikberg JES (2007) Bioclipse: an open source workbench for chemo- and bioinformatics. BMC Bioinformatics 8:59

8. Hanwell MD, Curtis DE, Lonie DC, Vandermeersch T, Zurek E, Hutchison GR (2012) Avogadro: an advanced semantic chemical editor, visualization, and analysis platform. J Cheminform 4:17

9. Guha R (2006) CDK descriptor calculator GUI. http://www.rguha.net/code/java/cdkdesc.html

10. Steinbeck C, Hoppe C, Kuhn S, Floris M, Guha R, Willighagen EL (2006) Recent developments of the chemistry development kit (CDK)—an open-source java library for chemo- and bioinformatics. Curr Pharm Des 12:2111–2120

11. O'Boyle NM, Hutchison GR (2008) Cinfony—combining Open Source cheminformatics toolkits behind a common interface. Chem Cent J 2:24

12. Rahman SA, Bashton M, Holliday GL, Schrader R, Thornton JM (2009) Small Molecule Subgraph Detector (SMSD) toolkit. J Cheminform 1:12

13. Hildebrandt A, Dehof AK, Rurainski A, Bertsch A, Schumann M, Toussaint NC, Moll A, Stockel D, Nickels S, Mueller SC (2010) BALL-biochemical algorithms library 1.3. BMC Bioinformatics 11:531

14. Hinselmann G, Rosenbaum L, Jahn A, Fechner N, Zell A (2011) jCompoundMapper: an open

source Java library and command-line tool for chemical fingerprints. J Cheminform 3:3

15. Hock S, Riedl R (2012) chemf: a purely functional chemistry toolkit. J Cheminform 4:1–19

16. Cao D-S, Xu Q-S, Hu Q-N, Liang Y-Z (2013) ChemoPy: freely available python package for computational biology and chemoinformatics. Bioinformatics 29:1092–1094

17. Cao Y, Charisi A, Cheng L-C, Jiang T, Girke T (2008) ChemmineR: a compound mining framework for R. Bioinformatics 24:1733–1734

18. Cao D-S, Xiao N, Xu Q-S, Chen AF (2014) Rcpi: R/Bioconductor package to generate various descriptors of proteins, compounds, and their interactions. Bioinformatics. doi:10.1093/bioinformatics/btu1624

19. http://wiki.chemkit.org/Main_Page

20. Herraez A (2006) Biomolecules in the computer: Jmol to the rescue. Biochem Mol Biol Educ 34:255–261

21. Krause S, Willighagen E, Steinbeck C (2000) JChemPaint—using the collaborative forces of the internet to develop a free editor for 2D chemical structures. Molecules 5:93–98

22. https://github.com/cdk/cdk/blob/master/AUTHORS

23. Bashton M, Nobeli I, Thornton JM (2006) Cognate ligand domain mapping for enzymes. J Mol Biol 364:836–852

24. Rojas-Cherto M, Kasper PT, Willighagen EL, Vreeken RJ, Hankemeier T, Reijmers TH (2011) Elemental composition determination based on MSn. Bioinformatics 27:2376–2383

25. Steinbeck C (2001) SENECA: a platform-independent, distributed, and parallel system for computer-assisted structure elucidation in organic chemistry. J Chem Inf Comput Sci 41:1500–1507

26. Steinbeck C, Kuhn S (2004) NMRShiftDB—compound identification and structure elucidation support through a free community-built web database. Phytochemistry 65:2711–2717

27. Yap CW (2011) PaDEL-descriptor: an open source software to calculate molecular descriptors and fingerprints. J Comput Chem 32:1466–1474

28. http://cdk.sourceforge.net/old_web/software.html

29. http://www.rdkit.org/docs/Overview.html

30. http://www.rdkit.org/docs/Overview.html#the-contrib-directory

31. http://rdkit.org/RDKit_Docs.current.pdf

32. http://sourceforge.net/projects/openbabel/files/stats/timeline?dates=2001-11-25+to+2014-11-14

33. http://scholar.google.co.in/scholar?hl=en&as_sdt=0,5&q=openbabel

34. http://www.eyesopen.com/toolkits

35. http://www.eyesopen.com/academic

36. http://openbabel.org/

37. O'Boyle NM, Morley C, Hutchison GR (2008) Pybel: a Python wrapper for the OpenBabel cheminformatics toolkit. Chem Cent J 2:5

38. http://creativecommons.org/licenses/by/3.0/

39. Pavlov D, Rybalkin M, Karulin B, Kozhevnikov M, Savelyev A, Churinov A (2011) Indigo: universal cheminformatics API. J Cheminform 3:P4

40. http://jcompoundmapper.sourceforge.net/

41. http://www.scala-lang.org/

42. https://github.com/stefan-hoeck/chemf

43. Jarvis RM, Broadhurst D, Johnson H, O'Boyle NM, Goodacre R (2006) PYCHEM: a multivariate analysis package for python. Bioinformatics 22:2565–2566

44. Wang Y, Backman TWH, Horan K, Girke T (2013) fmcsR: mismatch tolerant maximum common substructure searching in R. Bioinformatics 29:2792–2794

45. Cao Y, Jiang T, Girke T (2010) Accelerated similarity searching and clustering of large compound sets by geometric embedding and locality sensitive hashing. Bioinformatics 26:953–959

46. Hoksza D, Skoda P, Vorsilak M, Svozil D (2014) Molpher: a software framework for systematic chemical space exploration. J Cheminform 3:32

47. Schling B (2011) The boost C++ libraries. XML Press, Laguna Hills, CA

48. Hu B, Lill MA (2014) PharmDock: a pharmacophore-based docking program. J Cheminform 6:1–14

49. Plewczynski D, Lazniewski M, Augustyniak R, Ginalski K (2011) Can we trust docking results? Evaluation of seven commonly used programs on PDBbind database. J Comput Chem 32:742–755

50. Li X, Li Y, Cheng T, Liu Z, Wang R (2010) Evaluation of the performance of four molecular docking programs on a diverse set of protein–ligand complexes. J Comput Chem 31:2109–2125

51. Cereto-Massague A, Ojeda MJ, Joosten RP, Valls C, Mulero M, Salvado MJ, Arola-Arnal

A, Arola L, Garcia-Vallve S, Pujadas G (2013) The good, the bad and the dubious: VHE-LIBS, a validation helper for ligands and binding sites. J Cheminform 5:36

52. Sehnal D, Varekova RS, Berka K, Pravda L, Navratilova V, Banas P, Ionescu C-M, Otyepka M, Koca J (2013) MOLE 2.0: advanced approach for analysis of biomacro-molecular channels. J Cheminform 5:39

53. Petrek M, Kosinova P, Koca J, Otyepka M (2007) MOLE: a Voronoi diagram-based explorer of molecular channels, pores, and tunnels. Structure 15:1357–1363

54. Yaffe E, Fishelovitch D, Wolfson HJ, Halperin D, Nussinov R (2008) MolAxis: efficient and accurate identification of channels in macro-molecules. Proteins 73:72–86

55. Yaffe E, Fishelovitch D, Wolfson HJ, Halperin D, Nussinov R (2008) MolAxis: a server for identification of channels in macromolecules. Nucleic Acids Res 36:W210–W215

56. Chovancova E, Pavelka A, Benes P, Strnad O, Brezovsky J, Kozlikova B, Gora A, Sustr V, Klvana M, Medek P (2012) CAVER 3.0: a tool for the analysis of transport pathways in dynamic protein structures. PLoS Comput Biol 8:e1002708

57. Khashan R (2012) FragVLib a free database mining software for generating "Fragment-based Virtual Library" using pocket similarity search of ligand-receptor complexes. J Che-minform 4:1–6

58. Ekins S, Clark AM, Sarker M (2013) TB Mobile: a mobile app for anti-tuberculosis molecules with known targets. J Cheminform 5:13

59. Bienfait B, Ertl P (2013) JSME: a free mole-cule editor in JavaScript. J Cheminform 5:24

60. Gutlein M, Karwath A, Kramer S (2012) CheS-Mapper—chemical space mapping and visualization in 3D. J Cheminform 4:7

61. Le Guilloux V, Arrault A, Colliandre L, Bourg SP, Vayer P, Morin-Allory L (2012) Mining collections of compounds with Screening Assistant 2. J Cheminform 4:1–16

62. Sud M, Fahy E, Subramaniam S (2012) Template-based combinatorial enumeration of virtual compound libraries for lipids. J Che-minform 4:23

63. Cereto-Massague A, Guasch L, Valls C, Mulero M, Pujadas G, Garcia-Vallve S (2012) DecoyFinder: an easy-to-use python GUI application for building target-specific decoy sets. Bioinformatics 28:1661–1662

64. Huang N, Shoichet BK, Irwin JJ (2006) Benchmarking sets for molecular docking. J Med Chem 49:6789–6801

65. Irwin JJ (2008) Community benchmarks for virtual screening. J Comput Aided Mol Des 22:193–199

66. Wallach I, Lilien R (2011) Virtual decoy sets for molecular docking benchmarks. J Chem Inf Model 51:196–202

67. Durant JL, Leland BA, Henry DR, Nourse JG (2002) Reoptimization of MDL keys for use in drug discovery. J Chem Inf Comput Sci 42:1273–1280

68. Kerber A, Laue R, Gruner T, Meringer M (1998) MOLGEN 4.0. MATCH Commun Math Comput Chem 37:205–208

69. Peironcely JE, Rojas-Cherto M, Fichera D, Reijmers TH, Coulier L, Faulon J-L, Hanke-meier T (2012) OMG: open molecule gener-ator. J Cheminform 4:21

70. Brefo-Mensah EK, Palmer M (2012) mol2-chemfig, a tool for rendering chemical struc-tures from molfile or SMILES format to LATEX code. J Cheminform 4:24

71. Lawson KR, Lawson J (2012) LICSS—a chemical spreadsheet in microsoft excel. J Cheminform 4:1–7

72. Wilhelm J-H (2011) MyChemise: a 2D draw-ing program that uses morphing for visualisa-tion purposes. J Cheminform 3:53

73. Tosco P, Balle T, Shiri F (2011) Open3DA-LIGN: an open-source software aimed at unsupervised ligand alignment. J Comput Aided Mol Des 25:777–783

74. Norgan AP, Coffman PK, Kocher J-P, Katz-mann DJ, Sosa CP (2011) Multilevel parallel-lization of AutoDock 4.2. J Cheminform 3:12

75. Demir-Kavuk O, Bentzien J, Muegge I, Knapp E-W (2011) DemQSAR: predicting human volume of distribution and clearance of drugs. J Comput Aided Mol Des 25:1121–1133

76. Jimmy R, Laurence M, Serge P (2009) Shape: automatic conformation prediction of carbo-hydrates using a genetic algorithm. J Chemin-form 1:1–7

77. Rijnbeek M, Steinbeck C (2010) OrChem: an open source chemistry search engine for Ora-cle. J Cheminform 2:P28

78. Gramatica P, Chirico N, Papa E, Cassani S, Kovarich S (2013) QSARINS: a new software for the development, analysis, and validation of QSAR MLR models. J Comput Chem 34:2121–2132

79. http://www.vega-qsar.eu/index.php

80. http://www.oecd.org/chemicalsafety/risk-assessment/theoecdqsartoolbox.htm

81. http://www.chemaxon.com/free-software/

82. http://teqip.jdvu.ac.in/QSAR_Tools/

83. Wang X, Chen H, Yang F, Gong J, Li S, Pei J, Liu X, Jiang H, Lai L, Li H (2014) iDrug: a web-accessible and interactive drug discovery and design platform. J Cheminform 6:1–8

84. Oprisiu I, Novotarskyi S, Tetko IV (2013) Modeling of non-additive mixture properties using the Online CHEmical database and Modeling environment (OCHEM). J Cheminform 5:4

85. Walker T, Grulke CM, Pozefsky D, Tropsha A (2010) Chembench: a cheminformatics workbench. Bioinformatics 26:3000–3001

86. Zhang L, Zhu H, Oprea T, Golbraikh A, Tropsha A (2008) QSAR modeling of the blood-brain barrier permeability for diverse organic compounds. Pharm Res 25:1902–1914

87. Breiman L (2001) Random forests. Mach Learn 1:5–32

88. Wishart DS, Knox C, Guo AC, Shrivastava S, Hassanali M, Stothard P, Chang Z, Woolsey J (2006) DrugBank: a comprehensive resource for in silico drug discovery and exploration. Nucleic Acids Res 34:D668–D672

89. Olah M, Mracec M, Ostopovici L, Rad R, Bora A, Hadaruga N, Olah I, Banda M, Simon Z, Mracec M (2004) WOMBAT: world of molecular bioactivity. Chemoinf. Drug Disc., Wiley-VCH, New York, 223–239

90. Bradley J-C, Lancashire RJ, Lang ASID, Williams AJ (2009) The Spectral Game: leveraging Open Data and crowdsourcing for education. J Cheminform 1:1–10

91. http://www.acdlabs.com/resources/ilab/

92. Tiwari A, Sekhar AKT (2007) Workflow based framework for life science informatics. Comput Biol Chem 31:305–319

93. http://accelrys.com/products/pipeline-pilot/

94. http://www.inforsense.com/

95. Warr WA (2012) Scientific workflow systems: Pipeline pilot and KNIME. J Comput Aided Mol Des 26:1–4

96. Tan W, Madduri R, Nenadic A, Soiland-Reyes S, Sulakhe D, Foster I, Goble CA (2010) CaGrid Workflow Toolkit: a taverna based workflow tool for cancer grid. BMC Bioinformatics 11:542

97. http://www.myexperiment.org/

98. Kuhn T, Willighagen EL, Zielesny A, Steinbeck C (2010) CDK-Taverna: an open workflow environment for cheminformatics. BMC Bioinformatics 11:159

99. http://cdktaverna2.ts-concepts.de/wiki/index.php?title=Main_Page

100. Truszkowski A, Jayaseelan KV, Neumann S, Willighagen EL, Zielesny A, Steinbeck C (2011) New developments on the cheminformatics open workflow environment CDK-Taverna. J Cheminform 3:54

101. Fiannaca A, La Rosa M, Di Fatta G, Gaglio S, Rizzo R, Urso A (2014) The BioDICE Taverna plugin for clustering and visualization of biological data: a workflow for molecular compounds exploration. J Cheminform 6:1–6

102. Beisken S, Meinl T, Wiswedel B, de Figueiredo LF, Berthold MR, Steinbeck C (2013) KNIME-CDK: workflow-driven cheminformatics. BMC Bioinformatics 14:257

103. Ruusmann V, Sild S, Maran U (2014) QSAR DataBank—an approach for the digital organization and archiving of QSAR model information. J Cheminform 6:25

104. Weber J, Achenbach J, Moser D, Proschak E (2013) VAMMPIRE: a matched molecular pairs database for structure-based drug design and optimization. J Med Chem 56:5203–5207

105. Bolton E, Chen J, Kim S, Han L, He S, Shi W, Simonyan V, Sun Y, Thiessen PA, Wang J (2011) PubChem3D: a new resource for scientists. J Cheminform 3:32

106. Masciocchi J, Frau G, Fanton M, Sturlese M, Floris M, Pireddu L, Palla P, Cedrati F, Rodriguez P, Moro S (2009) MMsINC: a large-scale chemoinformatics database. Nucleic Acids Res 37:D284–D290

107. Schreyer A, Blundell T (2009) CREDO: a protein-ligand interaction database for drug discovery. Chem Biol Drug Des 73:157–167

108. Seiler KP, George GA, Happ MP, Bodycombe NE, Carrinski HA, Norton S, Brudz S, Sullivan JP, Muhlich J, Serrano M (2008) ChemBank: a small-molecule screening and cheminformatics resource database. Nucleic Acids Res 36:D351–D359

109. Chen J, Swamidass SJ, Dou Y, Bruand J, Baldi P (2005) ChemDB: a public database of small molecules and related chemoinformatics resources. Bioinformatics 21:4133–4139

110. Girke T, Cheng L-C, Raikhel N (2005) ChemMine. A compound mining database for chemical genomics. Plant Physiol 138:573–577

111. Milne GWA, Nicklaus MC, Driscoll JS, Wang S, Zaharevitz D (1994) National Cancer Institute drug information system 3D database. J Chem Inf Comput Sci 34:1219–1224

112. Pence HE, Williams A (2010) ChemSpider: an online chemical information resource. J Chem Educ 87:1123–1124

113. Irwin JJ, Shoichet BK (2005) ZINC—a free database of commercially available compounds for virtual screening. J Chem Inf Model 45:177–182

Methods in Pharmacology and Toxicology (2016): 297–305
DOI 10.1007/978-1-4939-3521-5
© Springer Science+Business Media New York 2016

# INDEX

Printed in the United States
By Bookmasters